PHYSIC

PAEDI

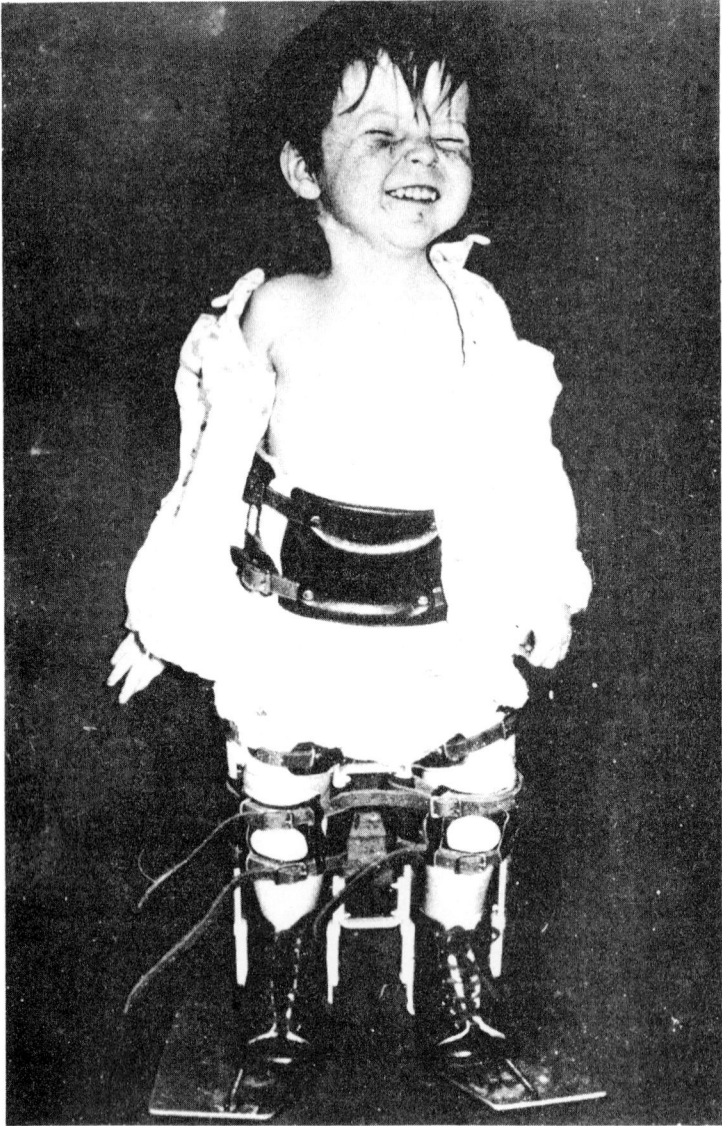

PHYSIOTHERAPY IN PAEDIATRICS

Roberta B. Shepherd Dip. Phty. (Syd.)

Fellow of the Australian College of Physiotherapists
Senior Lecturer, School of Physiotherapy,
Cumberland College of Health Sciences, Sydney

SECOND EDITION

WILLIAM HEINEMANN MEDICAL
BOOKS LIMITED
LONDON

Heinemann Medical Books

Heinemann Medical Books
An imprint of Heinemann Professional Publishing Ltd
Halley Court, Jordan Hill, Oxford OX2 8EJ

OXFORD   LONDON   SINGAPORE   NAIROBI
IBADAN   KINGSTON

First published 1974
Second edition 1980
Reprinted 1984
Reprinted 1985, 1986, 1987, 1989

ISBN 0 433 30131 7

Typeset by
Malvern Typesetting Services
Printed in Great Britain by
Antony Rowe Ltd, Chippenham, Wiltshire

PREFACE TO THE FIRST EDITION

This book has been written for undergraduates as a guide to physical treatment in the field of Paediatrics. I hope they will study in greater detail the subjects which interest them, and that they will have as teachers people who will demonstrate the use of practical techniques in the actual treatment of patients, something which a textbook can never do.

I have concentrated on relating pathology, anatomy and physiology to the problems found in sick and disabled children, suggesting the rationale for physical treatment. Actual techniques for treatment are outlined only briefly, in the belief that the acquisition of wisdom is not the collection of recipes for all occasions but the development of an understanding which makes possible an intelligent and imaginative planning of treatment for each particular patient. I hope the book will stimulate students to question many established practices in physiotherapy, and to seek out new and more effective methods of treatment.

I gratefully acknowledge the advice and encouragement given to me by friends and teachers, especially by Professor James McLeod, Drs. Janet McCredie, Corrie Reye and Edward Bates, and Mrs. Berta Bobath, Miss Nancie Finnie, Miss Janet Clarke, Miss Jennifer Harrison and Miss Janet Carr. To the latter I owe particular thanks for the patience with which she read and re-read the manuscript in its various forms, and for the kindness with which she gave praise and criticism where they were most needed. The Council of the New South Wales branch of the Australian Physiotherapy Association and the Director of the School of Physiotherapy, Miss Jeanette Salmon, were generous in giving me study leave.

I would also like to thank Mrs. Penny Eamer, Medical Artist, for the drawings and diagrams, and the Departments of Photography of the Royal Alexandra Hospital for Children and the Royal Prince Alfred Hospital for their help. Finally, I must thank the parents of the children whose photographs appear on these pages.

JUST A LITTLE MORE
AND WE SHALL SEE THE ALMOND TREES IN BLOSSOM
THE MARBLES SHINING IN THE SUN
THE SEA, THE CURLING WAVES.

JUST A LITTLE MORE
LET US RISE JUST A LITTLE HIGHER

—George Seferis (transl. Rex Warner)*

*Quoted from George Seferis, *Poems*, by kind permission of The Bodley Head

PREFACE TO THE SECOND EDITION

The purpose of the second edition, as with the first, is to provide the student with an outline of the most common problems which may be encountered in sick and disabled children and the rationale for treatment or intervention by the therapist. I have not included all the medical and surgical conditions found in children, preferring to illustrate to the student ways of going about problem-solving which she can apply to any child she may encounter in a clinical paediatric situation.

Several of the chapters have been completely revised, segments have been added on the blind child and the infant with developmental delay. Two new chapters have been written, one on the burnt child and the other on the child with minimal brain dysfunction.

I am grateful to numerous colleagues, reviewers and students who have pointed out errors and omissions in the first edition and who have suggested ways of clarifying certain points. I also wish to acknowledge with thanks the work of David Robinson, photographer at Cumberland College of Health Sciences, who is responsible for many of the new photographs.

CONTENTS

PREFACE   v

SECTION I

INTRODUCTION TO PAEDIATRICS
1. The Child, His Parents and the Physiotherapist   3
2. The Nature of Movement   13

SECTION II

DEVELOPMENTAL AND NEUROLOGICAL DISORDERS
   Introduction   51
1. Cerebral Palsy and Developmental Delay   66
2. Head Injuries   142
3. Minimal Brain Dysfunction   147
4. Mental Retardation   160
5. Infections of the Brain, Spinal Cord and Peripheral   182
   Nervcs
6. Brachial Plexus Lesions in Infancy   200

SECTION III

CONGENITAL ABNORMALITIES
1. Talipes Equinovarus   209
2. Talipes Calcaneo-Valgus   233
3. Congenital Dislocation of the Hips   237
4. Arthrogryposis Multiplex Congenita   251
5. Spina Bifida   255
6. Congenital Limb Deficiencies   288

SECTION IV

DISORDERS OF BONES, JOINTS, MUSCLES AND SKIN
Introduction   309
1. Duchenne-type Muscular Dystrophy   319
2. Muscular Torticollis   338
3. Structural Scoliosis   355
4. Inflammatory Disorders of Soft Tissues and Joints   366
5. The Burnt Child   384

SECTION V

DISORDERS INVOLVING THE RESPIRATORY TRACT
Introduction   403
1. The Development and Mechanics of Respiration   407
2. Respiratory Disorders in the Neonatal Period and in   416
    Infancy
3. Respiratory Disorders in Childhood   426
4. Specific Techniques of Physical Treatment   450

APPENDICES   485
INDEX   513

Section I

Introduction to Paediatrics

1.   *THE CHILD, HIS PARENTS AND THE PHYSIOTHERAPIST*

2.   *THE NATURE OF MOVEMENT*

Chapter 1

The Child, His Parents, and the Physiotherapist

The child is not a miniature adult. The period of development into a fully integrated human being which begins with the embryo does not cease until growth, mental and emotional, as well as physical, is complete. In the physical sense, development does not merely mean that the various parts of the child grow larger, but also that these parts change, adapting to some extent, according to the demands of the environment.

The infant's central nervous system is not fully developed at birth, and the development of the skills of movement follows upon a progressive change in his nervous system. He cannot therefore be expected to achieve skills in advance of his neurological development. Similarly, the infant's respiratory system is not fully developed at birth. There must be further structural development, including an increase in the number of terminal airways as well as an increase in their relative size, before he will acquire really effective respiratory function. These considerable changes which occur with growth and development must be appreciated in order that respiratory care can be appropriate to infant and child and not merely reflect treatment principles developed for the adult.

The effect of his environment upon the child cannot therefore be too highly emphasized. It is recognized that the child's emotional development may be impeded by a lack of maternal warmth and love, but it must be stressed that the child's physical development may also be retarded or deformed by many factors as he progresses from infancy. Retention of secretions within the lungs of an infant will have a far more disabling effect upon his ventilatory function than upon an adult's because the damage to these immature structures will prevent their normal development. Abnormal posture resulting from muscle imbalance will cause maldevelopment of bone in growing children which will result in far more severe and disabling deformity than a similar muscle imbalance in adult life. Bones develop as they grow according to the stresses placed upon them. If these stresses are abnormal, skeletal development will also be abnormal.

The drive towards development is strong, the child appearing to reach a stage when physically and mentally he is ready for the next developmental skill. Therefore a child with paralysis or even absence of lower limbs, who cannot pull himself to standing at nine months, may have lost the urge to stand and walk if he is encouraged to do so at a much later stage.

These factors bring an element of urgency to treatment. Those responsible for the treatment of infants and young children must have an understanding of the importance of early treatment, which should begin before interference with essential development can occur and before irreversible damage takes place.

This is why the physiotherapist working in the field of paediatrics must be aware of the nature of growth and development of the child, as this will require an approach to treatment which will not be quite the same as that for adult patients whose physical development is mature. This knowledge of the child may also help the adult responsible for him to understand and accept him for what he really is, to understand that the child's behaviour is to some extent the result of his physical, mental and emotional immaturity. A small child cannot sit still when asked to do so if he has a need to be elsewhere; he cannot speak quietly when he feels like shouting. He cannot conform to social and environmental pressures as can an adult.

In childhood the potential to understand all things and to be all things lies somewhere within the child's developing brain, but without considerable love and stimulation this potential will not become a reality. Hence the child who must live in an institution, or who is confined to hospital for a long period, may be deprived of both love and stimulation of the required kind and may as a result demonstrate considerable retardation as he develops.

The effects of separation of a child from his mother have been documented by many authors (Bowlby 1953, Winnicott 1964). The age at which a child is most likely to suffer from this separation is said to be between six and nine months and the effects will be particularly evident if the infant has had a close and loving relationship with his mother (Bowlby 1953). This infant will demonstrate his deprivation by becoming quiet, by moving and vocalizing less, and by failing to respond to the overtures of an adult. He seems withdrawn. Motor development is affected and the infant develops more slowly than his peers. This factor must be kept in mind when assessing the developmental milestones of a hospitalized or institutionalized infant as one may make the error of assuming him to be mentally retarded. However, a younger infant and a child in his second or third year will also suffer a marked emotional response. A substitute mother, someone who is personally responsible for his care, will allay some of these effects in the case of an infant in his first year, but a 2- or 3-year old child will usually reject this substitute, refuse to be comforted, refuse to eat, will cry inconsolably, and eventually may become apathetic and regress to bed-wetting and thumb-sucking. Bowlby (1953) suggests that at this age a violent reaction to another adult is a healthy reaction, and a quiet resigned attitude a sign of unhealthy emotional development. Between three and five years the child is beginning to grasp the idea that his mother will return in the future, and this probably helps him cope emotionally with the situation at least to some extent. An older child may still suffer considerable anxiety, worrying that his stay in hospital may be a form of punishment, or that he may not be wanted at home.

In an attempt to overcome these problems which it is thought may result in serious emotional difficulties in adult life, most paediatric hospitals allow free visiting for parents, and in many centres there are facilities for the admission of the infant's mother so she may continue to look after him. However, paediatricians try to limit the period of admission to hospital in the case of infants and small children and if possible will arrange for the child to be treated at home.

It is not only in an institution that a child may suffer deprivation as this may also occur in his own home. He may lack 'mothering', that is, a stable mother figure with whom he can form a bond (Rendle-Short 1971). The child who is deprived in his own home may also suffer physical abuse, and the physiotherapist should be aware of this possibility when a child she is treating presents with multiple bruising or burns, and must report this damage to the child's doctor. The abuse of young children by their parents is not uncommon and is more often a manifestation of neurosis in the parents than of calculated cruelty. The situation

5

can become very serious and the child may die as the result of such physical ill-treatment (Rendle-Short 1971). The beatings usually do not occur as isolated instances, hence the need for all responsible for the child's well-being to report their suspicions to the doctor in order that further attacks may be avoided. The handicapped child may also experience rejection within his family, and although this rejection may not be overt, the child may suffer emotionally as a result, becoming attention-seeking, manipulative or actually destructive. The situation may become so serious as to require psychiatric help. However, a very large number of parents of handicapped children come to terms with their child's disability, and develop a positive approach which communicates itself to the child giving him encouragement.

A child will develop no matter what his environment, whether it be good or bad, but for him to develop as well as possible, he will need guidance, good example and close bonds of love within his family. When his welfare is considered it cannot be thought of in isolation from the welfare of his family. He depends upon them for love and stimulation, and he is very much part of a unit. It is because of this that the physiotherapist treating children will concern herself with the child as he exists within the family. She will have the parents present when she treats the child wherever possible, which will be reassuring for him and will ensure that their handling of him at home provides a carryover of her treatment. She will concern herself with the family's affairs insofar as they relate to the child's disability, and this may consist of advice about caring for a severely handicapped child, about a suitable chair for a child who is mentally retarded, methods of toilet training or bathing a cerebral palsied infant, or she may need to provide an understanding ear for a depressed or anxious parent.

Care must be taken not to bombard the parents with suggestions for treatment and advice. Home treatment must be kept to a minimum. Most parents will be more able to carry out a short home programme which they understand than a lengthy one no matter how clearly it is explained. Many parents prefer to write down the home programme themselves as the therapist explains it to them, finding their own notes a better reminder than a printed sheet supplied by the physiotherapist. It is essential where the parents do not understand English, that the therapist seeks the help of an interpreter in discovering the child's and the parents' problems, and in explaining the reasons for treatment.

The child in hospital is kept as much as possible in touch with his home by a therapist who talks to him about his family and his pets, and who encourages his parents to bring in his favourite toy or doll. The child who is treated as an outpatient in a hospital or in the private rooms of a physiotherapist needs to be given time to adjust to his new surroundings and to this new adult in his life. The room in which he is first seen is uncluttered and quiet with a calm atmosphere. It should be a child's room with furniture suited to his needs and painted in simple bright colours. He may later prefer to be treated in a larger room in the company of one or two other children, but in the beginning this may be a confusing, and for the older child an embarrassing experience. Where possible, visits to the physiotherapist are kept to a minimum, the parents treating the child at home, returning to the therapist for supervision and further advice. In some cases, however, a period of intensive treatment will be required.

The therapist's approach to a child will depend to some extent on the child's age. An infant responds to someone who smiles and makes encouraging noises to him provided this person is close enough to him for her face to be clearly seen. A small child will resent being taken from his mother or being undressed by a stranger. If necessary this child can be assessed initially on his mother's lap, and he need not be undressed until he has had time to grow accustomed to the new atmosphere. It is wiser not to talk to a child as though to an inferior. Explanations and requests may have to be simplified, and will probably have to be repeated, but conversations can centre on the child's particular interests or on his task of the moment, in much the same way as in conversation with an adult. The child may not be able to express himself clearly yet, but his understanding is probably in advance of his speech, and his speech will develop by listening, so baby-talk is both unnecessary and regressive. Many adults find it difficult to play with a child, and a physiotherapist who must depend upon her skill and imagination to prevent her patient from becoming bored and distracted may find it beyond her to think of some activity which will both please the child and be appropriate to her treatment objectives. To play successfully with a child requires a knowledge of his stage of development as well as a real interest in

7

playing as an expression of the child's personality. Games may be too easy and therefore boring or too difficult in which case the child will not persevere. The child's insatiable curiosity, and, at certain ages, his need to imitate, may be used by the therapist to gain the movement she requires of him.

Disciplining of the child is the responsibility of the parents and not of the physiotherapist. However, if faced with a 'naughty' child the physiotherapist could consider what might be the reason for the child's behaviour. He may be uninterested in what he is supposed to be doing and will therefore fidget, throw everything on the floor or run away. He may be naughty because he is uncomfortable, too hot, too cold, or suffering from a pain. He may be hungry or thirsty. Of course, he may be pitting his wits against those of the adult or experimenting with a new form of behaviour. In this situation it is better for the therapist to avoid the impulse to threaten the child or to bargain with him, and instead she should distract him with a change of activity or scene which will fully occupy him. Parents must also be dissuaded from threatening the child if he does not meet their expectations of good behaviour while with the physiotherapist.

The therapist will need to adapt herself to the needs of the child as he will be unable to make this adjustment himself. An important means of obtaining active co-operation from a small child consists of putting him in such a situation that he performs the action required while playing a game, quite unaware that he is fulfilling the therapist's objective of treatment. Questions such as 'Would you like to do this?' when directed to a small child are likely to elicit a negative response and are better avoided until he is older. There is a stage when every suggestion or request is met with a negative reply although this reply does not necessarily indicate the child's real feelings. This sort of questioning can result in a remarkably negative treatment session.

Knowledge of the development of movement and of methods of stimulating automatic movements will help the therapist elicit the responses she requires from an infant or small child too young to understand what is required. For example, extension of the head and trunk will be stimulated by holding the child in ventral suspension and moving him slowly about. The scheme of infant gymnastics designed by Neumann-Neurode (1967) and the methods of facilitation evolved by Bobath and Bobath (1964) demonstrate the ease with which responses may be elicited where co-operation cannot be obtained.

It is the treatment of the child aged two to four years, who is active and incapable of remaining in one place or of concentrating for more than a few moments, which is most likely to strain the tolerance and patience of an inexperienced adult. If the child is made to remain still he will find this intolerable. He is mobile and his treatment must be mobile too. The therapist can, however, make use of his natural curiosity and his tendency to imitate and if she is mobile intellectually and physically herself, she will think of ways of amusing him which will also accomplish her objectives. It is at this stage that a child may be unable to tolerate being handled by a stranger and the therapist may have to treat him by remote control, his mother handling him while the therapist guides her. The rationale for this approach must be carefully explained to the child's parents lest they should fail to understand and be resentful.

At seven to eight years of age most children will be more interested in what is happening to them and will become more conscious of themselves in relation to other people. At this stage the therapist can begin to explain to the child why he is having treatment, and the reasons for each particular part of his treatment. However, in the case of children with progressively disabling conditions such as muscular dystrophy it will be necessary for these explanations to be modified in order that they may be encouraging. As the child grows older he becomes increasingly involved in his treatment, gradually taking over the responsibility for some of his home treatment, although under the discreet supervision of his parents.

It is possible in most cases to avoid upsetting or frightening a child if the therapist takes the time to allow him to make some adjustment. The therapist can usually anticipate the child's tears and by changing the emphasis of treatment avoid them. If he does cry it is often better for the therapist to try to console him herself and to return him to his mother when he feels happier. This may avoid a circle of events in which every time he cries he is given to his mother for consolation and every time he is handled by the therapist he cries.

Some situations, especially in hospitals, do pose a considerable threat to a small child, and particular care should be taken by the adults involved to avoid causing unnecessary fear. A child who must, for example, have a plaster cast removed, is under considerable strain unless he has been in this situation frequently enough to have become reconciled to it. The use of plaster shears is probably less frightening than an electric saw, but they must be carefully used to avoid painful pinching of the skin which will occur if the lower blade is not kept parallel with the skin while the top blade does the cutting. Unless the child is experienced there should be someone else, preferably a parent, to sit with him and reassure him. This can be a very unpleasant experience especially for a child who is too young to understand what is happening to him.

During treatment of the older, chronically and perhaps progressively disabled child it is important that he be allowed to feel successful in his activities. He should not be confronted with failure, as he is so often during his daily life, in the activities he attempts in treatment, and unfortunately this happens easily where he is severely handicapped and the therapist insensitive and unobservant. Techniques can always be modified to allow him to feel he is both exerting himself and realizing a goal, even if it is a small one. It is failing at the apparently small and unimportant things that so often frustrates a child. Treatment should always be fun and he should look forward to his sessions with the physiotherapist as times of achievement.

Parents of sick or handicapped children face considerable difficulty in coming to terms with the child's illness and require support from all those with whom they come in contact. Where the child requires long-term treatment it is the physiotherapist to whom he becomes close and she is often the person best able to understand the stresses placed upon him. It is important that those involved in the child's treatment do not add to the parents' stress by giving them conflicting advice, and this will be avoided if there is regular communication between the various people responsible.

SUMMARY

Growth and development are the key concepts for understanding the behaviour and the needs of the child. For example, lack of speech as a means of communication in the infant or young child, or in the brain-injured child, does not presuppose a lack of understanding, or an inability to communicate, and the adult treating such an infant or child must remember this and make every effort to communicate by facial expression and gesture as well as by vocalization. Even the small infant is sensitive to atmosphere and knows from the way he is handled whether or not he is cared for, and whether or not he will be safe.

Although it is the child who may need treatment, it is the parents who will require guidance and support, and the child treated in isolation from his family will not be treated effectively.

The atmosphere surrounding the child is important for his happiness and co-operation. Both infant and child will respond well to calmness and a lack of fuss. Treatment and play are inseparable in the young child, and with disabled children, treatment must enable the child to learn about the world and his relationship to it.

References

Bobath, K. and Bobath, B. (1964) The facilitation of normal postural reactions and movements in the treatment of cerebral palsy. *Physiotherapy,* **50,** 8, 246.

Bowlby, J. (1953) *Child Care and the Growth of Love.* London: Pergamon.

Neumann-Neurode, D. (1967) *Baby Gymnastics.* London and Oxford: Pergamon.

Rendle-Short, J. (1971) *The Child.* Bristol: Wright.

Winnicott, D. W. (1964) *The Child, the Family and the Outside World.* London: Penguin.

Further Reading

Axline, V. (1966) *Dibs: In Search of Self.* London: Gollancz.

Bowlby, J. (1969) *Attachment and Loss.* New York: Basic Books.

Bowley, A. and Gardner, L. (1969) *The Young Handicapped Child.* London and Edinburgh: Livingstone.

Brazelton, T. B. (1969) *Infants and Mothers.* New York: Delacorte Press.

Brazelton, T. B. (1970) *Doctor and Child.* New York: Delacorte Press.

Brazelton, T. B. (1974) *Toddlers and Parents.* New York: Delacorte Press.

Brazelton, T.B. (1976) Early parent-infant reciprocity. In *The Family—Can It Be Saved?*, edited by V. C. Vaughan and T. B. Brazelton. New York: Year Book Pub. Inc.

Collins, G. M. (1968) *The Secure Child.* Sydney: Hodder & Stoughton.

Easson, H. M. (1970) *The Dying Child.* Illinois: Thomas.

Forrester, R. M. (1967) Journey with a handicap. *Special Education*, **56**, 3.

Freeman, R. R. (1967) Emotional reactions of handicapped children. *Rehabilitation Literature*, **28**, 9.

Goffman, E. (1963) *Stigma. Notes on the Management of Spoiled Identity.* New York: Prentice-Hall.

Illingworth, R. S. (1975) *The Development of the Infant and Young Child.* 6th Edition. Edinburgh: Livingstone.

Illingworth, R. S. and Holt, K. S. (1955) Children in hospital; some observations on their reactions with special reference to daily visiting. *Lancet* **2**, 1257.

Klaus, M. H., Jerauld, R., Kreger, N. C., McAlpine, W., Steffa, M. and Kennell, J. H. (1972) Maternal attachment. *New Eng. J. Med.* **286**, 460.

Ounsted, C., Oppenheimer, R. and Lindsay, J. (1974) Aspects of bonding failure. *Develop. Med. Child Neurol. 16*, 447.

Reynell, J. K. and Martin, M. C. (1965) The response of children to physiotherapy. *Physiotherapy,* **51**, 186.

Richardson, S. A., Hastorf, A. H. and Dornbusch, S. M. (1964) Effects of physical disability on a child's description of himself. *Child Development*, **35**.

Robertson, J. (1958) *Young Children in Hospital.* London: Tavistock.

Robertson, J. (1968) The long-stay child in hospital. *Maternal and Child Care*, **4**, 40.

Schmitt, B. D. and Kempe, C. H. (1975) *Child Abuse.* Basle: Ciba-Geigy.

Sheridan, M. D. (1965) *The Handicapped Child and His Home.* London: National Children's Home.

Thomas, A., Chess, S. and Birch, H. G. (1970) The origin of personality. *Scient. Amer. 223*, 2, 102.

Chapter 2

The Nature of Movement

The following pages comprise an attempt to describe briefly the nature of movement. The attempt has unfortunately resulted in considerable over-simplification of what is a vastly complicated mechanism. However, the author has aimed here merely to indicate to the student the importance of sensation in the initiation and control of movement, to point out the automatic nature of movement, and to demonstrate, however briefly, the control exercised by the brain over movement and posture. The development of movement from birth through childhood is described briefly and some suggestions are made for the analysis of movement. The student is advised to consult the textbooks and articles listed at the end of the chapter in order to pass from this brief introduction to a more detailed understanding of the subject.

THE NEUROPHYSIOLOGY OF NORMAL MOVEMENT

Movement may be initiated within the brain by the mechanism of volition or intention, or reflexly via the peripheral nervous system from receptors in skin, joints and muscles. Movement is controlled by cells within the brain which send impulses via the spinal cord and the peripheral system to the groups of muscles involved in a particular movement or in the maintenance of a particular posture. Since Hughling Jackson's time it has been generally considered that the motor cortex contains the basic neuronal programme that controls movement. That is, the brain is more concerned with movements than with muscles. Recent evidence seems to indicate that discrete muscles are represented in the motor cortex. If this is so, movement controlled by the motor cortex must be achieved by the selective activation of the appropriate combinations of cortical efferent columns (Eyzaguirre and Fidone 1975).

Importance of the sensory system

The result, however, will only be controlled movement if the sensory part of the nervous system is intact. It has been suggested that the brain is an organ of *reaction*, not of action. It can only initiate and control movement in response to the messages it receives which describe the outside world and the body's relation to it, as well as such internal matters as the state of tone, position of one part of a limb in relation to another part. This sensory feedback from proprioceptors in joints, muscles and tendons, from skin receptors, from the eyes and from the labyrinths of the ears, gives the brain the information it needs for it to send off the appropriate impulses of reaction to the periphery of the nervous system. Without an intact sensory system there cannot be 'controlled' movement or 'controlled' postural adjustment. Lance (1971) suggests that the sensory input seems to supply a driving force for the sensori-motor cortex. Mott and Sherrington performed an experiment on a cat in which they severed all the afferent or sensory connections on one side of the animal. The animal appeared hemiplegic as a result. It was unable to balance in any position and was unable to move the limbs on the deafferentated side. Taub and Berman (1968), however, demonstrated with spinal deafferentation of monkeys, that peripheral inflow from receptors in the limbs is not required for the performance of complex movements. Jones (1974) and others have pointed out that the Mott and Sherrington experiment was a unilateral deafferentation, whereas Taub and Berman's experiment was bilateral. Taub and Berman explain the contradiction by suggesting that the movements of one arm have an inhibiting effect on the movements of the other. This effect is normally counteracted by the ipsilateral segmental afferent inflow. If this inflow is abolished to one side then the remaining active limbs would have an inhibiting effect on the movements of the deafferented side.

A central feedback system has been postulated to explain how motor learning can take place in the absence of sensation and including vision. Evarts (1971) comments that when sensory feedback is eliminated by deafferentation it may be possible that feedback generated internally or by knowledge of results is of great importance in motor control.

Bruner (1973) suggests that in the infant's growth of competence there are three central themes—intention, feedback and the patterns of action which mediate between them. He comments that 'feedback' is not as simple as is sometimes thought, but consists of internal feedback which signals an intended action within the nervous system.

The automatic nature of learned movement

Movements must become automatic before they can be completely effective. For example, basic movements have to become automatic in the baby before he is free to develop other skills which in their turn will become automatic. He must learn to balance when he walks so his hands are freed for carrying his toys from one place to another. The maintenance and regaining of balance against the pull of gravity must become automatic as man spends most of his life struggling to maintain himself against gravity. Kinnear Wilson (1925) described all our movements as ranging from least automatic to most automatic. If our movements and postures were not automatic we would be very ineffective, incapable of thinking of anything other than the movement we are trying to perform. Carrying out such a simple movement would demand our full concentration. However, with practice, this movement and thousands of others have become to a large extent automatic. It is probably because of this that movements are so difficult to analyse when this must be done by observation alone.

Man has developed a complex system for controlling posture and movement. An important part of this control comes from the regulation of equilibrium, exercised through balance reactions elicited according to the sensory stimuli received, and the regulation of tone, exercised through the effects of the supraspinal and internuncial pathways on the muscle spindle. Below is a brief description of what is thought to occur in the sensori-motor system in order to maintain a posture, or by changing it, to move.

Muscle tone

This term is used in the clinical sense to mean the subjective sensation of resistance or assistance felt by the examiner when he moves a limb passively. Muscle tone refers to the potential a muscle has for activity. It does not mean activity is present in the resting muscle. There is no active contraction of the muscle to be demonstrated electrically, that is, no tonic stretch reflex (Lance 1971).

The control of muscle tone, posture and movement

When a muscle is put on a stretch specialized muscle fibres called intrafusal fibres or spindles lying in parallel with the unspecialized or extrafusal fibres, are also put on a stretch. As a result the spindles fire off impulses via monosynaptic and polysynaptic reflex arcs, resulting in the reflex adjustments necessary for posture and movement. Other impulses travel via the posterior columns (figure 1) and the spino-cerebellar tracts, transmitting information to the brain about the situation peripherally.

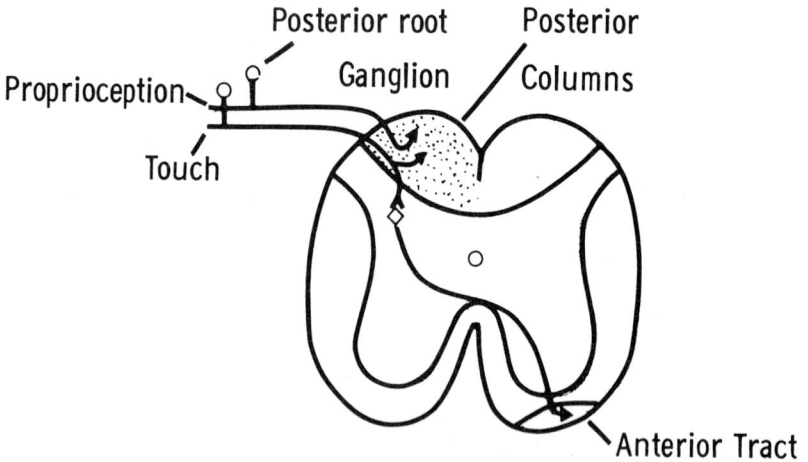

Fig.1 Cross section through the spinal cord showing the sensory pathways for proprioception and touch. (From Ranson, S. W. and Clark, S. L. (1959) *Anatomy of the Nervous System.* Philadelphia and London: Saunders.)

The impulse travels along these pathways to nuclei in the brain stem and cerebellum. The cerebellum is an important regulatory centre for control of motor activity. It uses the sensory information it receives to predict, judge and correct the motor activity. It has been likened to a comparator, comparing the state of affairs in the periphery with the desired motor act as signalled from the cerebral cortex (Eyzaguirre and Fidone 1975).

16

The final sorting out, interpretation and storage occurs in the more highly specialized cells in the cerebral cortex and the cerebellum. These cells receive all the relevant information from other specialized cells in the brain which will enable them to evolve the appropriate postural and movement patterns needed in response (figure 2). This response passes from the motor cells of the cortex via the pyramidal (corticospinal) and extrapyramidal tracts. The pyramidal tract is thought to be essential for the production of fine skilled movement, while the extrapyramidal tracts are responsible for the regulation of tone and postural adjustment. The extrapyramidal system is a vast, complex motor network arising from sub-cortical and cortical structures. The complicated number and arrangement of multisynaptic inter-connections throughout this system makes it difficult to analyse the motor effects of its neural activity.

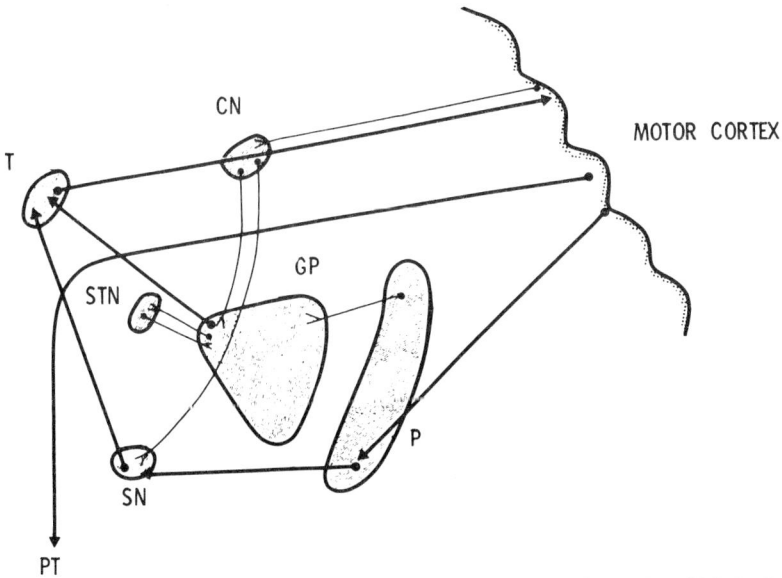

Fig.2 The connections of the basal ganglia. (From McLeod, J. M. (1971) Patho-physiology of Parkinson's Disease. *Aust. New Zeal. J. Med. Suppl.* 1, 1, 19.) CN — caudate nucleus. P — putamen. GP — globus pallidus. T — thalamus. STN — subthalamic nucleus. SN — substantia nigra. PT — pyramidal tract.

The most important of the extrapyramidal tracts are the reticulospinal tracts arising from the reticular formation which consists of cells spread throughout the brain from the cerebral cortex to the medulla, and the vestibulo-spinal tract arising from the vestibular nucleus in the brain stem (figure 3). Information about the position of the head in relation to gravity passes from the labyrinths of the ears, via the vestibular nerve to the lateral vestibular nucleus. Facilitatory impulses are then passed down the vestibulo-spinal tract to produce alteration in tone and consequent changes in posture, according to the response required (Lance 1971).

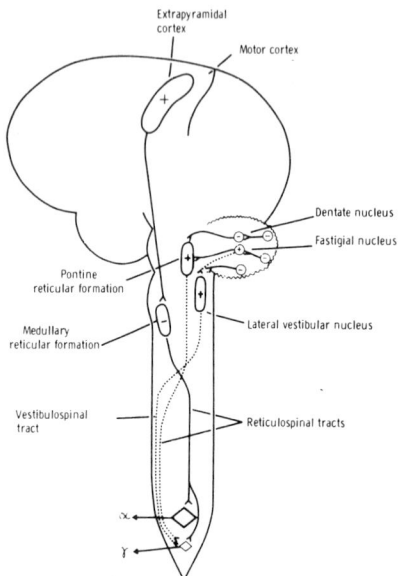

Fig. 3 Diagrammatic representation of the brain and spinal cord to show the extrapyramidal tracts responsible for controlling tone and movement. (From Lance, J. W. (1971) *A Physiological Approach to Clinical Neurology.* London: Butterworth.)

As impulses pass down through the brain they are further modified by postural reflexes such as the tonic neck and labyrinthine reflexes, which are mediated through the brain stem, and other postural and righting reflexes mediated through the midbrain, basal ganglia and thalamus (Lance 1971).

The impulses travel down the spinal cord in the tracts mentioned until they reach the appropriate segments in the spinal cord, where they synapse with the anterior horn cells, and pass via the efferent or motor part of the peripheral nerve to the spindles to maintain them in a state of controlled excitation or inhibition, and to the extrafusal fibres urging them to contract or lengthen, according to what is required by the posture or movement (figures 4 and 5). As well as the controlling effect of cells in the brain, there is also an internuncial system by which neurones within the spinal cord itself also exercise a regulating effect on the muscle spindle.

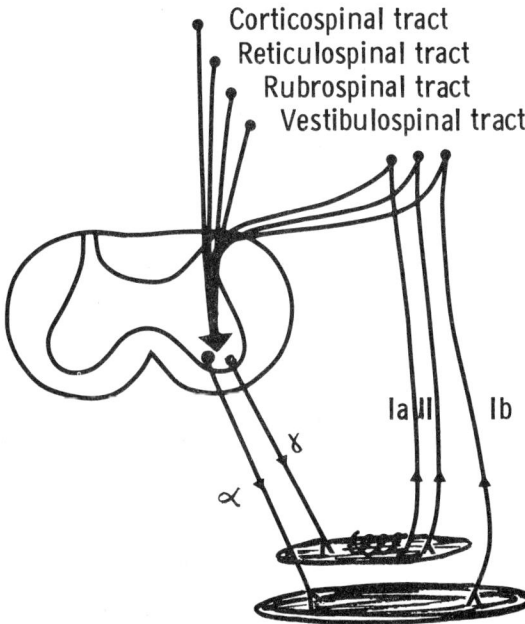

Corticospinal tract
Reticulospinal tract
Rubrospinal tract
Vestibulospinal tract

Ia II Ib

γ

α

Fig. 4 Efferent pathway to extrafusal and intrafusal muscle fibres. The alpha motoneurone innervates the extrafusal muscle fibres and the gamma motoneurone the muscle spindle. Group Ia afferent fibres from the muscle spindle synapse with the alpha motoneurone to form the afferent limb of the stretch reflex arc. Group 11 afferents have sensory receptors in the muscle spindle and group 1b in the Golgi tendon organ. (From McLeod, J. M. (1971) Pathophysiology of Parkinson's Disease. *Aust. New Zeal. J.Med. Suppl.* 1, 1, 19.)

To summarize, normally all reflex activity, whether tonic or spinal, is held in check by the higher centres in the brain acting through the pyramidal and extrapyramidal tracts, and dependent

19

upon the controlling influence of the basal ganglia and reticular formation (Lance 1971). These higher centres can only exert their influence upon movement at segmental level in the spinal cord, that is, through the gamma and alpha motorneurones.

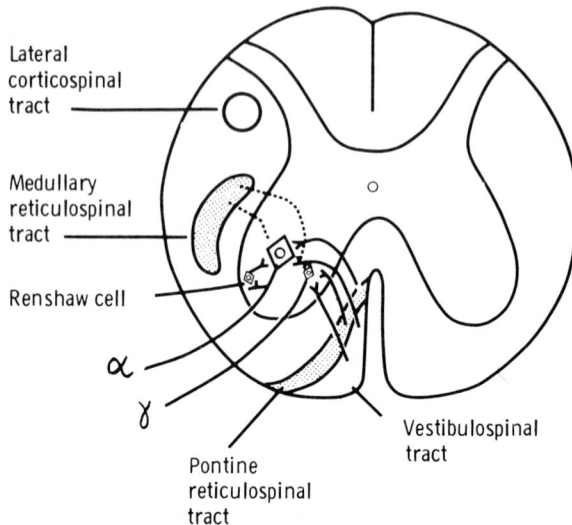

Fig. 5 Cross section through the spinal cord showing control over the alpha and gamma motoneurone. (From Lance, J. W. (1971) *A Physiological Approach to Clinical Neurology.* London: Butterworth.)

THE DEVELOPMENT OF MOVEMENT

The development of movement in a baby and young child is described in detail by many authors. It is not intended here to list all the stages through which a baby passes on the road to mature motor behaviour. For these details the reader is referred to the reading list at the end of the chapter. Appendix 7 lists the developmental reactions and the times at which they may be seen in the first two years of life.

For the physiotherapist involved in treating children with any disorder interfering with normal development, it is important to understand, not only what function develops at a particular chronological age, but how the baby prepares himself for each new step in his development. It is not so important in treatment to know, for example, that a baby can usually sit without support from his hands by eight months, but it *is* important to know *why* he can do this, that he has developed this ability *because* he has good head control and sufficient extension against gravity, and has developed effective balance in this position. It is important to know that until he can sit like this he will not be free to use his hands, therefore manipulation will not progress at a normal speed, and learning will be retarded.

Although the four major areas of sensori-motor development are discussed below separately, it will be seen that stages of development do not proceed in an arbitrary and unrelated manner, but that manipulative, locomotor, visual and oral functions all progress together, and depend upon one another, and that all these aspects of development in turn depend upon certain basic factors such as the development of head control, extension against gravity, symmetry, and on the gradual disappearance of the primitive movements found in the neonate.

The development of head control

Head control is an important prerequisite for the development of all functions. Until the position of the head in space and against gravity is established, the young baby cannot develop eye-hand control, visual acuity or balance against gravity. He cannot roll over, sit up or take his hands to his mouth. He cannot eat properly or vocalize effectively.

The development of head control infers the development of the labyrinthine righting reactions. These begin to develop first in prone, then in supine. Some element of head righting is present at birth as seen in the protective side turning of the head in prone, when the head is raised momentarily before it is turned, and in the small degree of correction of the head seen when the infant is pulled to sitting.

Before the infant's development can proceed from the immature reflex behaviour of the neonatal period towards the relatively sophisticated behaviour of the one-year old baby, the immature predominantly flexor activity must be inhibited, allowing the development of extension which will ultimately allow the baby to become antigravity. This extension begins at the head and progresses in a caudal direction with an important part of the development occurring in the first six months.

21

The newborn baby, when pulled to sitting, exhibits some head lag, but he does make some attempt to right his head, in contrast to the hypotonic, brain-damaged or mentally retarded infant, each of whom may demonstrate a complete head lag (figure 6). In the first four months the baby develops good head control, and at this stage when he is pulled to sitting, he will bring his head beyond the midline into flexion (figure 7). From the age of five months, when his mother puts out her hands to pull him up, he will initiate the head movement even before she grasps his hands (figure 8), and by six months he will be able to lift his head from the bed voluntarily and spontaneously and to look at his toes. It is

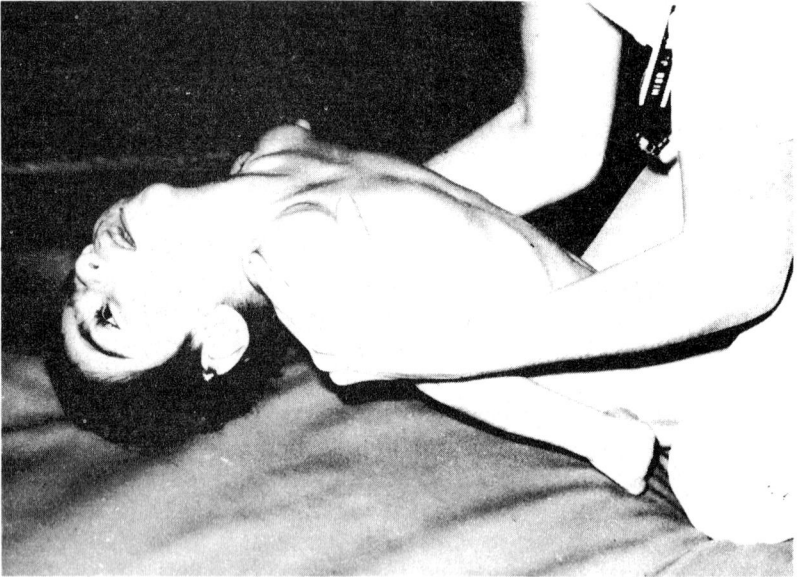

Fig. 6 Severe head lag in a floppy baby.

interesting and an example of the relatively rapid development of extensor compared to flexor activity, that it takes six months for the baby to develop movement of the head against gravity in supine, while in prone he moves his head against gravity by the time he is two months old.

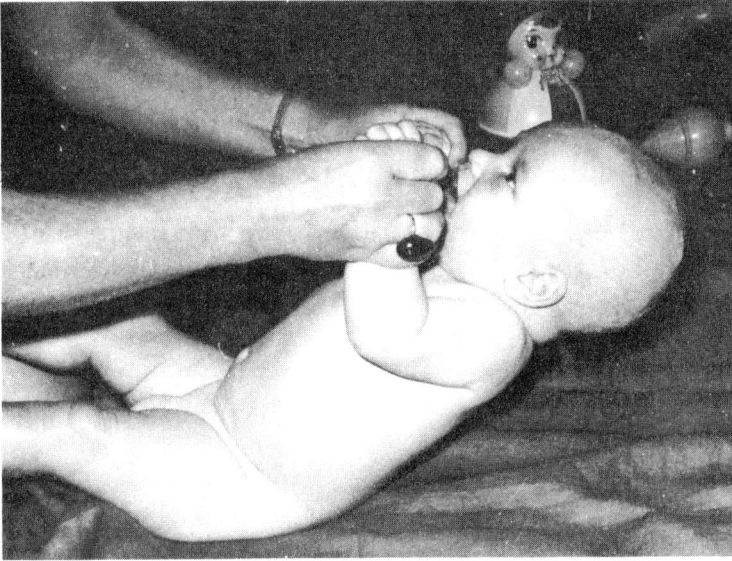

Fig. 7 Normal 3 month old baby pulled to sitting. Good head control.

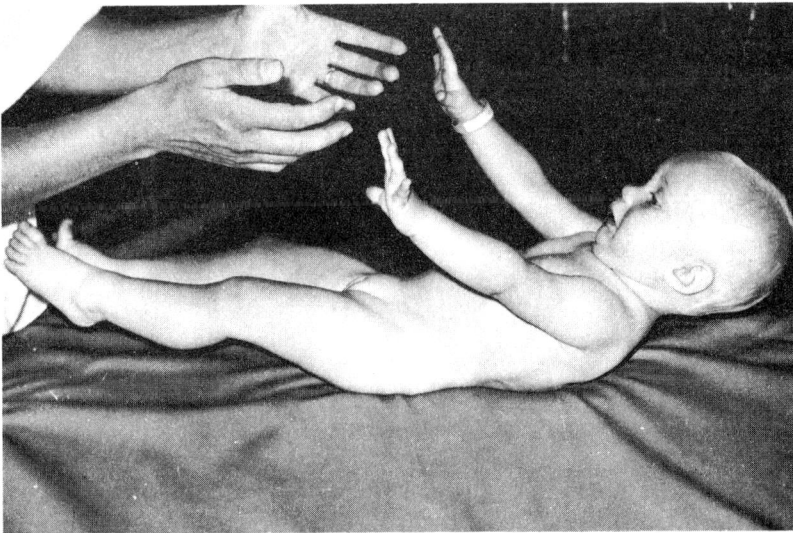

Fig. 8 Aged 9 months, lifting head and shoulders in anticipation of being pulled to sitting.

The development of locomotion

At birth, if the infant is held upright on his feet, he will stand (figure 9), and if his body is tilted forward he will walk. It is a parody of standing and walking, but a glimpse of things to come. These are stereotyped and primitive automatic movements but give an indication that, even at this reflex level, the potential for

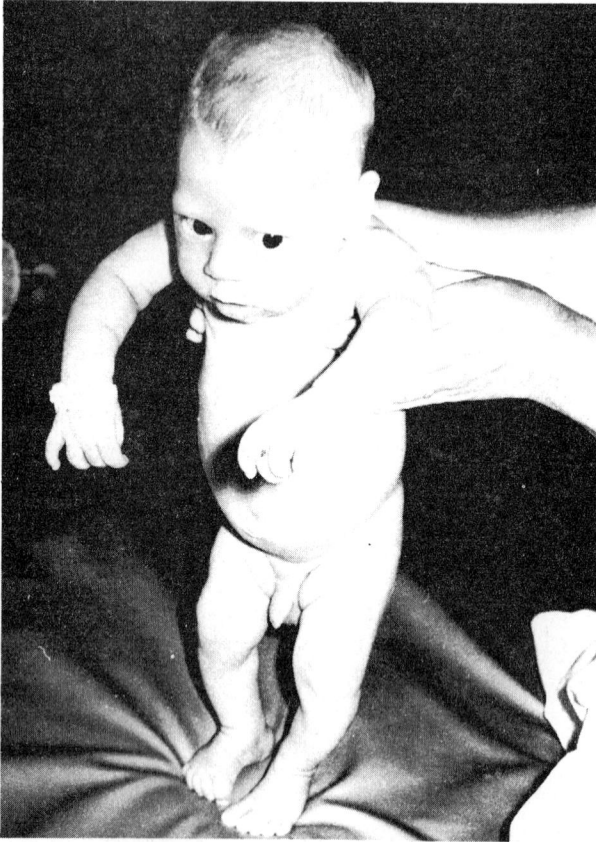

Fig. 9 Primary standing.

standing and walking is present in his brain, and will develop, with the acquisition of head control, extension against gravity and balance, into something freer, more mobile and less stereotyped, that is, into the normal controlled walking of the older baby. This development will take some five years to complete and even then the finer points of walking requiring perfect balance control will need further practice if they are ever to develop.

This reflex walking and standing occurs from birth to about eight weeks, then is lost. Now, when he is held in standing, his legs will collapse into flexion and he will not respond by straightening his legs and taking weight on his feet until he is approximately four months old.

The infant's ability to get from one position to another or from one place to another depends upon his developing the ability to shift his weight and to balance throughout each weight shift.

Locomotion does not develop as a separate entity, but as a result of development occurring in other areas. In order to stand the infant must hold himself erect against the force of gravity. He must develop extension and this occurs from birth in a cephalo-caudal direction. At birth the infant can only raise his head momentarily in prone in order to turn his head to one side to avoid suffocation. The ability to extend his head and trunk develops quickly until at six to eight weeks he can raise his head up and hold it there. By three months he can raise it to an angle of 90 degrees from the floor and a few weeks later he can hold it steadily there for an indefinite period. By this time he can take weight on his forearms with his back well extended (figure 10). As he develops even more extension he will take weight on his hands with his elbows extended. He has now almost completely developed his ability to extend against gravity. The final step comes at five months when he lifts his head, upper trunk and arms from the floor simultaneously and stays in this fully extended position for a few moments. When he is able to shift his weight from one arm to the other, he will be able to reach out with one hand for a toy (figures 11 and 12). Should he be held in standing at this stage he would show a great deal of extensor tone with difficulty getting his feet flat on the floor.

Shortly before this he attempts to crawl as a means of getting about on the floor. At this stage of maximum extensor activity he tries to get into four point kneeling but may fail because of his inability to combine the extension with flexion of his knees and hips. However, he pulls himself along the floor with his arms. As soon as he can get into four point kneeling he must develop equilibrium reactions in this position in order to transfer his

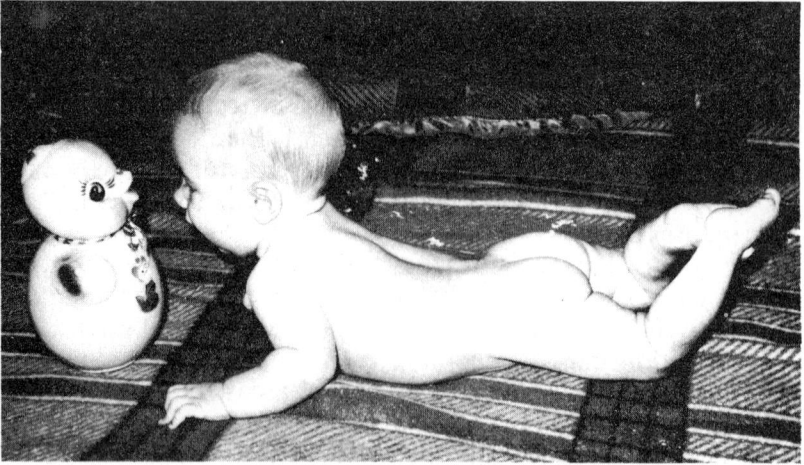

Fig. 10 Aged 4 months, weight-bearing on his forearms, head and upper trunk well extended.

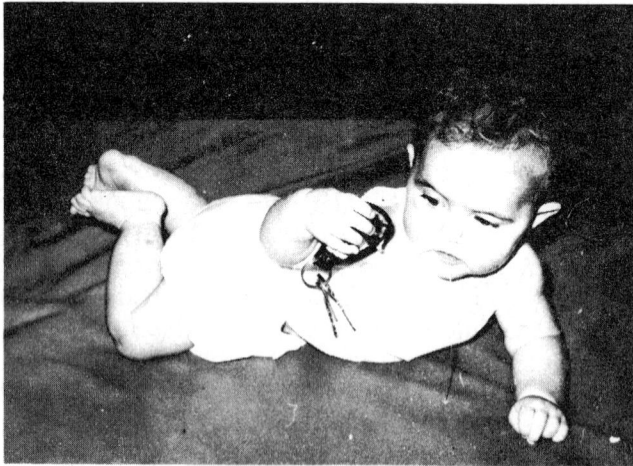

Fig. 11 Aged 6 months, weight-bearing on one arm with trunk rotation.

weight from one side to the other. He practises by rocking back and forth, lifting first one arm then the other. At approximately the same time as he is able to shift weight enough to lift one arm and grasp a proffered toy, he will begin to crawl. He will become expert at balancing in this position, and will be seen to stop,

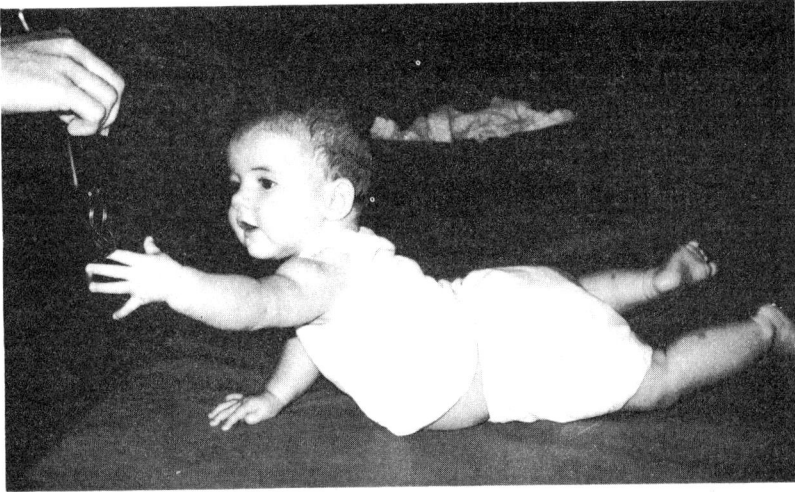

Fig. 12 Aged 6 months, weight transference on to one arm in order to reach forwards.

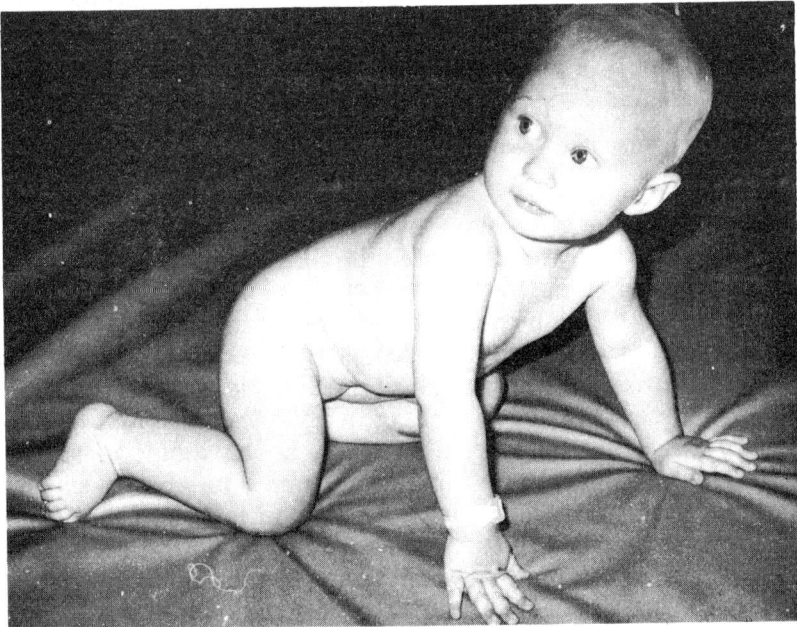

Fig. 13 Aged 10 months, demonstrating ability to transfer weight and turn the head in four point kneeling.

poised delicately on the hand and leg on one side, while he turns to look at what is happening behind him (figure 13). Some time between crawling and walking he may progress like a bear on his hands and feet (figure 14).

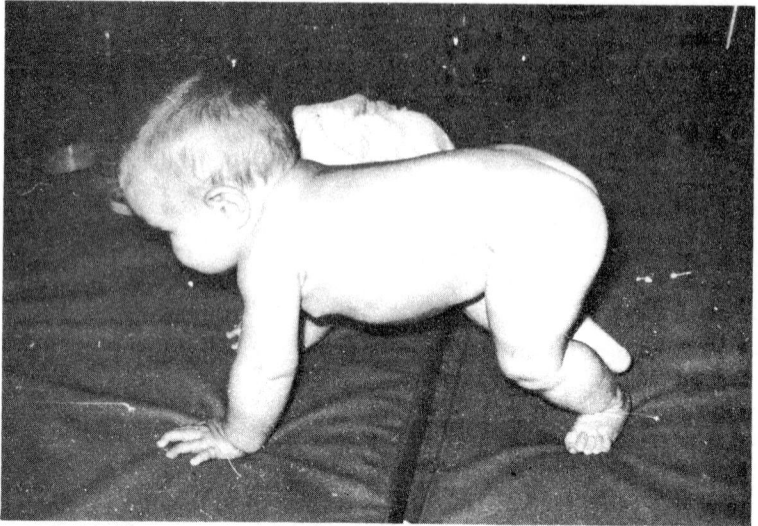

Fig. 14 Aged 6 months, extending knees in four point kneeling in preparation for bear walking on hands and feet.

At approximately eight months he begins to pull himself to standing, usually by holding on to the cot sides. He has developed good extension, at the hips as well as at the knees and trunk, so he stands well although he needs the support of his hands. However, he lacks again the ability to change from extension to flexion which he must do if he wants to sit down again. Also at this stage his grasp has progressed to the stage when he has a well-developed palmar grasp but no effective release. So he stands in his cot crying until his mother sits him down, or until he screams so hard he inadvertently lets go with his hands and falls into the sitting position. He repeats this performance several times, exhausting the patience of his mother, until he has learned the combination of movements which enables him to sit down of his own accord. Soon after this he will be able to stand from the crouch position and from a half-kneeling position (figures 15 and 16).

28

Some time before he can walk alone, he 'cruises', walking sideways around his bed and the furniture, holding on and occasionally falling down to the sitting position. He practises constantly, occasionally letting go and standing for a few moments with arms abducted. He is developing transference of weight laterally and the equilibrium reactions which he must have in order to balance alone in standing. He will not walk alone until he has developed equilibrium reactions in standing, and for his walking to become less wide-based, and for arm swing to develop, his balance must develop still further.

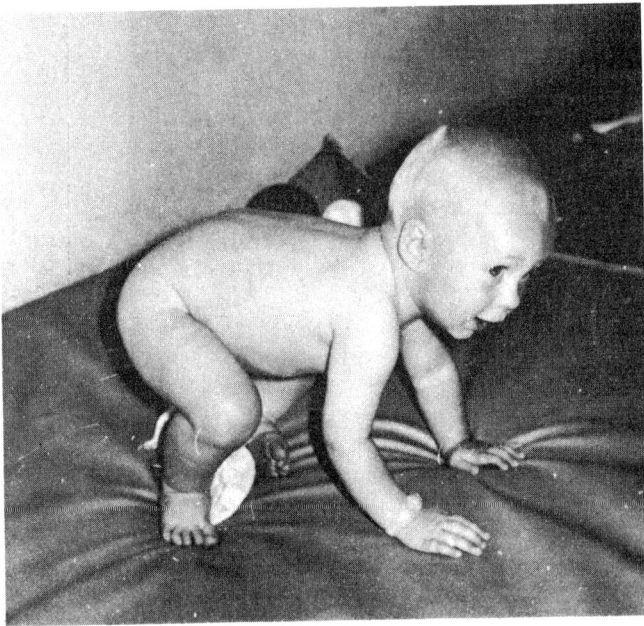

Fig. 15 Aged 11 months, standing up from sideways sitting through the crouch position.

Eventually, some time between eight and eighteen months, he walks alone, and he does this because he has developed head control, a postural reflex mechanism (comprising the automatic reactions of righting and equilibrium) that is efficient enough to enable him to balance fairly well in standing, and inhibition of the extension activity, strong at five months, sufficient to allow him

29

to develop the sophisticated motor patterns which comprise a bipedal gait.

His first walking is very tentative, a few steps, then a fall into his parent's arms. With more confidence, and much tenacity and practice, he will launch forth on his own, first in order to get from point A to point B, then to begin a detailed exploration of his

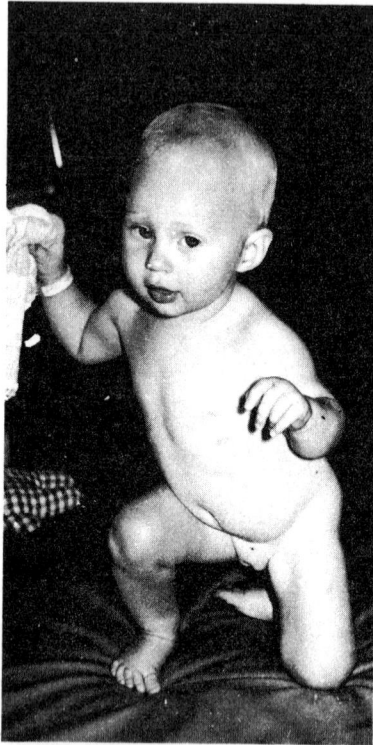

Fig. 16 Aged 13 months, attempting to stand up through half kneeling.

surroundings. At first he will walk with his arms abducted and flexed, feet wide apart, using his arms to compensate for his imperfect equilibrium reactions. He appears ataxic. His walking has many of the elements of ataxia because of its wide base, constant adjustments, inaccurate directional sense, and excessive ranges of motion. He lifts his feet too high and puts them down either too firmly or too tentatively. He over-balances which means he reacts to his threatened balance too vigorously and falls over. He cannot carry anything as he needs his hands to help him balance. He tries to carry a toy across the room to his father, but falls over, and either walks across without the toy or crawls over with it, depending on which seems the most important at the time.

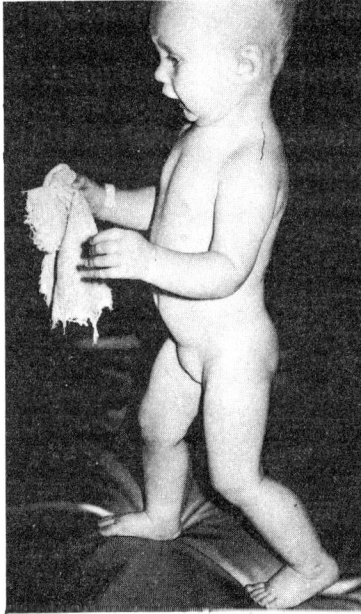

Fig. 17 Aged 13 months, walking.
Note the forward tilt of the pelvis.

As he practises and as his balance develops his base becomes less wide, his hands come down by his sides and he is able to trail his favourite blanket behind him. Eventually he will carry a large toy in both hands, indicating that his hands are now completely free and can be used to play and explore rather than to help him balance (figures 17 and 18). He may drive his mother to desperation as he continues his, by now, detailed and continuous exploration of everything within his reach. He is able to learn at an intense rate now that locomotion has opened up his area of

31

exploration. His walking becomes steadier and he is able to walk increasingly long distances. He will not be able to jump on both feet until three years, stand on one leg until four years, or hop until five years. Should he feel inclined when he is an adult he will be able to develop his balance and therefore his locomotor abilities to the fine precision needed to walk a tightrope, or traverse a snow-covered ridge in the Himalayas.

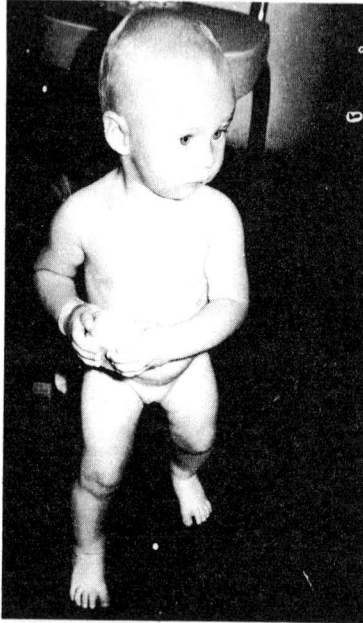

Fig. 18 Aged 13 months, walking. Note the wide base on which she walks. She can carry an object in both hands now. She no longer needs her arms for balance.

The development of prehension

A newborn baby has no ability to use his hands. He holds them fisted, thumbs either inside or outside the fist. This flexion of the fingers is part of the generalized flexor hyperactivity found in the neonatal period. Until the age of four weeks his hands are open only when he is relaxed, while being fed or when he is asleep. A reflex grasp can be stimulated by placing a finger across his palm. He will hold on, and in the first few weeks his grasp, although reflex in character, is strong enough to support his whole weight if he is lifted from the bed. His general flexor tone is so pronounced in this early period that he is unable to move his arms in any but the most stereotyped manner, lacking elbow extension and unable to reach out with his arms. He can stretch his arms only as part of the reflex Moro response, when his fingers and elbows almost fully extend.

The neonate will follow an object briefly with his eyes and he will follow a face from one side to the other, if it is close enough to him. It will be the conjunction of eye and hand control that will start the infant on the path to functional use of his hands. The development of manipulative skill can be said to date from this time.

Voluntary grasp cannot begin to develop until the immature grasp reflex is modified, which it does some time between fourteen and sixteen weeks. By three months the hands are brought to the midline, and the infant clasps and unclasps them. At twelve weeks the hands are mostly open, which corresponds to the general development of extensor tone throughout the body. At this stage he is lifting his head well up in prone. As extension activity in prone becomes even more pronounced, so finger extension is more evident, and at three months he begins to reach out toward an object hanging above him. Until this time he had looked at it with interest, but made no attempt to reach it, although he would grasp a rattle if it were placed in his hand and wave it around, sometimes looking at it, sometimes not. At this time he is waving his arms around in an apparently aimless manner, laughing and gurgling in evident pleasure, but eventually he 'catches' his hands with his eyes and this is the beginning of hand regard.

By four months he has made real progress. He will reach out to touch a brightly-coloured toy, but his successful attempts at hitting it will contain an element of luck because he is very incoordinate. However, he has been getting his hands to the midline, meaning that both hands at once can be regarded by the eyes. This is an important step in the development of prehension.

The baby puts his fist in his mouth in the early weeks, but this appears accidental and due to the flexed position of his arm as he lies with his head to one side. However, he appears to use his hand to comfort himself, even in the neonatal period, sucking on his fist when he is upset. Although he may at times lie in an asymmetrical tonic neck posture (see Appendix 1), this is never constant in a normal baby, and the relatively fleeting nature of the response is shown when he flexes the arm on the face side, bringing his fist in contact with his mouth. It is not until he develops more extension tone that he can put his fingers in his mouth, and not until his thumb comes abducted away from his hand that he will be able to suck his thumb separately.

It should be noted that throughout manipulative development the infant 'grasps' with his eyes before he grasps with his hands. By six weeks he is watching his mother's face intently, although he is probably unable to identify particular aspects of it apart from the eyes. By eight months he will have become fascinated with the different parts of her face and will watch her mouth when she talks and try to put his fingers in it. He will try to poke his index finger into her eye, her nose or her ear, an indication of his increasing ability to recognize the parts of her face plus the ability to use his index finger separately from the rest of his hand.

At five months, when he begins to grasp voluntarily, he grasps his toes when in supine, often transferring them to his mouth (figure 19). He has little control over the strength of his grasp, and will hold an object either too strongly or too gently. At this stage, he may grasp a handful of his mother's hair and it is not naughtiness that makes him hang on while she tries to wrest it from him, but an inability on his part to modify his grasp enough to let go. At nine months he cannot voluntarily release an object and it is interesting that this coincides with his inability to sit down from standing.

Development of manipulation suffers a temporary halt when the baby begins to sit, as his hands are needed for support. The first attempts at sitting occur at six months when he has developed head control and sufficient trunk extension. He takes weight with his hands between his feet (figure 20) and as his balance improves his hands are moved more laterally (figure 21). At seven months, with his hands well forward, he finds his feet again and plays with them briefly. At this stage he begins to transfer objects from hand to hand. It is the development of the parachute reaction between six and eight months which enables the baby to use his hands for propping in sitting.

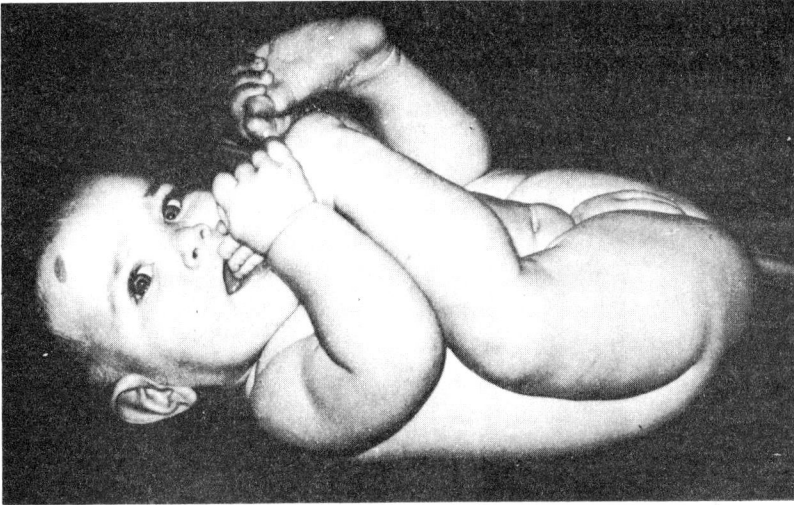

Fig. 19 Aged 5 months, she grasps her toes and puts them in her mouth.

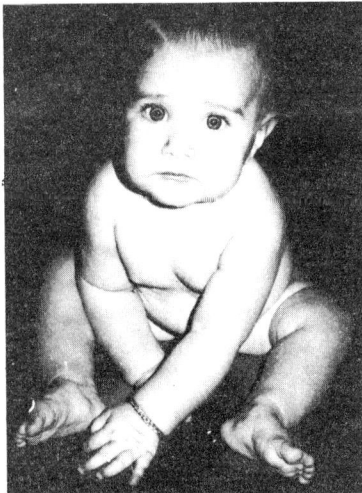

Fig. 20 Aged 6 months, propping forwards on her hands. At this stage the parachute reaction forwards is developing.

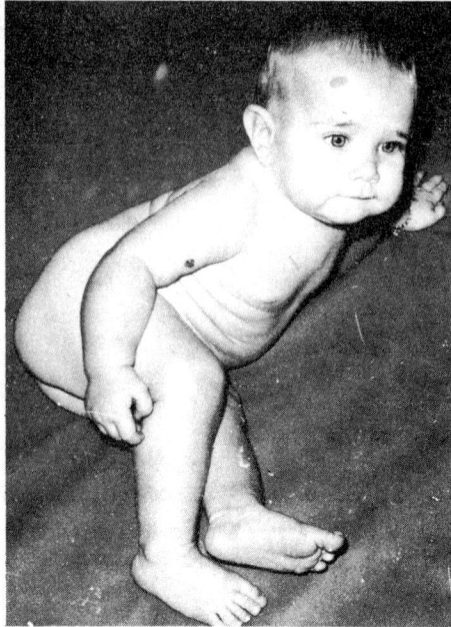

Fig. 21 Aged 7 months, sitting with support sideways.

At seven to eight months his balance improves still further as his equilibrium reactions develop in this position and he plays with other parts of his body, including his hair. As he now no longer needs his hands for support (figure 22), he can play with toys, and his manipulation will begin to progress once more (figure 23). At nine months, when he is handed an object, he will not release it again immediately. By twelve months however, he will hand the object back when asked to do so. By eight months his balance will be efficient enough for him to be able to rotate his trunk in sitting and reaching out for toys behind him, which enlarges his scope considerably (figure 24).

At six to seven months, when he is offered a biscuit, he will put it in his mouth. Chewing has developed so he will be able to eat it. Before this stage, if he is offered a biscuit, he will clutch it, and wave his arm about, then either drop the biscuit or hold it so hard it crumbles. Some babies begin to feed themselves with a spoon by

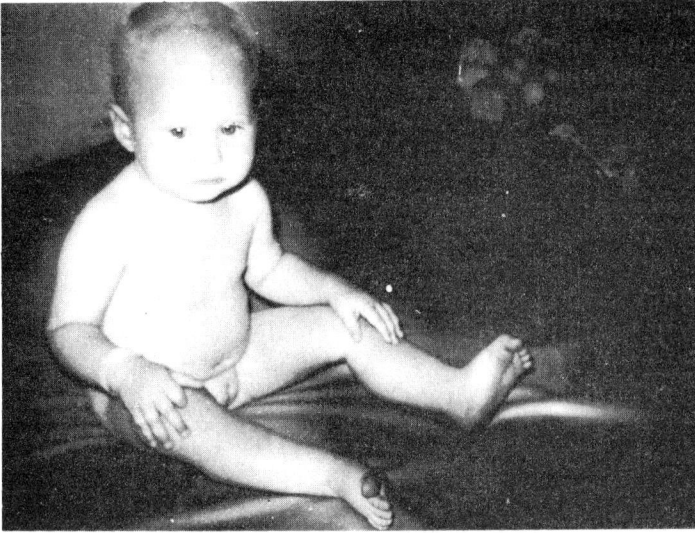

Fig. 22 Aged 11 months. The hands are not needed for support.

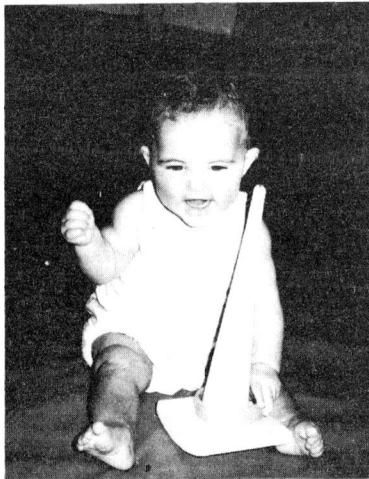

Fig. 23 Aged 7 months, hands can be used for playing now they are no longer needed for support.

nine months, but with a great deal of mess and inaccuracy. (Most babies will accomplish this by fifteen months.) He will bang the spoon on his table and much of the food will go into his hair and on to the floor. At this stage everything within reach goes into his mouth, and this mouthing of toys, clothes and hands continues until twelve months.

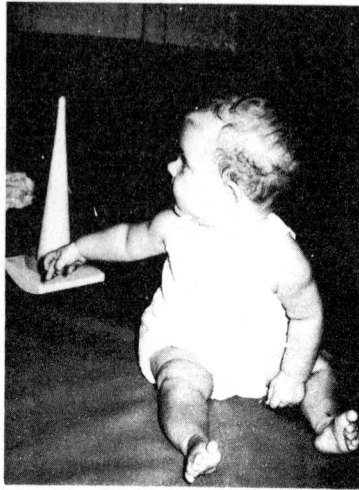

Fig. 24 Aged 7 months, sitting balance is well enough established to allow rotation within the trunk.

The first voluntary grasp is with the whole hand, tending more toward the ulnar side. The object is not held in the radial side of the hand until seven months, and he will not develop an immature pincer grasp until about nine months. At this stage he grasps, using the terminal phalanx of the thumb against the second phalanx of the index finger, in what is sometimes called a scissor grasp. The pincer grasp does not become mature until twelve months, when the baby can grasp effectively using the tip of thumb and index finger. The hand is then completely orientated, as is the adult's, toward the radial side (figure 25).

Mature voluntary grasp is preceded by a range of activities such as patting, poking, plucking and raking, which are practised diligently and repetitiously. These movements appear to be exploratory in nature, but there seems an element of perseveration in their being so constantly performed. Once mastered they combine to provide a more effective hand function, with grasp, release and manipulation.

Once the baby has developed an effective and mature grasp his manipulative ability develops very quickly. Handedness varies in its time of establishment, but most children show a hand preference by fifteen months. He will attempt to put one block on

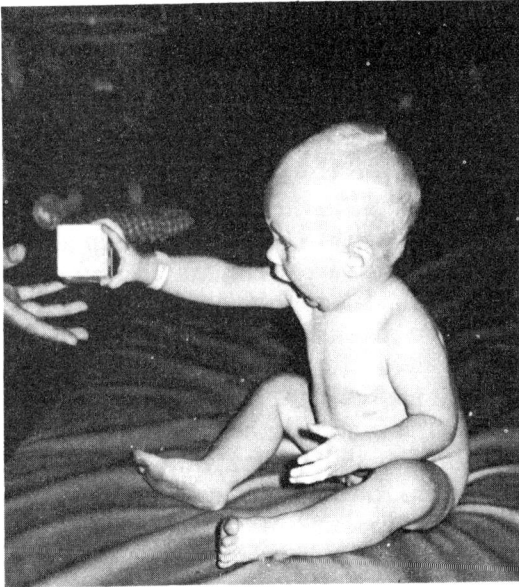

Fig. 25 Aged 11 months. Grasp is becoming more radially orientated. Note the extension of the fingers of both hands, plus the opening of the mouth which at this stage is often associated with finger extension. These are associated or synkinetic movements.

top of another at twelve months, if the action is demonstrated for him, and by the age of three he will build a tower of ten blocks. He begins to undress himself at eighteen months, by pulling off his vest. By two years he can put on his socks, by three his shoes, and by five he will be almost independent in personal care. At the age of two most children will imitate a vertical line, but not until two and a half can they imitate a horizontal line or circle. By four most will be able to draw a man.

The development of oral function, speech and communication

Speech also does not develop as a separate entity but as part of oral function, requiring normal tone throughout the body, the development of head control, and the opportunity of communicating with someone to whom the infant feels close. A baby learns to babble and then to talk depending upon those to whom he is able to talk. This is one of the reasons suggested (Luria and Yudovich 1959) for the poor speech development sometimes found in twins, since they mostly talk to each other. Babies in institutions are known to be slow to babble, and even when older tend to talk less than their peers who have had close relationships with their parents.

Crying is known to improve lung function in the first few days of life (Long and Hall 1961). It is also the earliest form of vocal communication, although it is triggered off by such basic feelings as hunger, cold and pain. In the neonate it is also triggered off by the startle response which is very easily elicited at this stage. The stages of preverbal and verbal communication are described in detail by Sheridan (1964) and include, as well as crying, smiling, frowning, nestling and pushing away. In the first few weeks, crying takes on a cyclic form and it is difficult to console the infant by the usual methods. At this stage the parents worry that the crying represents a failure in their nurturing, not realising that it is usually self-limiting and unavoidable. The tension engendered by their anxiety seems to communicate itself to the baby who may cry for even longer periods.

A baby may vocalize as early as four to six weeks, making small throaty sounds, which reflect to some extent his physiological and emotional state. By twelve weeks he makes these sounds as a means of communication with the person closest to him, obviously deriving pleasure from this. The baby laughs aloud at three to four months. By eight months he makes repetitive sounds such as 'da-da' but at irrelevant moments. This babbling is an essential prelude to speech, and adults instinctively reinforce this by making babbled sounds back to the child. At twelve months he knows one or two words, although if he is intelligent and in a stimulating environment he will probably know more.

The various oral reflexes are described in Section II, Chapter 1. The development of normal tongue movement, of normal swallowing and of normal co-ordination between respiration and oral function are all essential elements in the development of speech. It is thought that the muscular action involved in feeding is an essential preparation for babbling and speech.

It is interesting to consider the association between vocalization and movement. In the baby vocalization tends to be associated with movement and the infant may reach a crescendo of babbling with jerky bouncing movements of his limbs and trunk, speech and movement reinforcing each other. In the older child, speech is used in play to reinforce the action, and the child can be heard describing aloud to himself the story behind the game he is playing.

The acquisition of motor skill

In considering the development of motor activity in childhood it is necessary to consider also the acquisition of skill in movement. The term 'development of movement' is usually used to describe the effects of maturation of the brain in the early years of life. It is also important to consider how the child builds upon his basic motor development the skills he will need eventually for adult life, recreation, sport and work.

Annett (1971) defines skill as any human activity which becomes better organised and more effective as the result of practice. Learning a motor skill requires, according to Singer (1968), monitored practice, motivation, awareness of goal, and a knowledge of results. Motor skill is learned by breaking the skill down into its component parts, practising each part separately, then putting them together in the appropriate order necessary for the skill.

Inhibition is considered to play an important role in the development of motor co-ordination in both childhood and adult life. Motor learning and control are said to depend more on the progressive inhibition of unwanted muscular activity than on the activation of additional motor units (O'Connell 1972, Basmajian 1977). The following example will illustrate the importance of being able to inhibit unwanted activity. A toddler, having un-wrapped a chocolate, walked over to a litter bin in order to throw away the wrapping paper. He held the chocolate between his thumb and index finger and the paper was held in his palm by his remaining fingers. As he released his fingers, his thumb and index finger also opened, and he dropped both paper and chocolate. In order to execute this motor task with skill, that is, with control, he will need to inhibit all muscular activity which is unnecessary.

There are many other factors involved, and the reader should consult the relevant references at the end of this chapter.

The premature infant

Any infant born before term can be called premature. A foetus can survive after 25 weeks gestational age if temperature and nutrition are adequate. A more rational use of oxygen (not causing either ocular damage or intellectual retardation), monitored by frequent blood gas estimations, reduces the risks usually associated with prematurity. Nevertheless, the more advanced the infant's maturity the better his chance of survival. The infant matures in an identical manner whether in an incubator or in utero. Therefore at 41 weeks his neurological status is approximately the same as that of the full term infant.

The premature infant has certain characteristics. He is somnolent and hypotonic. He demonstrates tremorous athetoid movements of his arms. The Moro reflex and placing reactions are present, the latter from 32 weeks. Tone gradually increases in a caudo-cephalic direction and the infant assumes to some extent the flexed posture of the neonate. The development of the premature infant is described in detail by Dargassies (1968). Carter and Campbell (1975) describe the progress of one premature infant aged 34 weeks for the first eight weeks of postnatal life.

ANALYSIS OF NORMAL MOVEMENT

Having seen how movement develops in a baby, the next step is to develop an understanding of movement itself. It is only by understanding normal movement that the therapist will recognize abnormal movements as they occur in neurological disorders and in other disorders affecting the locomotor system. Similarly, it is only by understanding normal movement that the therapist will be able to assess which elements are necessary in order for her patient to develop a particular function, and which elements are missing or abnormal. For example, she must know the relevance of weight transference in the action of standing from sitting if she is to understand why her patient, who lacks this essential element, is unable to perform the action.

It is not intended to describe here the anatomical mechanism of movement. For movement to be normal there must be normal ranges of movement at the individual joints involved in the movement, and a normal musculo-skeletal and nervous system. The various movements occurring at individual joints should be studied simultaneously with the anatomy of the area as this knowledge is important in the assessment of disability. However, to understand movement requires in particular the ability to see the important elements of normal movements, and to correlate this knowledge with a knowledge of the development of movement and the acquisition of skill in the infant and child.

A description of two basic movements is given here in the hope that this will stimulate the physiotherapist to make further discoveries on her own.

Walking forward

Walking has been described as a constant losing and regaining of balance, which refers to the transference of weight laterally and forward, the basic elements of the movement. This transference of weight causes balance to be momentarily lost, but it is regained by the swinging forward of the free leg, with lateral movement of the head and trunk, and the transfer of weight forward and laterally on to this leg. Movement forward and laterally on to the leg is accomplished as much by extension at the weight-bearing hip as by flexion of the other. Without this extension a normal step cannot be taken. A small degree of rotation occurs within the trunk itself and at the hips. There is a small degree of posterior then anterior tilting of the pelvis as the leg is swung forward and weight is taken over it. Lateral pelvic movement takes place, to an extent which is variable in different people, as weight is transferred laterally on to one leg. The hip of the weight-bearing leg moves into extension as weight is transferred forward, a movement the importance of which is often underestimated. The knee of the weight-bearing leg remains potentially mobile as weight is transferred on to it, enabling balance to be more effectively maintained during the brief period when all the weight is maintained on the one leg.

Sitting to standing

The important components in this movement are the initial

shifting of the feet to an appropriate position and the symmetrical shifting of the extended trunk and head forward by flexion at the hips.

These are very simplified descriptions, but the aim of such simplification is to indicate the relative importance of particular components which are frequently missing in patients with disorders of movement and to stress the importance of balance throughout each shift in the body's centre of gravity. It is suggested that the student analyse for herself other basic movements such as rolling over and standing up from prone or supine, as well as such functions as dressing and undressing. This method of observing basic movements is intended as an introduction to the study of the complexities of movement, which can only be explored with a detailed understanding of skeletal, muscular and neurological anatomy, and function. Electromyographic studies are adding to our knowledge of muscular activity during movement but such information is of little value unless coupled with the awareness of the importance of the *sequence* of the components within a movement, of the most *important components* in each movement, and of the *necessity for balancing* the body throughout all movements.

SUMMARY

For the physiotherapist, understanding the nature of movement involves knowledge of the anatomy and physiology of sensorimotor function, appreciation of the details of child development (particularly as related to the development of movement) plus the ability to analyse the movements used by the normal child and adult as he goes about his daily activities and demonstrates his various motor skills.

References

Annett, J. (1971) Acquisition of skill. *Br. Med. Bull.*, **27** 3, 266–271.

Basmajian, J. V. (1977) Motor learning and control. *Arch. Phys. Med. Rehabi.*, **58**, 38–41.

Bruner, J. S. (1973) Organisation of early skilled action. *Child Develop.* **44**, 1–11.

Carter, R. E. and Campbell, S. K. (1975) Early neuromuscular development of the premature infant. *Phys. Ther.*, **55**, 12, 1332.

Dargassies, S. SA (1968) *The Development of the Nervous System in the Foetus*. Geneva: Nestlé.

Evarts, E. V. (1971) Feedback and corollary discharge: a merging of the concepts. *Neurosciences Res. Proj. Bull.*, **9**, 86–112.

Eyzaguirre, C. and Fidone, S. J. (1975) *Physiology of the Nervous System*. Chicago: Year Book Medical.

Jones, B. (1974) The importance of memory traces of motor efferent discharges for learning skilled movements. *Develop. Med. Child Neurol.* **16**, 620–628.

Kinnear Wilson, S. A. (1925) The Croonian lectures on some disorders of motility and muscle tone with special reference to the corpus striatum. *Lancet* **2**, 169.

Lance, J. W. (1971) *A Physiological Approach to Clinical Neurology*. London: Butterworth.

Long, E. C. and Hull, W. E. (1961) Respiratory volume flow in the crying newborn infant. *Pediat.* **27**, 373

Luria, A. R. and Yudovich, F. la (1959) *Speech and Development of Mental Processes in the Child*. London: Staples Press.

O'Connell, A. L. (1972) *Understanding the Scientific Basis for Human Movement*. Baltimore: Williams and Wilkins.

Sheridan, M. D. (1964) Disorders of Communication in Young Children. *Monthly Bull. of Ministry of Health Lab. Service*, **23**, 20.

Singer, R. N. (1968) *Motor Learning and Human Performance*. New York: MacMillan.

Taub, E. and Berman, A. J. (1968) Movement learning in the absence of sensory feedback. In *The Neuropsychology of Spatially Oriented Behaviour*, edited by S. J. Freedman. Homewood, Illinois: Dorsey Press.

Further Reading

Abercrombie, M. L. J. (1968) Some notes on spatial disability, movement, intelligence quotient and attentiveness. *Develop. Med. Child Neurol.* **10**, 206.

Anthony, E. J. (1968) The child's discovery of his body. *Physical Therapy,* **48**, 10, 1103.

Bilodeau, E. A. (1969) *Principles of Skill Acquisition.* New York: Academic.

Bower, T. (1966) The visual world of infants. *Scientific American*, **215**, 80.

Brazelton, T. B. (1962) Crying in infancy. *Pediat.*, April.

Carr, J. H. (1979) Oral function in infancy. *Aust. J. Physiother.* In press.

Cashdan, A. (1969) The role of movement in language learning. In *Planning for Better Learning.* London: Heinemann.

Connolly, K. (1975) Movement, action, skill. In *Movement and Child Development*, edited by K. S. Holt. London: Heinemann.

Critchley, M. (1966) *The Parietal Lobes.* New York: Hafner.

Davis, J. A. and Dobbing, J. (1974) *Scientific Foundations of Paediatrics.* London: Heinemann.

Denny-Brown, D. (1929) On the nature of postural reflexes. *Proc. Roy. Soc. Med.* **3**, 104, 252.

Denny-Brown, D. (1966) *The Cerebral Control of Movement.* Liverpool: University Press.

Gatev, V. (1972) Role of inhibition in the development of motor co-ordination in early childhood. *Develop. Med. Child Neurol.* **14**, 336.

Gesell, A. and Ilg, F. L. (1937) *Feeding Behaviour of Infants.* Philadelphia: Lippincott.

Gesell, A. and Ilg, F. L. (1949) *Child Development.* New York: Harper and Row.

Gordon, I. J. (1973) *Baby Learning Through Baby Play.* London: Sidgewick and Jackson.

Granit, R. (1970) *The Basis of Motor Control.* New York: Academic.

Held, R. (1966) Plasticity in sensori-motor systems. *Scientific American* **213**, 5, 84.

Holt, K. S. (1975) *Movement and Child Development.* London: Heinemann.

Illingworth, R. S. (1975) *The Development of the Infant and Young Child*, 6th Edition. Edinburgh and London: Livingstone.

Isaacs, N. (1961) *The Growth of Understanding in the Young Child. A Brief Introduction to Piaget's Work.* London: Ward Lock.

McGraw, M. B. (1945) *The Neuromuscular Maturation of the Human Infant.* New York and London: Hafner.

Martin, J. P. (1967) *The Basal Ganglia and Posture.* London: Pitman.

O'Doherty, N. J. (1971) Neurological foundations of motor behaviour in infancy. *Physiotherapy*, **57**, 4, 144.

Paine, R. S., Donovan, D. E. and Hubbell, J. P. (1964) Evolution of postural reflexes in normal infants and in the presence of chronic brain syndromes. *Neurology,* **14**, 1036.

Peiper, A. (1963) *Cerebral Function in Infancy and Childhood.* London: Pitman.

Robinson, R. J. and Tizard, J. P. M. (1966) The central nervous system in the newborn. *Brit. Med. Bulletin,* **22**, 1, 49.

Robinson, R. J. (1969) *Brain and Early Behaviour.* London: Academic.

Rorke, L. B. and Riggs, H. E. (1969) *Myelination of the Brain in the Newborn.* Philadelphia and Toronto: Lippincott.

Rosenbloom, J. and Horton, M. (1971) Maturation of fine prehension in young children. *Develop. Med. Child Neurol.* **13**, 3.

Schulte, F. J. (1974) The neurological development of the neonate. In *Scientific Foundations of Paediatrics*, edited by J. A. Davis and J. Dobbing. London: Heinemann.

Sheridan, M. D. (1968) *The Developmental Progress of Infants and Young Children.* London: Ministry of Health.

Sherrington, C. S. (1913) Reflex inhibition as a factor in the coordination of movements and postures. *Quart. J. exp. Physiol.* **6**, 251.

Stone, L. J., Smith, H. T. and Murphy, L. B. (1974) *The Competent Infant.* London: Tavistock.

Van Blankenstein, M., Welbergen, U. R., de Haas, J. H. (1975) *The Development of the Infant.* London: Heinemann.

Weisz, S. (1938) Studies in equilibrium reaction. *J. Nerv. and Mental Dis.* **88**, 150.

Section II

Developmental and Neurological Disorders

INTRODUCTION

1. *CEREBRAL PALSY and DEVELOPMENTAL DELAY*

2. *HEAD INJURIES*

3. *MINIMAL BRAIN DYSFUNCTION*

4. *MENTAL RETARDATION*

5. *INFECTIONS OF THE BRAIN AND SPINAL CORD*

6. *BRACHIAL PLEXUS LESIONS IN INFANCY*

Introduction

This Section describes the disorders of movement which result from abnormal development of or interference with the nervous system. In children, the commonest sites of these disorders are the brain and the spinal cord. The peripheral system may be involved in certain hereditary diseases which will result in poor motor development, but in children this system is not commonly subject to trauma. Nevertheless, a child who falls over with a glass in his hand may sustain a median or ulnar nerve lesion as would an adult, a child with a complicated supracondylar fracture may suffer a Volkmann's ischaemia of the nerves and muscles in the forearm, and an infant may sustain a brachial plexus lesion during a difficult birth.

The poliomyelitis virus may destroy anterior horn cells in the spinal cord. Guillain-Barré's syndrome is an acute polyneuritis of uncertain origin and peripheral neuropathy may also result from such factors as vitamin deficiency or lead poisoning. Failure of the spinal cord of the embryo to develop normally causes malformation of the spinal cord as occurs in spina bifida cystica.

Cerebral palsy is a broad term indicating abnormal development of or injury to the foetal or infant brain, and the area involved may be relatively circumscribed and confined to the cerebral cortex in its motor or sensory parts, to the cerebellum or the basal ganglia, or more generalized and involving many areas in the brain. Trauma may occur to the brain due to accident, with motor vehicle accidents being an ever-increasing cause. In these cases the damage tends to be more generalized than specific. Infection may cause an encephalitis or a meningitis which injures the brain in a diffuse manner. Genetic factors may cause a baby to be born with Down's syndrome (mongolism) or with a developmental disorder which makes him mentally deficient with clumsy movements. Microcephaly will result in mental deficiency and abnormalities of tone through the failure of the skull to develop adequately. An abnormal increase in cerebrospinal fluid or a failure of its absorption will result in hydrocephalus which, if uncontrolled, will also lead to sensori-motor disorders and mental retardation. Tumours developing within the brain or spinal cord will cause symptoms depending upon the area involved. Cerebrovascular accident or stroke may occur as a result of occlusive vascular disease or congenital anomalies, such as aneurysms or vascular malformations. The sequelaé will depend on the area of brain involved.

In this Section, the overall management of cerebral palsy is described in some detail, the author hoping that this will act as a guide for the treatment of other disorders of movement, whether due to traumatic lesions of the brain, to encephalitis or meningitis, or following surgery for the removal of tumours. The techniques of physical treatment itself are described only briefly. The author is concerned to avoid a situation in which 'recipes' for treatment may be noted by the student and applied to patients without consideration of their particular problems. Techniques of treatment are more effectively learnt by practical application and it is hoped that such details as are given here will give the student a background which will enable him to learn and develop the necessary practical skills under expert guidance.

The management of poliomyelitis is also described in detail, as the problems arising from muscle paralysis and weakness in this disease provide a good example of the problems which will arise in patients with other lower motor neurone disorders, and the methods of treatment used for the rehabilitation of more normal movement in all patients with lower motor neurone lesions will be similar.

THE DEVELOPMENT OF THE NERVOUS SYSTEM

The development of the nervous system through the fetal and embryonic periods is briefly outlined in figure 26. A period of rapid brain growth, called the 'brain growth spurt' begins in mid-gestation. However, 85% of brain growth takes place post-natally. Certain periods involve more active growth than others, and the brain is thought at these times to be particularly sensitive to changes in the environment and to internal influence, thus demonstrating its plasticity (Timiras 1972, Dobbing 1974).

There are thought to be considerable individual variations in the time of development of sensori-motor reactions in early childhood (Dekaban 1970). The primitive reflexes of infancy disappear as the cerebral cortex matures anatomically and functionally and takes over control of the lower centres of the brain (Langworthy 1933). The cerebral cortex seems to contribute little to the function of the nervous system before this maturation occurs (McGraw 1945).

At birth the part of the brain posterior to the pre-central sulcus is better developed than the part anterior to it. The convolutions of the brain are partly developed. The cerebral cortex of the full-term neonate is only half its eventual adult thickness. The increase in thickness will result from an increase in size of nerve cells and sprouting of their processes. The dendritic processes of cortical neurones begin to develop a few months before birth but are still rudimentary in the brain of the newborn. During the first year of post-natal life, these dendritic processes develop to establish their connections with other neurones. The cerebral capillaries are relatively permeable at birth. Therefore, in infants with jaundice, serum bilirubin may penetrate the brain, damaging the basal ganglia.

It is interesting to note that the ascending afferent fibres in the spinal cord are relatively well myelinated at birth, while the descending corticospinal tracts and the white matter of the cerebral and cerebellar hemispheres are to a large extent unmyelinated. The descending motor tracts do not become fully myelinated until years 1 and 2. The olfactory tracts are unmyelinated, the optic tracts partly and the remainder of the cranial nerves are well myelinated. The early myelination of the cranial nerves is related to the infant's well developed ability to suck and swallow. The cerebellum itself is immature and remains relatively immature until the child is two years old.

At six months of age, when the infant is gaining more cortical control over his activities, the frontal and temporal lobes are becoming more mature, most of the tracts in the spinal cord are well myelinated, and the optic nerve is completely myelinated. The immaturity of the cerebellum at this stage can be demonstrated by the infant's lack of control over attempted grasping (Dekeban 1970).

THE DEVELOPMENT OF THE CENTRAL NERVOUS SYSTEM

	STRUCTURE	FUNCTION
WEEK 2	Blastocyst (future embryo & placenta) embedded in the uterine mucosa & begins its specific development.	
WEEK 3	Ectoderm thickens to form neural plate. Neural plate develops neural groove. Neural crest cells form. Neural groove deepens ⟶ formation of neural folds.	
WEEK 4	Fusion of neural folds ⟶ neural tube. Neural tube dilates ⟶ forebrain vesicle, midbrain vesicle, hindbrain vesicle. Remainder of tube elongates ⟶ spinal cord. Neural crest cells differentiate into various sensory and autonomic ganglia.	Heart beats
WEEK 5	Forebrain & hindbrain vesicles divide. Their cavities form lateral, third & fourth ventricles & aqueduct of Sylvius. Cerebral hemispheres begin to expand.	
WEEK 6	Thalamus indicated. Cerebellum appears. Cerebral commissures appear. Motor & sensory nuclei of cranial nerves 9, 10, 11, 12 originate in medulla oblongata. Capillary system formed (cerebral vascular system).	
WEEK 8	Corpus striatum differentiates into caudate nucleus & lentiform nucleus. Lentiform nucleus divides into putamen & globus pallidus. Expansion of cerebral hemisphere ⟶ overlapping of mid & hindbrain. Formation of frontal, temporal & occipital lobes. Spinal cord same length as vertebral column. Development of sense organs progressing. Meninges (pia, arachnoid, dura matera) are distinct. Brain has a human appearance.	First reflex arc functional. Reflex responses to tactile stimulation Irritation of upper lip ⟶ withdrawal of head. Neck & trunk movement.
WEEK 10	Corpus callosum appears & connects R & L cerebral hemispheres. Epithalamus, thalamus & hypothalamus developing from forebrain.	Spontaneous movements observable & stereotyped. Tactile stimulation of lips ⟶ swallowing movement

Fig. 26 Table showing the development of the nervous system. (From Carr, J. H. and Shepherd, R. B. (1980) *Physiotherapy in Disorders of the Brain.* London: Heinemann. In press.)

WEEK 12	Vermis & cerebellar hemisphere recognisable. Anterior commissure develops and connects R&L cerebral hemispheres. Taste buds appear. Inner ear developing adult configuration.	Less stereotyped movements becoming more individuated. Movements increase in force. Mouth opening & closing. Chest muscles contract. Tactile stimulation of face head turning, contraction of contralateral trunk muscles, trunk extension, rotation of pelvis to other side.
WEEK 14	General sense organs (pain, temperature, deep pressure & tactile endings, chemical endings, neuromuscular spindles & neurotendinous end organs) begin to differentiate.	
WEEK 16	Characteristic folia of adult cerebellum gradually develop. 3 small apertures (F. of Luschka & F. of Magendie) appear → free passage of CSF between ventricles & subarachnoid space. Cervical spinal cord developing myelin. Cervical & lumbar enlargements form.	Tongue movements. Abdominal muscles contract.
WEEK 20	Main components of middle & external ear have assumed adult form. Pacinian corpuscles appear. Muscle spindles in almost all muscles. Golgi endings & rudimentary joint endings present.	Effective but weak grasp. Protrusion & pursing of lips. Contraction of diaphragm. Sucking.
WEEK 24	Myelination in brain begins in basal ganglia, pons, medulla, midbrain. Spinal cord extends to SI vertebrae Posterior columns myelinated. Vestibulo - spinal, reticulo - spinal tracts myelinated.	Temporary respirations if born.
WEEK 28	Cerebral & cerebellar connections myelinated. Spino - cerebellar, spino - thalamic tracts myelinated.	Permanent respiratory movements established on birth. Eye sensitive to light. Maintained grasp. Olfactory perception.
FINAL 12 WEEKS	Differentiation of some sense organs completed. Taste buds reach functional maturity.	Reflex mechanisms for sucking, swallowing, well established.

55

Myelination commences near the nerve cell and spreads along the fibre (Hamilton, Boyd and Mossman 1972). All structures in the spinal cord, brain stem and cerebellum are myelinated by two years and the peripheral nerve roots by three years. By five years myelination of all cerebral structures seems to be completed, and from the development point of view in a six-year-old has reached its optimum (Dekeban 1970).

Although the maturation of the nervous system is little understood, there appears to be a direct relationship between the development of myelination within the nervous system and the development of neural function, and a stimulus to myelination seems to occur from activity within the various systems (Dekeban 1970). Certainly it appears that tracts may become myelinated at approximately the same time as they become functional. Fibres appear to be able to conduct impulses before they have developed myelin but these impulses are conducted at a slower pace.

SOME RELEVANT PATHOPHYSIOLOGY

The Brain

When the cortical sensori-motor system of the brain is damaged there may be a release of primitive reflexes such as the grasp and sucking reflexes normally only seen in the young infant. There may also be a release of the phylogenetically older brain stem tonic reflexes from the control normally exercised by the more specialized cells of the cortex and by their pathways, the pyramidal and extrapyramidal tracts. In this case there will also be *hypertonus* (*spasticity, rigidity*) occurring in certain patterns or synergies throughout the body. When the patient moves he will do so in abnormal patterns. A typical pattern, approximating to that of decorticate rigidity, is found in many patients. It is a pattern of extension of the legs and flexion of the arms, with the trunk in extension (figure 27). The extension pattern in the legs includes the elements of adduction and internal rotation at the hip, and plantarflexion of the feet. The flexion pattern of the arms includes retraction of the shoulder girdle, internal rotation and adduction at the shoulder, pronation of the forearm with ulnar deviation at the wrist, and thumb adduction. Most patients show some modification or variation of these patterns and it is unusual to find two patients with a similar distribution of hypertonus or with completely similar patterns. There is always some degree of asymmetry evident, particularly in the trunk which is flexed to whichever side demonstrates the most hypertonus. However, it is only the severely brain stem injured patient who demonstrates an unmodified decerebrate rigidity pattern, with extension of the arms and legs, and opisthotonus.

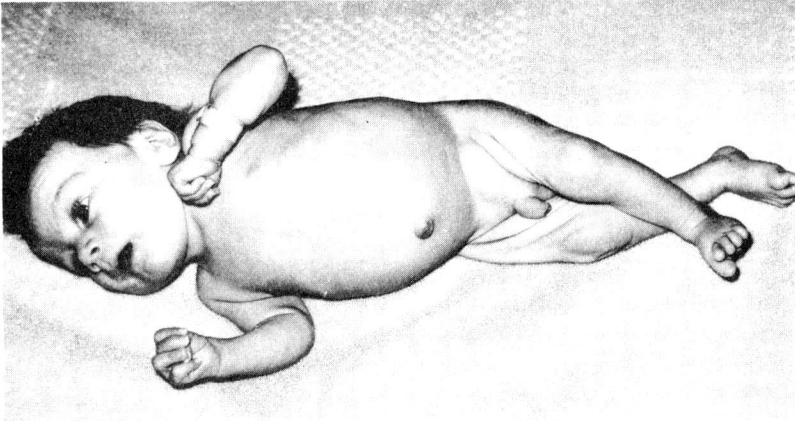

Fig. 27 Spastic quadriplegia. Note flexion pattern of arms with adducted thumbs and extended 'scissoring' posture of the legs.

The *release of tonic neck reflexes* means that movement of the head with consequent stretch to the neck muscles alters the state of tone throughout the body in either a symmetrical or an asymmetrical manner (Bobath 1971). Similarly the position of the head in space, actually the position of the otoliths of the labyrinths in space, will also cause a certain state of tone throughout the body. The effect of the asymmetrical tonic neck reflex is seen, for example, in the spastic or athetoid quadriplegic patient who is able to extend his affected arm and take weight on his hand only when his head is rotated towards this side, the extension being lost when his head is turned to the other side. Another patient may be able to maintain a grasp with his affected hand only when his head is turned away. It will be seen in the description of treatment that it is necessary to inhibit this abnormal tonic reflex activity before the patient will be able both to grasp an object and to look at what he is grasping.

The distribution of abnormal tone throughout the body results in abnormal patterns of movement as well as abnormal patterns of posture. Movement has been described as being a series of changes of posture. The child can only move in the abnormal

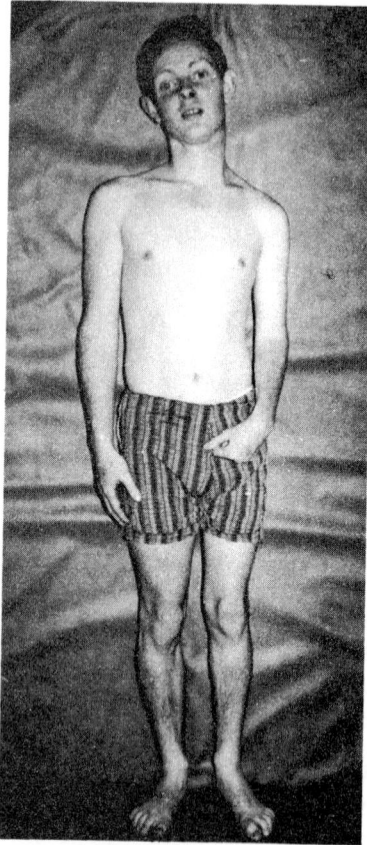

Fig. 28(a) Spastic hemiplegia. Note marked asymmetry of the trunk, head and limbs.

patterns allowed him by his spasticity, which will result in his movements becoming very stereotyped. If, for example, he manages to reach out his arm, despite his flexor spasticity, to grasp an object, his arm will be internally rotated, and he may not be able to extend his wrist and fingers at the same time in the first stage of a normal grasp (figure 35). If his spasticity is mild enough to allow him to do the various parts that make up the whole movement of reach and grasp, he will still reach inaccurately and

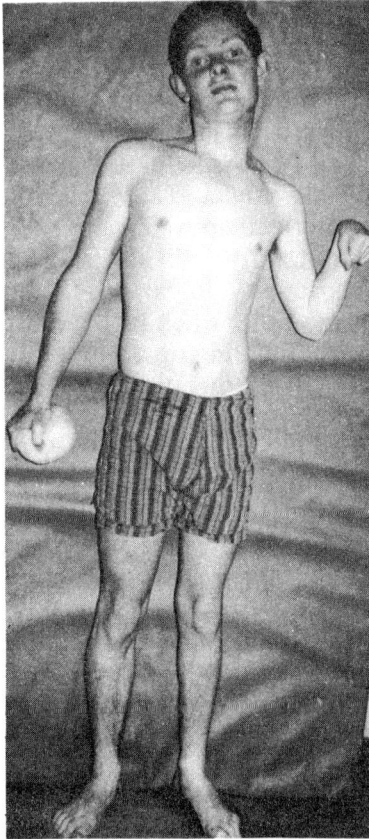

Fig. 28(b) Associated reactions. A strong grasp with the right hand results in an increase in tone in an abnormal pattern on the left side of the body, most evident in the left arm.

grasp clumsily or ineffectively because, although his hypertonus may only be mild, and may not be evident at rest, the attempt at performing what normally requires considerable neurological co-ordination, results only in an inferior type of movement, moderately effective perhaps, but clumsily executed.

In the brain-damaged patient, effort and excitement, speech and sometimes even the contemplation of a movement will cause a further increase in tone if he is hypertonic, or if he has intermittent spasms. This increase occurs throughout the body, not just in the part being moved (figure 28). It may not be so marked as to cause an actual movement, but may be discerned as an increased resistance to movement, made obvious by the patient's inability to move, and felt by the physiotherapist as an increased resistance to passive movement. These reactions will occur in the abnormal patterns described above.

In the normal person, effort will also cause an increase in tone, an overflow of reflex activity, in parts of the body not involved in the movement. For example, when lifting a heavy object, we grit our teeth and grimace, building up an overflow of activity which results in movement of another part of the body which occurs automatically reinforcing that movement. This increase in tone is variously described as *associated movement* (Fog and Fog 1963) *associated reaction* (Walshe 1923), *synkinetic movement* or *overflow*. It does not normally interfere with movement. However, it may seriously interfere with movement in a hypertonic patient who has apparently only a moderate degree of spasticity at rest.

It is important to consider the involvement of the trunk in hypertonic patients. Frequently emphasis is placed on the spasticity and abnormal patterns evident in the limbs, with little reference made to the effect of the spasticity upon the trunk. In the brain-damaged patient, it is usually the lack of postural control (inability to regain balance) or of postural stability within the trunk which is the major reason for ineffective function.

Increased tone occurs throughout the body and the spasticity of the muscle groups which act on the limb girdles and the abnormal patterns of this spasticity must have an effect on the trunk. Flexion spasticity of the hips results in extension of the lumbar spine and a forward tilted pelvis, due to the pull of the spastic psoas muscle. If this occurs unilaterally, as in the hemiplegic patient, the lumbar spine will be pulled into an asymmetrically extended and laterally flexed position, and some mobility of this part of the spine will be lost, interfering with such activities as walking and other movements which require transference of weight. If there is flexion spasticity of the upper limb with associated depression of the shoulder girdle the trunk will be flexed to that side with the pelvis hitched up and pulled back by the action of latissimus dorsi. Spasticity involving this extensively attached muscle will effectively prevent movement within the trunk and will therefore interfere with normal movement and postural adjustment. This same flexor pattern, if it contains the element of shoulder girdle retraction, will prevent him from reaching out with his arm, elevating his arm above the head, and rolling over. It is this mechanism that results in the painful shoulder frequently found in adult hemiplegic patients, and sometimes in children. As the arm is passively abducted or flexed at the shoulder there is no reciprocal lengthening of the scapular retractors and internal rotators, and when the head of the humerus comes in contact with the acromion process of the scapula which cannot rotate laterally in the normal scapulo-humeral rhythm, there is damage to the soft tissues around the gleno-humeral joint. If the action persists, a permanently painful shoulder will result.

When certain cells of the brain including the basal ganglia are involved in the injury, the patient will demonstrate a disorder of movement called *athetosis* (figure 29). Athetosis is characterised by writhing movements which tend to alternate between two extremes of posture. These changes in posture appear to result from an intermittent build-up of muscle tension in antagonistic muscle groups. The postures underlying the athetoid movements are sometimes extreme and are called dystonic postures. These patients may demonstrate spasticity as well as athetosis, in which case the athetoid movements are slowed and more restricted in range.

Harris (1971) suggests that athetoid movements may arise from defective sensory feedback from the moving limb. He sees the problem as a 'control system failure'. Faulty feedback from peripheral sense organs, which does not accurately represent actual limb position, may cause the postural instability seen in athetosis.

When the cells and their pathways in the cerebellum are damaged, movement becomes inco-ordinated as the control normally exercised by the cerebellum through its connections with the labyrinths, the reticular formation, the cerebral cortex and the vestibular nucleus is lost. The neurones of the cerebellum with their connections are essential in the regulation of the normal postural background to movement, and without the postural stability which is required particularly in the proximal areas of the

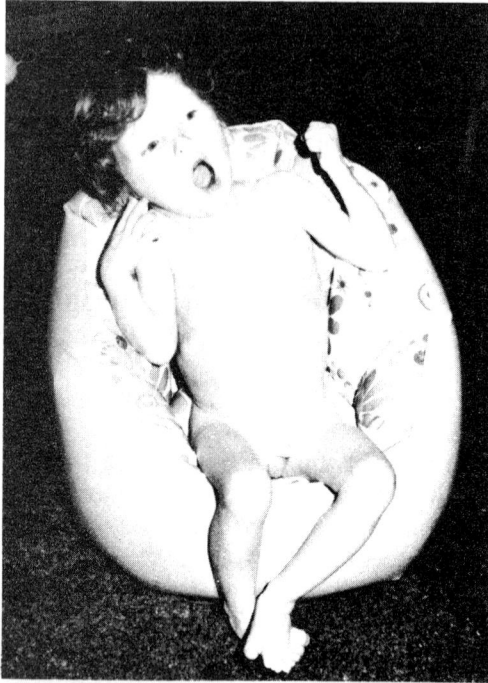

Fig. 29 Athetoid quadriplegia. Note the lack of postural control, the bizarre postures of the limbs, the lack of head control, and jaw thrust.

trunk and limb girdles, and without the ability to make the fine postural adjustments which result from this regulation, the patient is unable to perform a smooth co-ordinated movement. His inco-ordination and his poor balance are called *ataxia*. The patient with ataxia may not be able to maintain a posture against gravity without making continuous gross adjustments, which instead of compensating for his lack of balance further increase this lack.

The abnormal patterns of movement of the spastic patient and the inco-ordinated movements of the athetoid and ataxic patients tend to be reinforced within the brain by their repetition through the feedback system.

When the brain is damaged, the area specifically responsible for sensori-motor integration may be damaged, leading to disorders of movement such as agnosia and apraxia (Appendix 4). Similarly, areas whose cells are concerned with personality and intellect, mathematical and conceptual reasoning, speech and hearing, may also be affected.

The spinal cord

When the spinal cord is injured by trauma or by disease, the disorder of movement which results depends on the severity of the lesion (whether partial or complete) and on its site (whether cervical or thoracic). The spinal cord, that is, the pathways and cells which make up the spinal cord, ends at the level of the first lumbar vertebra in the older child and adult, and at the level of the fifth lumbar vertebra in the infant at birth. Below these levels is the cauda equina, made up of the peripheral sensory and motor pathways.

A complete lesion involving a segment of the cord itself will therefore result in a loss of descending control from the brain to the anterior horn cell, and a loss of ascending sensory feedback from the periphery to the brain. The monosynaptic stretch reflex arcs are therefore without control from higher centres, and stretch of the muscle spindles will result in uncontrolled reaction by the extrafusal fibres of the muscle group. The spindle itself will only be facilitated or inhibited by the intraspinal pathways which normally act to inhibit extensor tone and the result will be loss of movement and uncontrolled spinal reflex activity. The patient will be at the mercy of crude and gross reflexes such as flexor withdrawal, and may demonstrate uninhibited extensor activity upon, for example, the pressure of the sole of the foot against the floor. Interneurones within the spinal cord are responsible also for control of the crossed extensor reflex, so the patient with spinal cord injury may demonstrate this reaction uninhibited by the higher centres of the brain.

The peripheral system

If the anterior horn cells are damaged by disease such as poliomyelitis, or if the peripheral pathways (the cauda equina or peripheral nerve) between the anterior horn cells and the muscle fibres are involved in injury, dysplasia or disease, tone will be flaccid and no movement will be possible. This indicates the essential part played by the peripheral pathways in movement. The brain, for all its complexity, can only exercise control via the final common pathway, and this control can only result in effective movement if it receives accurate information via the sensory system.

References

Bobath, K. (1971) The normal postural reflex mechanism and its deviation in children with cerebral palsy. *Physiotherapy,* **57,** 11, 515.

Dekaban, A. (1970) *Neurology of Early Childhood.* Baltimore: Williams and Wilkins.

Dobbing, J. (1974) The later development of the brain and its vulnerability. In *Scientific Foundations of Paediatrics,* edited by J. A. Davis and J. Dobbing. London: Heinemann.

Dobbing, J. and Sands, J. (1973) Quantitative growth and development of the human brain. *Arch. Dis. Childhd.* **43,** 757.

Fog, E. and Fog, M. (1963) Cerebral inhibition examined by associated movements. In *Minimal Cerebral Dysfunction,* edited by M. Bax and R. C. MacKeith. London: Heinemann.

Harris, F. A. (1971) Inapproprioception: a possible sensory basis for athetoid movements. *J. Amer. P. T. Association.,* **51,** 7, 761–770.

Langworthy, O. R. (1933) in *Contributions of Embryology,* **24,** 139. Washington: Carnegie Institution of Washington.

McGraw, M. (1945) *The Neuromuscular Maturation of the Human Infant.* New York: Hafner.

Schulte, F. J. (1969) Structure — function relationships in the spinal cord. In *Brain and Early Behaviour,* edited by R. J. Robinson. New York: Academic Press.

Sinclair, D. (1973) *Human Growth After Birth.* 2nd Edition. London: Oxford University Press.

Timiras, P. S. (1972) *Developmental Physiology and Aging.* New York: MacMillan.

Walshe, F. M. R. (1923) On certain tonic or postural reflexes in hemiplegia with special reference to the so-called associated movements. *Brain I,* **46,** 2.

Further Reading

Conel, J. L. (1939) *The Postnatal Development of the Human Cerebral Cortex, Vol. I: The Cortex of the Newborn.* Cambridge, Mass.: Harvard University Press.

Gatz, A. J. (1972) *Manter's Essentials of Clinical Neuroanatomy and Neurophysiology.* Philadelphia: Davis.

Hamilton, W. J., Boyd, J. D. and Mossman, H. W. (1973) *Human Embryology.* Cambridge: Heffer.

Jacobson, M. and Hunt, K. (1973) Origins of neuronal specificity. *Scient. Amer.,* 26–35.

Lance, J. (1975) *A Physiological Approach to Clinical Neurology.* 2nd Edit. London: Butterworth.

Langman, J. (1969) *Medical Embryology.* Edinburgh and London: Livingstone.

Martin, J. P. (1967) *The Basal Ganglia and Posture.* London: Pitman.

Chapter 1

Cerebral Palsy and Developmental Delay

INTRODUCTION

AETIOLOGY

CHARACTERISTICS OF TYPES

> The spastic child
> The athetoid child
> The flaccid child
> The ataxic child

MANAGEMENT

> Developmental assessment of the infant
> Developmental assessment of the child
> Physical management
>
> > The concept of neurodevelopmental treatment
> > General points in treatment
> > Relationship between development and treatment
> > Involvement of parents in treatment
> > Specific points in treatment
> > Treatment of oro-facial dysfunction
> > Splinting and surgery
> > Other methods of treatment

THE DEVELOPMENTALLY DELAYED OR AT-RISK INFANT

THE BLIND INFANT

SUMMARY

INTRODUCTION

Cerebral Palsy is a term used to cover a variety of clinical features resulting from brain damage or developmental abnormality in fetal life or earliest infancy. In some cases the cause of the brain damage is known, but in many others it is not. However varied the aetiological factors may be the resulting abnormality of the central nervous system is not progressive. The clinical features appear to progress but this apparent progression is due to the effects of the child's development. As he learns to move about, sit up, develop postural reactions, manipulate, stand and walk, he does so in an abnormal manner, and as he learns, his only guide is his sensory system which feeds back to his brain information about an abnormal state of tone and about abnormal patterns of movement. It is these abnormalities therefore, which, through repetition, become learned and further reinforced within the brain. This mechanism probably accounts for the progressive motor disability which these children demonstrate over the first few years, particularly in the absence of treatment.

The variety of problems in cerebral palsy is considerable. Those responsible for the management of these infants and children come from many different fields, neurology, psychology, social work, physiotherapy, speech therapy, occupational therapy, education, orthopaedics, ophthalmology and otorhinolaryngology. All must have as complete an understanding as possible of all the problems of their patient, whether or not these seem at first sight to be relevant to the particular field in which the specialist works. Each disability, whether of speech, manipulation, hearing or of the balance mechanism, is the result of the damage to or the maldevelopment of the child's brain, and is therefore closely related to the others. One disability cannot be isolated and treated separately from the rest. This situation is recognized in most countries, and cerebral palsied children are frequently treated in special centres, staffed by specialists in the fields listed above. To attempt to understand the wide range of problems encountered in these children is a difficult undertaking. Hence the tendency of many of these specialists to make a further specialty of cerebral palsy.

A detailed description of the problems of these children and of their management is well beyond the scope of this book, and the author has concentrated on the methods of assessment of these infants and children, in the hope that this will stimulate the student physiotherapist to be observant when confronted with a cerebral palsied child or any child with brain damage. If she will take the time to observe him carefully, and if she has a good understanding of normal movement and its development, she will gain some understanding of his problems, and this understanding will give her a base upon which she can develop her treatment.

There have been many systems of treatment developed over the years by Collis, Phelps, Temple Fay, Bobath, Kabat, Rood, Pëto and Vojta, some of these people working specifically in the field of cerebral palsy, others working with patients with other neurological abnormalities. It seems that each new method has learned something from the methods which came before as well as from those which developed concurrently. The temptation for the individual when surrounded by such a variety of therapeutic means is to develop an eclectic approach, that is, an approach which takes techniques from each of several therapeutic ap-proaches and applies them to the problems of a particular child. Two problems arise from this temptation. Therapists will try to apply techniques from these different approaches without un-derstanding their background, the framework in which they have been designed. Moreover, many of the techniques devised would have conflicting objectives. Unfortunately, many physiotherapists are still very technique-oriented and so tend to seek for new tech-niques without always understanding the problems which they will be used to correct. The result of all of this is unlikely to be a treat-ment which is consistent for the problems of the particular child.

The above names have all made contributions to our un-derstanding of cerebral palsy and of movement. However the author agrees with Scrutton and Gilbertson (1975), who point out that '. . . one approach to the treatment of these disorders is in a category by itself and not to single it out would be to present an unbalanced picture. The work of Dr and Mrs Bobath challenged the established treatments and influenced physiotherapy more than is often appreciated. Perhaps the highest compliment paid to them is that their teaching, once considered controversial, is now generally accepted and commonly incorporated in treatments bearing other names'.

It must be stressed that there are two major objectives which the physiotherapist must keep in mind whatever treatment techniques she will use. The first is to understand thoroughly the infant's or child's problems, how they affect him and his parents, and, as far as possible, their physiological or behavioural cause. The second is to plan treatment which will help the child develop effective function.

The criteria for using a particular technique are as follows. The reason for using the technique should be understood, it should be effective, and it should not conflict with the general broad aims of treatment for that particular child. For example, if the broad aim for a spastic quadriplegic child is to stimulate more effective movement, it is unwise to give resistance to movements of the lower limbs and trunk which will result in an increase in tone in abnormal patterns in the upper limbs. The child will be gaining movements of his lower limbs at the expense of greater abnormality, perhaps increased flexor tone, in the upper limbs. In this example, the technique used is not appropriate to the broad aims of treatment, neither is it effective, as it increases abnormality rather than modifying or changing it.

The techniques of Bobath are considered to be particularly effective in the treatment of infants and young children, and in the treatment of patients with spasticity in particular (Bobath 1966, Shepherd 1968, Köng 1971). Some of the techniques of Kabat are effective in the treatment of children with ataxia as they aim to increase stability (Kabat 1952, Voss 1966). The techniques of Pëto and Vojta must be further studied before their place in the treatment of these children is fully understood, but it appears that the techniques of Pëto may have particular relevance in the education and group treatment of children with athetosis (Hari 1968, Cotton 1970, Clarke and Evans 1973). The techniques developed by Rood for the local stimulation of muscle groups may be of use wherever a more local response is required (Stockmeyer 1966, Goff 1969). However, it would be a mistake to consider that only the above people have contributed treatment techniques which may be useful for a brain-damaged child. Techniques of mechanical vibration (Eklund and Steen 1969, Bishop 1975), behaviour modification (Kolderie 1971) and biofeedback (Kukulka and Basmajian 1975), for example, all have their place in the management of certain movement problems. It must be stressed that the therapist, rather than considering what approach to treatment, what technique she will apply, should be more concerned with analysing the child's particular movement problems in detail, then seeking whatever way she can of enabling him to learn how to move more effectively.

It is the author's opinion that an understanding of the importance and the details of normal movement and a thorough system of assessment of the difference between normal and abnormal movement, of normal and abnormal postural reactions and their effect on a child's development, is necessary as a basis upon which to build treatment. This Chapter therefore emphasises these aspects and contains only a relatively brief outline of some important points to be considered in treatment. The student should study the problems of brain damage in greater depth if she intends to specialize in the treatment of the brain-damaged child.

AETIOLOGY

The series of disorders of the central nervous system known as cerebral palsy may occur as a developmental defect due to genetic breakdown, or as the result of insult or trauma to the fetal or infant brain. Many cases of cerebral palsy are inexplicable, in others the causative factors are known, and the commonest of these are intrauterine anoxia, anoxia from prolonged convulsions in early infancy, anoxia or trauma to the brain during a prolonged or difficult delivery, or as the result of the degeneration of the basal ganglia resulting from rhesus incompatibility. For a detailed description of the aetiology the student is referred to the reading list at the conclusion of this chapter.

CHARACTERISTICS OF TYPES

The cerebral defect commonly results in disorders of movement and tone referred to as spasticity, rigidity, flaccidity, athetosis and ataxia. These children show arrested or retarded motor development with a poorly developed postural reflex mechanism and many retain the primitive total movements of early childhood (Bobath 1966). All these children demonstrate abnormal tone. It may be increased, as in hypertonic children, probably as the result of the release of brain stem mechanisms from higher inhibitory control; it is fluctuating or decreased in those children with athetosis; it tends to be decreased in ataxic children. Both spastic and athetoid children may demonstrate flaccidity in early infancy.

Affected children are classified into groups but the classifications vary a little, some authorities suggesting one series of groups while others advocate their own variations. No matter what system of classification is used, in practice it is often impossible to categorize a child, so great is the overlap from one group to another. Some children are spastic and athetoid, some are ataxic and athetoid, some show rigidity, others are merely clumsy. Most children with the above motor disorders have associated abnormalities which may include one or more of the following: apraxia, high frequency deafness, visual defects, receptive aphasia, dyslexia, intellectual retardation, agnosia, dysphagia, dysarthria (Appendix 4). Intellectual retardation may occur as a primary defect, but may also be secondary to motor and sensory disability. Assessment of intelligence may be very difficult, intelligence frequently being masked by the physical disability. Some children do not demonstrate any marked motor disorder but have an evident learning defect with difficulty in reading and writing, or apraxia and agnosia. The latter two defects may result in some of the difficulties of the so-called 'clumsy child'. Perceptual defects may be secondary rather than primary problems, due to the child's inability to explore his world through the normal development of movement, and sometimes due to his visual defects. Some children are so mildly affected in comparison with other cerebral palsied children as to appear normal until it is realized that their failure to achieve physical and mental equality with their peers is due to what is called minimal brain dysfunction (Chapter 3), rather than to a low mentality or to laziness. Most of these children have a sensori-motor defect of some type.

Cerebral palsied children are further categorized, according to the distribution of their motor involvement, into quadriplegic, diplegic and hemiplegic. A true monoplegic probably rarely occurs. A child may appear to have involvement of one lower limb only, but as he matures he will be found to have clumsy, poorly developed manipulative function of the hand on the same side, and his diagnosis will be more obviously that of hemiplegia.

Similarly, an apparently paraplegic child may be found to have clumsy hand function, and be in reality diplegic. Both the diplegic and quadriplegic child are involved in all four limbs and trunk, but the diplegic is more affected in the lower limbs and trunk and may only have mild upper limb involvement, whereas the quadriplegic may have more generalized involvement, although the upper limbs may be involved more than the lower.

Cerebral palsied children are described below under the headings of their principal motor abnormality of spasticity, ataxia, flaccidity, and athetosis. This is a classification used merely as a guide to treatment and makes no claim to represent all the variations found in practice. For example, children demonstrating rigidity are not discussed in a separate category as they will be treated in the manner described under spasticity, both these groups having as their main problem an increase in tone.

THE SPASTIC CHILD

The characteristics of these children are described according to the severity of their spasticity, as there are considerable differences between the severely and the moderately spastic.

Severe spasticity

A child with severe spasticity demonstrates little change in the state of his tone when his position is changed. His muscles are in a state of co-contraction, which means that all the muscles encompassing the limbs and trunk are spastic, although some groups will usually be more spastic than others. Children with rigidity come into this category, the hypertonus in these cases being more of the plastic type.

This severe degree of co-contraction prevents any but the slightest movement from occurring. If, for example, the child is moved from supine to prone some change in tone may occur because of the influence of the tonic reflexes (tonic labyrinthine and tonic neck reflexes), but it may not be obvious as a movement since the severe degree of spasticity surrounding the limbs and trunk prevents any marked reaction from occurring.

In the normal person it is co-contraction, especially proximally, which gives us stability. For example, when we stand on one leg there is simultaneous contraction (co-contraction) of agonists and antagonists in the standing leg (Riddoch and Buzzard 1921). Co-contraction in the normal person means the contraction of the muscles around a limb in order to keep that limb in a stable position. The degree of tone in the various muscle groups can, however, be varied in order to allow postural adjustment to occur, while in the severely spastic child co-contraction is not controlled and cannot be modified. Being too extreme and unchangeable it prevents movement from occurring and allows no postural adjustment. It usually occurs more proximally than distally.

Where there is severe co-contraction the child will have to use a great deal of effort if he attempts to move. This effort may itself cause a further increase in tone, making movement even more difficult. If he moves at all it will be in a very small range. The child will show little spontaneous movement. He may use his tonic reflexes in order to move, for example, using his tonic labyrinthine reflex in order to roll over.

There are certain typical patterns (synergies) of spasticity seen in these children, with a pattern of total flexion in the upper limbs and of extension in the lower limbs (figure 26). However, in practice there are many variations. The upper limb may be flexed at the elbow, wrist and fingers, retracted and depressed at the shoulder girdle, internally rotated and adducted at the shoulder, and pronated at the radio-ulnar joints. The elbow is extended rather than flexed in some children, and the shoulder girdle may be protracted rather than retracted. In the lower limb a pattern of extension is seen at the hip and knee joints, internal rotation and adduction at the hip, and plantarflexion and inversion in the foot. However, it is not only the limbs which are affected. Spasticity involving the limb girdles must affect the trunk. The spastic muscles such as latissimus dorsi with its attachments to the spine, upper limb, shoulder and pelvic girdles, are responsible for the marked side flexion of the trunk, with the shoulder pulled down and back and the pelvis pulled up and back (figure 27). A lack of trunk movement results. A spastic psoas muscle not only pulls the leg into flexion but also pulls the lumbar spine forward causing a marked lumbar lordosis and inhibition of the abdominal muscles.

When the child moves, if he does, it will be within these patterns. He may be able to move his leg into flexion but it will be a pattern of flexion, with external rotation, abduction and dorsiflexion. These patterns are ineffective because they are stereotyped. The child has no choice in his movements. He must do what his spastic muscles dictate.

He may demonstrate abnormal associated movement or reactions in response to stimuli such as effort, excitement, loss of balance, fear or anxiety, and these will mean a further increase in tone in abnormal patterns. If tone is low enough to allow movement to occur, associated movements may be seen on these stimuli, but usually the severely spastic child reacts by an increase in tone rather than in a movement. A spastic hemiplegic child, if asked to squeeze a ball in his unaffected hand, will demonstrate associated reactions on the affected side, with an increase in tone in an abnormal pattern of total flexion or extension (figure 28).

Primitive responses such as the Moro reaction and the neck righting reaction may persist in these children, interfering with the development of movement and of the more mature reactions of balance. The child may develop the ability to balance by using the least affected part of his body. Of course, his balance will not be really effective. Furthermore, his attempts at regaining his centre of gravity will be made only at the expense of effort which will cause associated reactions and a further abnormal increase in tone. A diplegic child may, for example, maintain and regain his balance by using his arms, and a hemiplegic will use his unaffected limbs, but a quadriplegic child may not develop equilibrium reactions at all.

Contractures and eventually deformity will develop in the severely spastic child if spasticity cannot be reduced. Contractures develop because of muscle imbalance. The muscles antagonistic to the spastic group are either inhibited by the spastic contraction of the opposing group, or lack cortical drive, and will be unable to contract actively. They will gradually lengthen thereby making their mechanical disadvantage even greater. The spastic group will continue to shorten lessening still more the chance of active contraction in their antagonists. The mechanism is similar to that which occurs in lower motor neurone lesions in the presence of a paralysed group of muscles opposed by a group of normal strength. This is seen particularly in the calf muscles in those spastic children whose anterior tibial muscles are inhibited by the spastic contraction of the calf muscles and are therefore unable to contract. Muscles and other soft tissues become contracted as an adaptive measure as they are never required to lengthen beyond a certain point.

Moderate spasticity

In these children, spasticity is mild or moderate at rest. It should be noted that 'at rest' does not necessarily mean in the supine position. A child with a positive tonic labyrinthine reflex will show a marked increase in extensor hyperactivity in this position and therefore his tone will appear much higher than if he was, for example, lying on his side.

A marked increase in tone occurs when the child attempts to move, particularly if he is moving in response to a threat to his balance. The changeability in tone is much more marked in these children than in the severely spastic. If he is doing a movement which is easy for him his tone may remain relatively normal, but as soon as he must use effort, or if he becomes excited or anxious, his tone will increase and may become very high indeed. Similarly, if a muscle is put suddenly on the stretch the hyperactive stretch reflex will be elicited and tone will again increase considerably. It is partly because of this that an intelligent child may make himself move more slowly than necessary. Quick movements result in increased tone because of the hyperactive stretch reflex, and this he will find out from experience. Unfortunately this type of child often appears lazy or even retarded mentally, when he has really made an intelligent response.

Primitive reactions may also be present in this moderately spastic child. He will usually develop some equilibrium reactions although they may be relatively ineffective. For example, the child may put out his arm to save himself when falling sideways but he may not be able to take weight on it. Tonic reflexes may also be present but are not so easily elicited as in the severe spastic. For example, the asymmetrical tonic neck reflex may only be elicited by turning the head quickly and not by turning it slowly.

Associated reactions are usually very strong and obvious. Whereas in the severely spastic child they may be evident only as an increase in tone, in this child they will be evident as movements. If the child clasps his hands together his legs will adduct and internally rotate. These reactions interfere greatly with the child's movements, particularly with his attempts to regain balance.

Contractures and deformities tend to be more severe in these children.

THE ATHETOID CHILD

These children are classified in groups in order to point out the principal differences in type. Many athetoids vary enough in their clinical features to make up a separate group, but for the purposes of treatment this classification covers the main clinical features found in these children. Most athetoid children are quadriplegic, many have an associated hearing loss. Their true intelligence is often not apparent because of the severity of the motor disability.

All these children have certain features in common. Tone is abnormal and varies in character and intensity, ranging in the one child from hypotonia to hypertonia, frequently with surprisingly sudden fluctuations. Involuntary movements occur which may not be movements at all but really tonus changes, and the lower the tone the greater the fluctuation appears to be. They have been described as being not movements in the physiological sense although they are movements in the physical sense. These tonus changes may occur as intermittent tonic spasms occurring in recognizable patterns, or as repetitive rhythmical movements, or as fleeting, irregular and localized contraction of muscle groups, muscles or muscle fibres (figure 29). It is these latter which may produce the grotesque facial grimacing seen in many athetoids. These involuntary movements are reinforced by any attempt at volitional activity or by excitement, even by the desire to move. The response to stimulation is very unpredictable in some of these children, as there is a changeable threshold of excitation.

Head control is always slow to develop. Tonic spasms or hypotonus make it difficult for the child to get stability around the neck and shoulders. Unfortunately the child cannot sit or stand or develop eye–hand control until he has developed some head control, and as this develops late, the child's general development will be correspondingly very delayed.

These children show little or no co-contraction, therefore are unable to maintain a posture or develop enough fixation for a moving limb. There is poor grading between the agonists and antagonists during a movement or if a posture is to be maintained. The defect seems to be an excess of reciprocal inhibition. When the child attempts to move a limb there is an immediate relaxation of the lengthening group of muscles (Bobath 1966). Control over middle ranges of movement in particular is very poor.

Joints are often hypermobile, the soft tissues surrounding them appearing lax. There is a tendency to dislocation, particularly in those children with intermittent tonic spasms. Persistent spasms into an asymmetrical tonic neck pattern result in persistent flexion and adduction of the leg on the occiput side, and eventually this hip will dislocate. Extension spasms of the jaw will result in subluxation of the temporo-mandibular joint if they are persistent and severe. Deformities do not usually occur in the very mobile athetoid, but they may be of great severity in those patients with dystonia, due to the extreme postures maintained. Scoliosis is common in these patients.

Breathing and vocalizing abnormalities are common. Breathing is often irregular with a small respiratory excursion. It is difficult to co-ordinate speech with breathing and difficult to sustain a sound. Sometimes the co-ordination of speech is better at an automatic level than at a voluntary level, and the child may be able to cry out for his mother, although he may not be able to vocalize when she comes to him.

Athetosis with spasticity

In this group of children either the athetosis or the spasticity is usually predominant. If spasticity is severe little movement occurs and athetosis will not be very evident. This group therefore covers the child who has minimal spasticity and obvious athetosis. There is usually some spastic co-contraction proximally so athetoid movements tend to occur more distally. Tone fluctuates in these children but is rarely low.

Dystonic athetosis

This group of children usually demonstrates very marked fluctuations in tone, ranging from considerable hypotonia to hypertonia. Increases in tone occur as spasms often in the pattern of the tonic reflexes, occurring proximally rather than distally. The child may appear fixed in a bizarre posture for a few moments and involuntary movements may be seen distally. Between these spasms the child may appear hypotonic.

77

Choreo-athetosis

These children demonstrate marked involuntary movements which have been called purposive movements to no purpose. These movements are continuous and choreiform or writhing in appearance. They occur against the patient's will. There is no stability proximally, but if this can be achieved the child may have surprisingly good hand function. He appears constantly mobile, his movements are loose, wide in range and uncontrolled. Tone is usually low, which is the reason for stability being so hard to attain. The child maintains and regains his balance by moving constantly.

THE FLACCID CHILD

Flaccidity is usually a transient stage in cerebral palsied children. It is seen in infants and young children, although it may last for the first two or three years. It is frequently possible to produce some degree of hypertonus if sufficient stimulation is given, and the transition from the stage of flaccidity to one of hypertonus may be very rapid and the change of tone itself considerable. Eventually many of these children develop athetosis, although some develop spasticity.

In the early stages it is often difficult to differentiate between the flaccid stage of cerebral palsy and the flaccidity seen in children with other disorders which feature flaccidity, such as Tay-Sachs Disease and Werdnigg-Hoffman's Disease. Hypotonus is also found in premature infants, and in some mentally retarded infants including those with Down's syndrome. Dubowitz (1969) has described the floppy infant in detail.

The child has no ability to move against gravity. Even respiratory movement occurs more as a lateral movement than an elevation of the thorax or abdomen when the child is in supine. He responds little to stimulation, appearing to have a high threshold. His postures are primitive. He lies with his arms and legs abducted and externally rotated and flexed. When he is pulled to sitting he shows a considerable head lag. In prone he may lack protective side turning of his head and risk suffocation. Kicking is absent or very feeble.

This child suffers considerable respiratory difficulty. Respirations are shallow. He has difficulty feeding, being unable to suck or swallow effectively. Feeds are frequently aspirated, coughing is ineffective because of poor muscle tone, and respiratory distress is common.

As he begins to react to his environment increased postural tone develops. He may demonstrate intermittent fluctuations in tone, throwing himself backwards into extension, in what Ingram (1955) has called dystonic attacks.

THE ATAXIC CHILD

Pure ataxia is not commonly seen in cerebral palsy, and is more commonly the result of hydrocephalus, head injury, infection (encephalitis) or cerebellar tumour. If ataxia occurs in the cerebral palsied child it may be associated with spasticity, in which case the ataxic element usually involves the upper limbs and is not severe, or associated with athetosis. Twitchell (1959) suggests that there is always an element of ataxia in athetoid patients.

These children may have tone which ranges from decreased to normal. There seems to be insufficient postural tone to hold a position, and the child makes constant adjustments, particularly when standing, in order to maintain his position. There is a lack of fixation proximally in the trunk and limb girdles, and this makes co-ordination difficult.

Movements, especially of the limbs, are dysmetric, which means that when the child attempts a movement there is a degree of inco-ordination and frequently overshooting (hypermetria). The middle range of movement is the most uncontrolled. Sometimes an intention tremor is present. Equilibrium reactions are ineffective as they are influenced by tremor and dysmetria. Reaction to loss of balance is excessive and unreliable.

The child, when he learns to walk, which will be later than normal, will walk on a wide base, staggering, with poor direction, and with an inability to put the feet on the floor without either excessive force or overshooting.

Eventually he may learn to limit his own movement, and by using less trunk rotation and by moving slowly and deliberately he may become more controlled. He will then appear to move stiffly, and care must be taken during assessment to describe this voluntary limitation of activities and the ataxia which underlies it.

MANAGEMENT

A detailed description of the management of the cerebral palsied child, with all his variety of problems, is beyond the scope of this book. In the author's opinion the physical treatment of these children should be in the hands of therapists trained at post-graduate level in the problems associated with brain damage. With the undergraduate in mind, however, the author has attempted to describe briefly some of the problems seen in cerebral palsied children. Assessment is described in some detail, in the hope that the reader may learn to see the difference between normal and abnormal motor activity and as a preparation for a more detailed understanding of treatment to be developed at postgraduate level. Assessment can be said to be basically subjective (usually qualitative in style) or objective (tends to be quantitative). The assessments described below are almost all subjective and are designed to give an analysis of problems which would act as a guide to treatment. On the whole, objective assessments are used for evaluating the effects of treatment, but as various tests become better documented and supported by normative data, such tests will also prove a reliable guide to treatment.

It is important for the student to appreciate that emphasis in treatment should be on gaining effective function, not merely on the treatment of spasticity or athetosis. It is necessary to understand these manifestations of brain damage and their effect upon function, but it is more useful in treatment to concentrate on a particular problem, such as inability to stand up from a chair, and the reasons for the problem (such as inability to flex the hips sufficiently) rather than to think generally about how to alter tone.

DEVELOPMENTAL ASSESSMENT OF THE INFANT

It is important to assess the motor development of babies who are considered, because of adverse prenatal or birth history to be 'at risk' developmentally and neurologically (Köng 1967), as well as those whose feeding difficulties, slow development, or apparently abnormal tone and motor behaviour make them suspects for a diagnosis of cerebral palsy or mental retardation. These assessments must be done by physiotherapists who have specialized training and experience in this field. The physiotherapist will summarize her findings and discuss them with the baby's doctor, who will endeavour to draw conclusions from these, and from the results of his own and other tests.

The criteria for judging normal motor behaviour and development in young babies are not established clearly enough for any assessment of a young baby of less than three or four months to be *conclusive* proof of neurological abnormality or normality. It may give information about the baby's present state, but it has uncertain predictive value. Although signs of motor retardation may be present in the early weeks, abnormal tone associated with abnormal patterns of movement may not be evident until the baby is a few months old.

Nevertheless, early assessment, even in the neonatal stage, is of great value for two particular reasons. It gives information about the baby which will enable therapists to help the parents with their handling of the infant and it gives information which will be essential data for the therapist intending to perform clinical trials.

With the assessment of both infants and children, it is important to discriminate between primitive motor behaviour and abnormal motor behaviour. Primitive motor patterns are those patterns present in early infancy and inhibited in the normal child as his central nervous system matures. Abnormal or pathological patterns, however, are patterns which are never present in the normal infant. For example, the neck righting reflex demonstrates a primitive pattern of motor behaviour which is present until approximately three months of age, while the pattern of adduction, internal rotation and extension of the lower limbs is a pathological pattern.

The physiotherapist commences treatment of the baby if there is any doubt about his being normal, and carries out reassessments at intervals until it becomes certain whether he is normal or not. Even if he is thought to be normal after a period of time, he is kept under observation, with testing at six-monthly intervals, in case any specific manipulative or learning disability becomes evident, particularly when he goes to school. On the other hand, if he is found to have definite abnormalities, treatment will continue and his parents will at least have the consolation of knowing that treatment will be more effective for having begun so early in the infant's life.

This routine of assessment, reassessment and treatment may result in some babies being treated whose neurological signs are only transient, and due to delay of maturation or minor brain damage. These babies would probably have overcome their problems without treatment (Köng 1967, Illingworth 1970). However, because of the greater effectiveness of treatment of cerebral palsy if it is begun early in the baby's life, and because of the uncertainty involved in the assessment, it is better to commence treatment, which in babies under three months of age consists in showing the parents correct methods of handling the baby (bathing, feeding, dressing and playing with him), and continue until he is shown to be developing normally.

Neurological assessment of infants is described by André-Thomas, Chesni and Dargassies (1960), and Prechtl (1977), behavioural assessment by Brazelton (1973). The method of assessment detailed below will act as an aid to diagnosis, making it possible to recognize the early signs of mental subnormality and cerebral palsy, and as a guide to treatment, which by beginning early, before maturation of the infant's nervous system, will probably be more effective (Bobath 1967).

Record of assessment

The form outlined in Appendix 2 is suggested as a guide to treatment. It is not, as it may appear, a number of tests done with little relationship to each other. There is no particular value in finding out whether one or two isolated reflexes can or cannot be elicited. Instead the examiner tries to get a general picture of the baby's development. In testing reflex responses and automatic behaviour and reactions, importance lies not so much in the baby's ability or inability to respond, but in *how* he responds. If he responds with consistent asymmetry, for example, this may be more relevant than if he does not respond at all.

It is essential that time is spent observing and handling the baby. It is only by watching him while he moves that the quality of his movements can be seen, and the many fleeting signs of normality or abnormality that would be missed if the physiotherapist were not both patient and observant.

The testing of the reflexes and reactions listed below and in Appendix 1 is unreliable if taken in isolation from the following 3 points:

1) Asymmetry.
2) Abnormal or stereotyped patterns of posture and movement.

The presence of either of these is an important clue to the diagnosis of cerebral palsy, as they will be accompanied by

3) Significant gaps in development.

These gaps may not be evident in the young baby, but usually become more evident after the baby reaches 4 months, when his activities usually become more varied. The examiner should beware of suspecting abnormality in a baby who has achieved better control in supine than in prone. She should enquire whether he spends many of his waking hours on his back in a bouncinette. Similarly, a baby who is put on his tummy most of the time, will develop well in prone, but his development may lag behind in supine. It must therefore be kept in mind that these and other environmental factors play a part in infant development.

When the tests and observation are completed, the relevant details must be summarized, then if a picture of abnormality has emerged, the summary must clearly indicate this picture and suggest briefly the main points to be dealt with in treatment.

One assessment is not sufficient initially, as babies vary from day to day in their responses. Two or three assessments should be made over a period of a few days before any conclusions can be drawn. If after these initial assessments there is doubt about the baby's condition, treatment is commenced and he is reassessed at intervals. Köng (1967) and Bobath (1967) have pointed out that abnormal signs will tend to increase in a cerebral palsied baby, as the uninhibited tonic reflexes grow stronger, and abnormal behaviour is constantly reinforced, whereas in the normal baby the apparently abnormal signs will become less evident and will eventually disappear.

The assessment

The infant is assessed in a warm room with his parents present. The assessment may be done on a mat on the floor or on a padded table. He must at some point be undressed, and this can be done by his mother, giving the physiotherapist a good opportunity to see how she handles the baby. The mother's behaviour when handling her child always gives important clues to the baby's condition. If she looks awkward it may be because the baby is awkward. A hypotonic baby is difficult to hold because he slips through the hands. A hypertonic baby is difficult to hold because he is stiff and handling him awkwardly makes him stiffen even more.

The assessment is done if possible approximately two hours after his last feed. It is difficult to get a realistic impression of his tone or his stage of development if he is hungry and agitated, or well-satisfied and sleepy. On the other hand, as Tronick and Brazelton (1975) point out, seeing a crying or fussing baby gives the therapist the chance of seeing how he comforts himself and pulls himself together. He should not be assessed while under the influence of certain drugs, particularly muscle relaxants or sedatives.

History-taking

The baby's doctor will have taken a thorough history, and the physiotherapist notes the following details for her own records.

Family history, including history of congenital or developmental abnormalities.

Relevant details of pregnancy-trauma, illness, threatened miscarriage, Rh incompatibility.

Hospital at which the baby was born.

Details of labour.

Baby's condition at birth or Apgar rating (Appendix 3).

Date of discharge from hospital.

Relevant details of baby's history since birth.

The therapist should not just look for negative factors in the baby's history but for the positive ones. She should look for the baby's and the parents' strengths and not just for their weaknesses.

Observation of posture, movement and reflex activity

It is important to observe not only what movements the baby can do, but also the manner in which he lies and moves about. Attention should be paid particularly to persistent asymmetry of posture and movement, and for stereotyped movements, as well as for abnormal patterns of movement and posture. Certain reflexes and reactions should be tested. The methods of testing are to be found in Appendix 1.

In supine certain signs may indicate abnormality:
1. Extended, adducted legs with plantarflexed feet; kicking into extension and adduction (figure 26).
2. Persistent asymmetry of posture. A normal newborn baby lies asymmetrically but can move his head to the opposite side and change his trunk posture.
3. Movement of one arm or leg persistently more than the other.
4. Failure to open one hand more than the other.
5. Persistent adduction of the thumb across the palm, or fisting of the hand.
6. A frequent Moro reflex on minimal stimulus after the age of four months.
7. Stereotyped movements. It is only in the neonate that one sees a relative lack of variety of movement.
8. Tremor on movement after the first few days.
9. Retraction of the head and trunk, or opisthotonus (figure 30).
10. Reaching out for an object with the arm always in internal rotation and pronation.
11. Complete head lag. Not even a neonate allows his head to fall completely uncontrolled when he is pulled to sitting (figure 6).
12. Well-sustained ankle clonus.

In supine these milestones in particular should be noted:
1. Head control (labyrinthine righting reaction).
2. Hands to midline.
3. Rolling to prone.
4. Raising head from bed.

Reflexes
1. Crossed extension response.
2. Moro reflex.

3. Asymmetrical tonic neck reflex.
4. Neck righting reflex.
5. Body righting reflex (after 5 months).

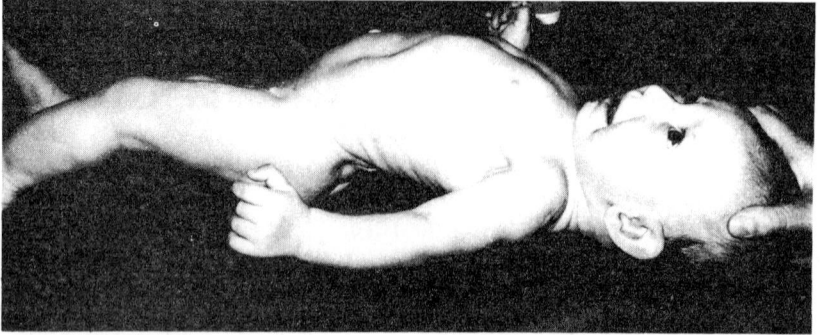

Fig. 30 Opisthotonus. This baby is so extended he cannot remain in supine but rolls to his right side.

In prone certain signs may indicate abnormality:
1. Lack of protective side turning of head.
2. No raising of head from bed.
3. Pelvis flat on bed in newborn period, or too high when it should be flat (figure 31).
4. Inability to bring arms out from under body.

In prone these milestones in particular should be noted:
1. Development of head control (labyrinthine righting reaction).
2. Weight taken on forearms and later on extended arms.
3. Rolling to supine.
4. Reaching out with one hand in prone and later in four-foot kneeling.
5. Pushing up to four-foot kneeling.
6. Getting to the sitting position.
7. Creeping and later crawling on all fours.

Reflexes — Reactions
1. Protective side turning of the head.
2. Automatic crawling.
3. Amphibian reaction.

In sitting certain signs may indicate abnormality:
1. Head and trunk retraction when supported in sitting. The examiner's hand must not be placed behind the head as this will stimulate a head thrust even in normal babies.
2. Inability to support himself with one or both hands. Supporting himself with one arm internally rotated and flexed, with hand fisted.
3. Adducted legs.
4. Sitting with weight persistently on one side.
5. Sitting with a wide base.

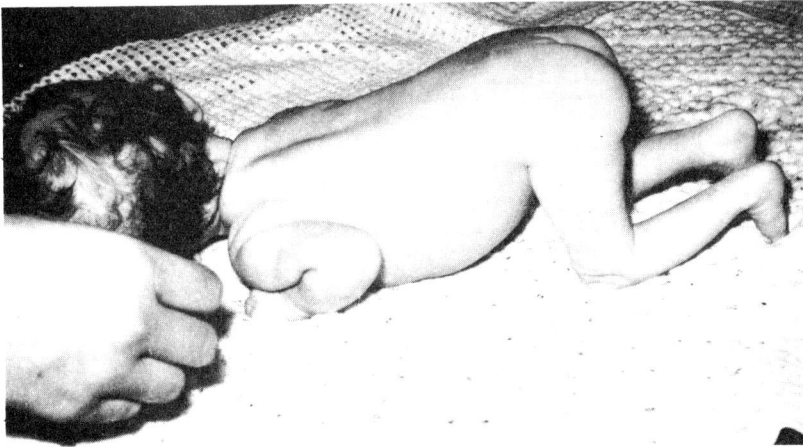

Fig. 31 Abnormal posture of baby aged 3 months. Pelvis should be flat on the table.

In sitting these milestones in particular should be noted:
1. Head control. Sitting and rotating to look behind.
2. Sitting without support.
3. Sitting sideways.
4. Getting from sideways sitting to four-foot kneeling and back again.
5. Pulling to standing.

Reflexes — Reactions
Parachute reaction forwards, then sideways, and later backwards.

In ventral suspension certain signs may indicate abnormality:
1. Complete head lag.
2. Complete dependency of arms and legs (figure 32).
3. Persistence of Galant reflex (figure 165).
4. Intermittent and asymmetrical raising of head.

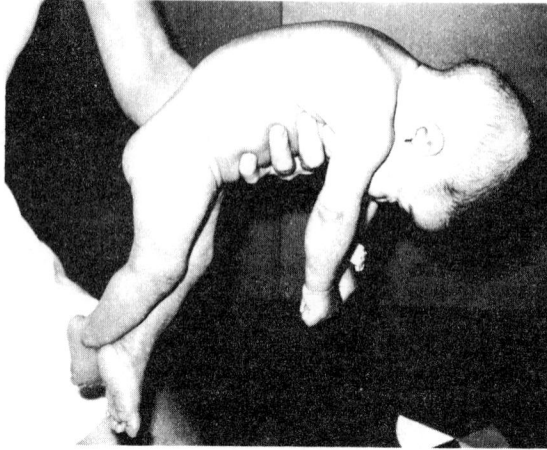

Fig. 32 Spastic baby in ventral suspension. Note flexion of head and trunk, internally rotated arms with fisted hands, and extended, adducted legs.

In ventral suspension this milestone in particular should be noted:
The ability to extend the head and trunk against gravity.

Reflexes — Reactions
1. Galant reflex.
2. Landau reaction.
3. Parachute reaction with arms.

Other Reflexes — Reactions
1. Automatic standing.
2. Automatic walking.
3. Placing reaction.
4. Parachute reaction with legs.
5. Labyrinthine righting reaction laterally.

Assessment of tone

The physiological mechanism of tone is described in Section 1, Chapter 2. The term 'muscle tone' is used clinically to mean the active resistance felt from muscle contraction when a joint is passively flexed or extended (Lance 1971). This term gives the impression of tone being a phenomenon found in isolated muscle groups on movement of one part of the body. Therefore some authorities prefer the term 'postural tone' to describe the situation which is found clinically to exist throughout the body during movement or the maintenance of a posture. That is to say, when tone is abnormally high the situation exists in certain patterns throughout the body and not just in isolated muscle groups.

Tone is estimated *throughout the entire assessment* by a combination of the following methods:

Handling

The physiotherapist will learn a certain amount about the baby's tone by picking him up and by her handling of him throughout the testing. A floppy hypotonic baby is difficult to hold. He slides through the hands that hold him under the arms. His head and limbs flop about, and he is hard to control and difficult to nurse. A spastic baby feels stiff and resists movement, and he does not fit comfortably into the arms of the person holding him.

Observation of abnormal patterns

Some of these abnormal patterns are described on previous pages. These patterns indicate the presence of hypertonus and are observed in all spastic babies. The baby's posture at rest is observed, as well as the way he moves his limbs and body. Persistently overactive tonic reflexes may act upon one group of muscles more than another, causing the limbs and trunk to maintain an abnormal pattern and to move in an abnormal manner (Lance 1971). The presence of the tonic labyrinthine reflex, for example, may dominate the motor behaviour of a baby with cerebral palsy. This reflex originates in the otolith organs of the labyrinths. Therefore, it is the position of the head in space which determines the distribution of tone throughout the body. In supine he suffers a generalized increase in extensor tone, while in prone there is an increase in flexor tone. This means that he cannot raise his head in

89

either supine or prone, neither can he roll from supine to prone, or from prone to supine.

Passive movement

A normal limb may offer resistance or assistance to passive movement, in contrast to a hypotonic limb which feels heavy and uncontrolled, and a hypertonic limb which resists the movement in one or both directions. A normal person controls his limb to some extent while it is being passively moved, unless he is asleep or capable of total relaxation. This limb feels light to move in contrast to the heavy hypotonic limb and to the resistance offered by a hypertonic limb. This resistance may be more marked in the beginning of the movement than at the end, although it may be noticeable throughout the range of movement in babies with a rigid form of hypertonus.

Tone is tested in the neck and trunk by raising the baby's head from the table in supine and prone. There should be no resistance to the movement. Where there is resistance, as there may be in a spastic or athetoid baby, this will be due in part to the influence of the tonic labyrinthine reflex.

Tone is tested in the upper limbs by moving the arms forward across the chest in supine to estimate whether there is increased tone in the scapular retractors, and in prone by raising the arms above the head to test for flexor hypertonus. The head should be in the midline to avoid an asymmetrical increase in tone due to the presence of an asymmetrical tonic neck reflex.

Tone is tested in the lower limbs by flexing and extending them in supine, and by testing for adductor blocking by abducting the extended legs. There are two other tests which may be useful. In a normal baby, passive flexion of one leg is followed by flexion of the other leg. A baby with spasticity will extend the contralateral leg, adduct, internally rotate it and raise it from the table (figure 33). Similarly, when both legs are flexed on to the baby's chest and then released they will normally remain flexed or drop down into a crook lying position. In a spastic baby the legs may extend and adduct with the feet plantarflexed and with internal rotation at the hips. In prone when the knees are passively flexed the normal baby of more than two or three months will hold his pelvis flat. The spastic baby, however, may flex at the hips, being unable to break up this flexor pattern (figure 34).

The assessment of tone is essentially subjective. It is necessary to spend much time in studying the reactions of normal babies to passive movement and watching their active movements before it is possible to appreciate the shades of difference between normal and abnormal. Even then the assessment remains subjective and therefore liable to error.

Tests for normal postural reflex activity and automatic reactions to being moved, are described in Appendix 1.

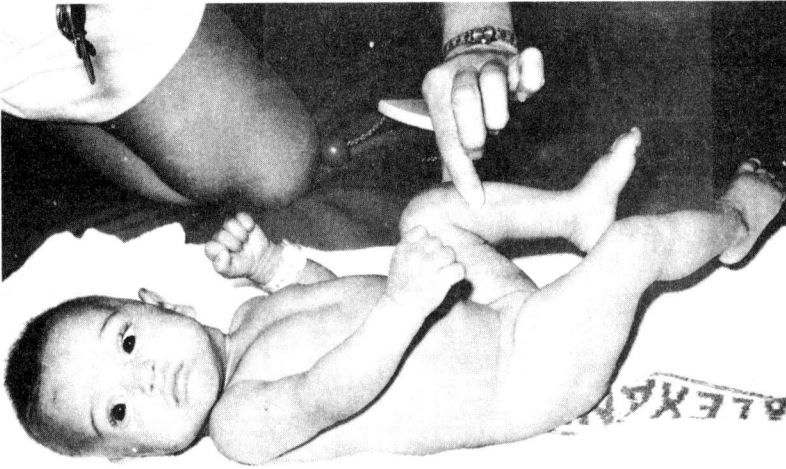

Fig. 33 Spastic baby. On flexion of the left leg the right leg lifts from the table and adducts. Note the influence of the asymmetrical tonic neck reflex.

Test for hand function

Tonic reaction of the finger flexors (grasp reflex)
This is tested in supine with the head in the midline to avoid the effect of the asymmetrical tonic neck reflex. The examiner places his finger in the baby's palm and presses down gently. This stimulates the reaction and the fingers flex. In a newborn baby the reflex action is so strong and constant that if traction is applied to the fingers the baby can be lifted from the table while maintaining the grasp. A similar response can be elicited in the toes. This reaction is present at birth, and can be elicited for approximately three months (André-Thomas *et al* 1960). Pathology is suspected

if the reflex cannot be elicited in this period, or if it persists, as it will do in the presence of spasticity, beyond its normal span. The response may be asymmetrical in a hemiplegic baby, and absent in a floppy baby.

Manipulation

Athetoid movements may be evident as the baby approaches an object with his hand, although this should not be confused with the inco-ordination normally found until five months of age in babies when they reach out towards an object. A spastic baby may reach out with his arm in an abnormal pattern of internal rotation and pronation.

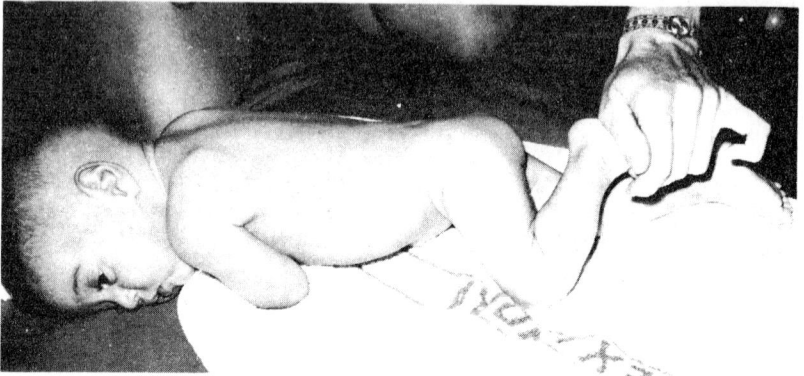

Fig. 34 Spastic baby. Passive flexion of the knee results in a total flexion pattern of the leg.

A spastic baby may grasp with his wrist in ulnar deviation, but this should not be confused with the normal ulnar-sided grasp of a baby of four months. It should be noted with which part of the hand the baby grasps, with the whole hand, the ulnar side or the radial side in the mature pincer grasp of a 12 month old baby.

It is as important to assess release as it is to assess grasp. There is a typical spastic release shown by a baby with hypertonus, in which there is excessive extension at the metacarpo-phalangeal joints of the fingers while the wrist remains flexed (figure 35). An athetoid baby may release an object prematurely or may fail to release it at all because of the fluctuations in his tone.

In hand function these milestones in particular should be noted:

Hands to mouth.
Hands to midline.
Transfer from hand to hand.

It should be noted whether the baby looks at his hand. However, persistence of hand regard is usually an indication of mental subnormality.

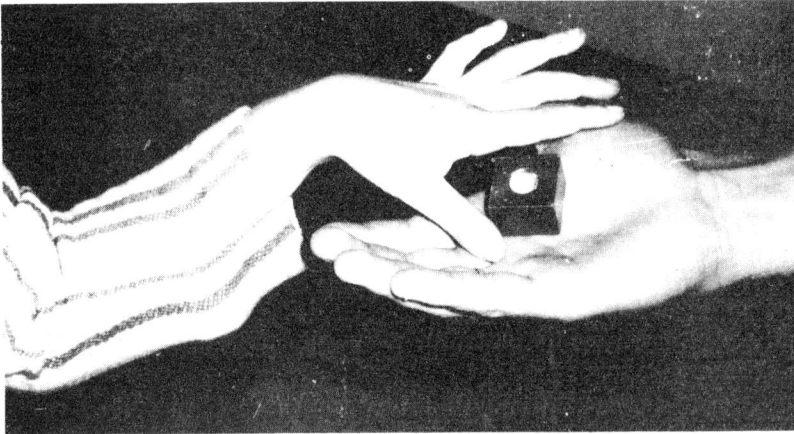

Fig. 35 A pattern of grasping associated with spasticity. Note the flexed wrist and excessive extension of the fingers and thumb, particularly at the metacarpophalangeal joints.

Tests for oral function

The following tests are done with the baby in supine or in the physiotherapist's or speech therapist's lap.

Rooting reflex

The examiner places her finger on the perioral skin at the corners of the mouth, the upper lip and the lower lip. The baby responds by turning his head towards the stimulus, moving his mouth laterally and attempting to take the finger into his mouth. This reflex is present at birth and enables the baby to find the nipple without guidance. Its absence in the neonatal period is usually indicative of severe pathology.

Suckling reflex

The examiner places her index finger in the mouth against the hard palate. The infant will immediately begin to suck, the tongue pushing the finger up against the roof of the mouth. This reflex is present at birth. Absence or persistance of this reflex indicates abnormality. If it persists the tongue does not develop the normal mature combinations of movements required for swallowing and will remain too far forward in the mouth to be effective when solids are eaten.

Bite reflex

The examiner places her finger inside the baby's mouth to touch the biting surface of the gums. The baby will respond by biting down firmly on the finger. This reflex is present at birth and persists until chewing starts at six months. It is absent in severe pathological states, or it may be very strong and persistent. Its persistence may be associated with increased flexor tone. It makes feeding difficult as the baby reflexly bites down on any object which enters his mouth. Chewing cannot develop until the reflex is inhibited.

Gag reflex

The examiner moves her finger backwards on the baby's tongue towards the soft palate until the reflex is elicited and the baby gags. The reflex is present at birth and continues throughout life. It is partly protective, preventing food and fluid being aspirated instead of swallowed. The reflex may be absent in hypotonic babies, causing great problems in feeding. In some hypertonic babies it is very over-active, being elicited even on the approach of the examiner's finger towards the mouth, or on a finger touching the lips. Feeding again becomes very difficult, as it is impossible for the bottle or spoon to approach the mouth without eliciting the reflex.

Testing tone

To test tone, the examiner puts a finger inside the baby's mouth and gently moves it between the gums and the cheek. A hypertonic baby may show hypertonus of all the muscles around the mouth, indicated by resistance to passive movement of the tissues. The examiner should test the tongue in a similar manner, and watch its movements, as asymmetry and tongue thrusting are frequently found in spastic babies and athetoid babies with intermittent tonic spasms. The face itself should be closely studied, as babies with hypertonus frequently show localized spasm of the muscles around the mouth and nose.

Vocalization

Absence of vocalization which normally begins at seven weeks and sometimes earlier, indicates the presence of abnormality. A mentally subnormal baby will not develop a varied repertoire of sounds but will perseverate on one or two. Crying may also sound abnormal in these babies. Illingworth (1970) describes the different types of crying. A spastic or athetoid baby may not make sounds, or may lack variety of sounds because he lacks co-ordination of oral function with breathing. A speech therapist will assess in detail the baby's ability to vocalize, and as the child grows older will assess his attempts at speech.

Feeding

The therapist should watch the infant drinking, and, when he is old enough, eating solids. She should check that there is adequate lip sealing around the teat preventing fluid from escaping, that he sucks effectively and strongly, shows no signs of hypersensitivity in the oral area, swallows without choking, takes solids from a spoon and swallows without pushing the food out with his tongue.

Parent's comments

As the physiotherapist talks to the baby's parents about any difficulties they may have in feeding, dressing, bathing or playing with him, she will be able to assess to some extent their reactions, and in this way will learn more about the baby himself.

Feeding

It is not enough to ask the parents if they have any problems feeding the baby. Often a mother will accept as normal the difficulties she has with her baby, or she may feel that these difficulties are her fault because she is not feeding him properly.

However, it is important to find out the answers to the following questions:

How long does it take to feed the baby? It may take a long time to feed a baby with abnormal reflex activity around the mouth.

Does he push the food out of his mouth with his tongue? This may indicate a tongue thrust, although it is seen in normal babies when they are not hungry or are playing with their food. It will also occur in young babies if the food is placed too far forward on the tongue.

Does he suck well? He may have a weak or absent suckling reflex.

Does he choke or gag, or vomit after meals? This, if persistent, may indicate abnormal swallowing or abnormal reflex activity, although it may also indicate other abnormalities.

Does he push his head back into her arm? A baby with extensor spasms, or with increased extensor tone will do this, although so also will an upset cranky baby.

Does the mother find it difficult to keep the food in his mouth because it does not close properly? An open mouth may be associated with extension hyperactivity.

Having asked the parents about feeding, the physiotherapist, if she has any doubts about oral function, should arrange to feed the baby herself with food and milk brought in by the parents at their next visit.

Dressing
Mothers of hypertonic and hypotonic babies frequently notice that the baby is difficult to dress and undress. It is often awkward to change the nappy of a spastic baby because of the adductor spasticity in his legs. The stimulation of the adductor stretch reflexes as the mother tries to abduct his legs, further increases the tone in these muscles, and makes nappy-changing even more difficult.

The mother of a baby with flexor hypertonus in the arms experiences difficulty when pulling his arms through his jumper. As she pulls on the already flexed arms, she stimulates the hyperactive stretch reflexes in the flexor groups, again causing an increase in tone.

A floppy hypotonic baby is difficult to dress because he is so difficult to control.

Sleeping
It is important to find out the following:

How long does he sleep?

A brain-damaged or retarded baby may sleep for long periods.

Does he sleep well, or does he wake up crying at frequent intervals?

A hungry baby will wake up crying, but he will also do this if he is uncomfortable. Hypertonic and hypotonic babies tend to wake up often because they become fixed in one position and cannot move out of it, the spastic baby because his abnormal reflex activity prevents him moving freely, the hypotonic baby because he lacks sufficient tone to move.

Bathing
Is it difficult to hold the baby in the bath? Does he enjoy playing in the bath, or does he become tense and stiff and cry?

Playing
What are his favourite toys? Does he play with his body? With his toes for example? Does he reach out for toys? Is he able to get his hands to the midline to hold a toy?

It is also important to find out whether the baby lies in his cot for most of the day, and whether he lies in prone or supine. This and other information gathered from the parents is a useful aid to assessment and a guide to treatment, should it be necessary. Correct handling of the infant by his parents is an important part of treatment.

Note on Assessing Premature Babies

In order to understand the development of a baby who was born prematurely and to assess him the examiner takes note of the time at which the baby actually becomes full-term. That is, a baby born four weeks prematurely is full-term when he reaches four weeks of age.

Illingworth (1970) notes the difference between full-term babies and premature ones, stressing particularly the differences in tone and degree of activity. The premature baby reaches his milestones in a more unpredictable manner, achieving some before and some after his full-term peers.

To summarize:

It is necessary to observe the baby's development very closely over a period of time, but there are certain signs which should be looked for by the physiotherapist assessing motor development:

Persistent asymmetry.
Stereotyped or persistently abnormal postures and movements.
Opisthotonus combined with abnormal patterns.
Persistent grasp or Moro reflex beyond the time when they should disappear.
Failure to develop a Landau reflex, righting reactions, equilibrium and protective reactions.
Feeding difficulties — disorders of suckling and swallowing.

DEVELOPMENTAL ASSESSMENT OF THE CHILD

The assessment of a young child follows closely the procedure suggested in the preceding pages on the assessment of the infant. It is usually easier in the child to see any abnormalities of reflex activity and of movement, as the older the child is the more established any abnormal patterns will be. However, because of the range of activities in the child compared to the infant, there will be far more to see and the assessment will take correspondingly longer. A severely handicapped child is much easier to assess than one who is mildly handicapped, whose abnormalities may be so minimal that only the most detailed assessment will discover them.

Procedure

He is assessed in a warm room with his parents present, and he must eventually be undressed. He should have a chair to sit on, and some toys, and a mat on the floor, and the atmosphere should be as relaxed and unhurried as possible. The young child may not want to leave his mother and he should not be taken from her. She can undress him, again with the physiotherapist watching in order to assess any difficulties she has, and she should play with the child herself, with the physiotherapist included if possible until he feels happy and secure. It is worth taking time, waiting for him to explore this new room, and for him to get to know this stranger a little, before beginning the part of the assessment that requires her to handle him. Before she can take hold of him to test reflex activity and his response to being handled, the physiotherapist will accomplish much of her assessment by observation of the child as he moves about the room and plays.

The form, outlined in Appendix 2, is suggested as a guide. As in the infant assessment, it is important to see the results as a whole. For example, it is not only necessary to see that the child demonstrates a positive asymmetrical tonic neck reflex when this reflex is tested, but also, and this is probably more important, to see the effect of this tonic reflex activity upon his movements.

This assessment is a guide to treatment and to progress, but the child is also reassessed as he is handled by the therapist. Not only does his motor behaviour change as he grows but it will also change while he is being handled during treatment and the therapist will have to adjust her treatment as she assesses the child's response.

It is important to assess not only *what* he can do but also *how* he does each movement and activity. Then it is necessary to discover *why* he can do some things but not others. It is a qualitative assessment rather than a quantitative one, and is intended as a guide to treatment.

History-taking

Details of the child's birth history and progress since birth are noted as before. The parents are asked not only for the times at which various milestones were passed, but also to describe if they can the details of such activities as crawling or progression along the floor. For example, a diplegic may have bunny-hopped along the floor, while a hemiplegic child may have bottom-shuffled, weight-bearing on one hand. Eating, speech and interest in surroundings are among the activities parents are asked to describe. Comparison of the child with siblings is often interesting, although not always relevant or to be depended upon. If the child is at school, any difficulties described by his school-teacher are noted, and it is frequently necessary for the physiotherapist to visit the school to see for herself what the child's problems may be. In the case of a mildly handicapped child attending a school for physically normal children, the physiotherapist must be discreet enough not to embarrass a child who is passing for normal among his peers.

Observation of posture and movement

The physiotherapist has two main aims in assessing the young cerebral palsied child.
1. To discover any gaps in his development.
2. To recognize the signs of abnormal postural reflex activity, i.e. abnormal tone and abnormal postural and movement patterns, and assess how these interfere with his development (Bobath 1967).

She will need to find out from her assessment what stage of development the child has reached in, for example, locomotion and manipulation, and compare this with his chronological age. She must differentiate between primitive and abnormal patterns. Having discovered his abnormal postures and movements she will have to estimate what, if any, contractures these may cause in the future. In movement, it is important to look for symmetry and variety.

During the assessment, the following abnormalities of movement may be noted. Only the most obvious deviations from the normal are mentioned. The student will need a thorough knowledge of normal movement and its development to be able to identify abnormalities especially in the more mildly handicapped child.

Rolling over

In all spastic children, there is an inability to rotate sufficiently within the trunk due to spasticity involving the trunk, therefore rolling, if indeed the child can roll, will occur all in one piece. A spastic hemiplegic child will prefer to roll to one side only. Spasticity around the shoulder girdle will make it difficult to reach forward with that arm, and a forward movement of the upper limb is essential for rolling from supine to one side. A spastic diplegic child will roll using his arms and upper trunk, but associated reactions will occur in his lower limbs and the increase in tone will cause them to remain extended and adducted, following almost passively after the trunk and arms. A spastic quadriplegic child may not be able to roll over. If he has a strong tonic labyrinthine reflex, increased extensor tone in supine and flexor tone in prone will prevent his rolling in either direction. An athetoid child will probably be able to roll over if he has sufficient tone to move against gravity but the movement will be ungraded and exaggerated. If he has spasticity and tonic reflex activity he may be in a similar predicament to the spastic quadriplegic child. A child who has retained the primitive neck righting reflex without developing the body righting on body reflex (Appendix 1) will roll all in one piece, as he lacks rotation within the trunk.

Sitting up from supine
A spastic diplegic child may sit up asymmetrically, leaning or rolling to one side, then pushing himself up by his arms. If he can sit up symmetrically, all the movement will occur in his upper trunk and arms, his hips remaining more extended than flexed. Associated movements of his legs and pelvis may be marked, and his extended, adducted legs may make it impossible for him to get up without pushing hard on his hands. A spastic quadriplegic child may be able to sit up only if he rolls to one side, but his inability to push himself up by extending his arms may make it impossible for him to get up to the sitting position. An athetoid child will sit up using his hip flexors strongly if he can learn to stabilize his legs.

Sitting up from prone
A spastic diplegic child may push himself up to four foot kneeling with his arms, pushing back until he sits between his feet with his legs internally rotated. A spastic hemiplegic child will push himself up to sideways sitting in an asymmetrical manner, using the unaffected hand for support.

Crawling
A spastic child will crawl with his legs internally rotated using flexion of his legs with minimal extension. Mobility of his trunk and weight transference will also be minimal. If his arms are moderately involved he may not be able to crawl at all, but will pull himself along the floor using his flexed arms, his legs dragging behind in extension. A spastic hemiplegic child will probably not crawl because of difficulty weightbearing on the affected limbs. He will prefer to shuffle along in side sitting,

propelling himself with his unaffected arm and leg. A spastic diplegic child may not be able to dissociate his legs one from the other, and instead of crawling will hop along with his head extended, using his extended arms to propel himself, and hopping forwards on his knees. An athetoid child may bunny-hop rather than crawl because of his inability to weight-bear effectively through his arms, and because he lacks stability of his pelvis.

Sitting

A spastic child whose spasticity prevents him developing and using his equilibrium reactions will be able to maintain a long sitting position only if he can use his hands to support himself. This means that he cannot use them for playing. He is also, because of extension spasticity, unable to flex his hips sufficiently, and again may only be able to sit by using his hands for support. As his hips are insufficiently flexed, his thoracic spine will be rounded in order to bring his weight forwards over his legs (figure 36). A spastic diplegic child may get over the problem by sitting between his feet with his legs internally rotated and flexed. In this way he has a stable broad base and his hands are free for whatever activity he chooses. However, it should be noted that this is also

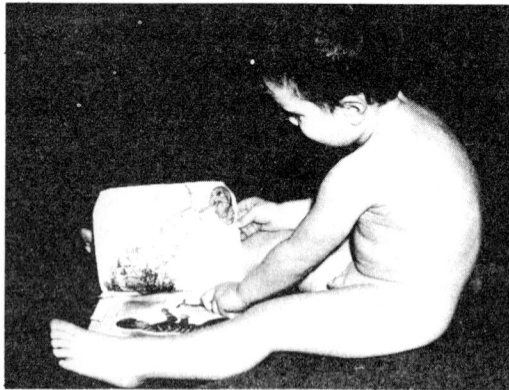

Fig. 36 Spastic diplegia. Note the inability to flex the hips sufficiently and the flexion of the trunk to compensate.

the favoured sitting posture of a number of normal children. Spastic children find sitting sideways a difficult position to maintain because of limitation in trunk rotation and side flexion and therefore seldom adopt it, although a spastic hemiplegic child will sit to his unaffected side, taking weight on that hand. A floppy child sits asymmetrically, collapsed between his feet, and cannot push himself erect with his arms.

Four-foot kneeling

A spastic child will find this difficult. As soon as his balance is disturbed, associated reactions with resultant increase in tone will inhibit normal equilibrium reactions and he will not, for example, be able to transfer weight in order to raise one arm and reach out to play. A spastic hemiplegic child will bear weight more on his unaffected side and be unable to transfer weight to the affected side. Both the athetoid and the ataxic child will have difficulty maintaining this position because of a lack of trunk and pelvic control.

Four-foot kneeling to upright kneeling

This movement involves weight transference backwards and extension of the hips while the knees remain flexed. Both these movements are difficult for the spastic child, and he may be unable to get to the upright kneeling position. The extension of the hips is difficult because it involves an alteration in the flexion pattern in the legs. The spastic diplegic child will accomplish the movement by using his head and trunk extensors, and by pushing off with his arms, but his hips will remain flexed to some extent and he will have a marked lumbar lordosis as a result. The athetoid child will perform the movement only if he has sufficient tone to move against gravity, in an uncontrolled manner, demonstrating his inefficient reciprocal innervation. He may shoot to the upright position then collapse down again because he lacks stability.

Upright kneeling

This is a most precarious position for the spastic child, and therefore one he will rarely attempt voluntarily. The effort of remaining in this flexor-extensor position causes associated reactions and any attempt to maintain equilibrium results in a further increase in tone. The child lacks all effective balancing ability. The diplegic child may manage better as he can use his arms and head to preserve balance to some extent. The ataxic child maintains balance by constant adjustments, and he will not be able to remain still in this position. The athetoid also will lack stability, although by excessive movement or by fixing his hips in hyperextension or flexion he may be able to maintain some semblance of balance.

To standing from upright kneeling

This movement is impossible for most spastic children unless they can use their hands to pull themselves up. The movement involves the ability to transfer weight completely to one side, and to dissociate one leg from the other. A spastic hemiplegic child will prefer to put the unaffected leg forwards. If he puts the affected one in front he will be unable to transfer weight far enough forwards, and will stand up quickly, bringing the other leg through to bear weight as soon as he can. A spastic diplegic child will stand up from a crouch position as this is easier than trying to dissociate

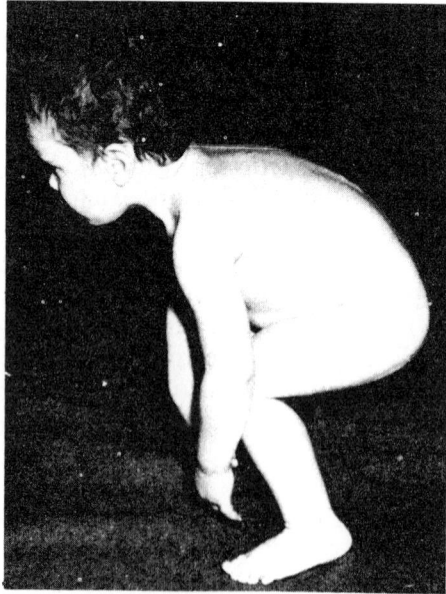

Fig. 37 Spastic diplegia. Standing up from the crouch position. Note the internally rotated, adducted legs, the inability to keep the heels on the ground and the flexion of the thoracic spine.

one leg from the other in upright kneeling (figure 37). The movement requires a great deal of stability, so the ataxic and athetoid child will also need to use their arms to help.

To standing from sitting

The spastic child also has difficulty transferring his weight forward when he is sitting on a chair because he has difficulty flexing his hips sufficiently due to extensor spasticity. He may therefore not be able to stand up without help, unless he uses this extensor spasticity. If he stands up this way he is not able to maintain balance in the standing position on his extended adducted legs and plantarflexed feet. A diplegic child will stand using his hands to push or pull himself up, and by extending his head and trunk. He will use his legs minimally.

Walking

Gait is a complicated activity to assess and the problems that may occur are so varied and numerous that only a few of the most common will be described here. The spastic child lacks the appropriate body alignment, the ability to move one leg independently of the other, effective equilibrium reactions and weight transference forwards and laterally.

He may walk, if he is diplegic, by using his arms and upper trunk to maintain balance. It will be easier for this child to walk quickly as he then spends less time on one leg and has therefore less chance to lose his balance. The diplegic child barely moves his hips and pelvis and has minimal trunk rotation. His hips remain adducted and internally rotated and in a semi-flexed position, and he may appear to be moving only from the knees (figures 38 and 39). His heels may not touch the ground and he may be so precariously balanced that he cannot stand still without holding on to a piece of furniture. The spastic child lacks stability around the pelvis, although the marked co-contraction of the muscles around the hips, pelvis and lower trunk may make this instability less apparent. The normal co-ordinated relationship between the hips and pelvis, and pelvis and trunk is absent, and when the child stands on one leg his pelvis may be seen to drop to the opposite side, a definite sign of instability and inco-ordination. A primitive gait is frequently noticed in young children with spasticity, who walk using the positive supporting reaction, giving a mechanical

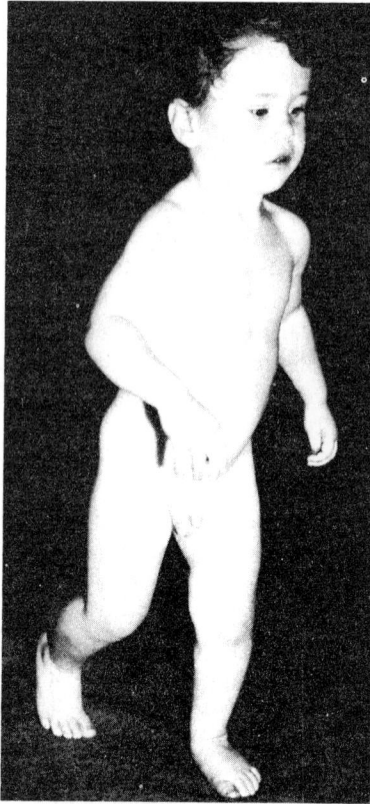

Fig. 38 Spastic diplegia. Note the internal rotation particularly of the left leg, the inability to dorsiflex at the left ankle and the resultant valgus position of the foot with the use of the arms for balance.

flexion-extension of the legs in which both the flexion and the extension are exaggerated. Athetoid children walk in a disorganized fashion, demonstrating the defective lengthening reaction which causes the muscles contracting to do so in an uncontrolled manner with a chaotic result. An ataxic child walks with a wide base, putting his feet down either too gently or too hard, stepping backwards or sideways if his balance is threatened, constantly attempting to stay on his feet.

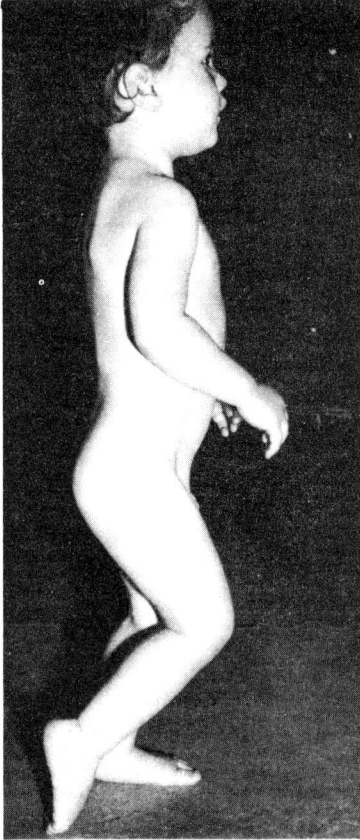

Fig. 39 Spastic diplegia. Note the inability to control the pelvis laterally, the forward tilt of the pelvis, the lack of extension of the standing leg, indicating the difficulty the child has in dissociating one leg from the other.

Assessment of tone

Tone is tested in basically the same way in the young child as in the infant, that is, by passive movement, by assessing the effects of handling, and by observing abnormal patterns, but more emphasis will be on observing the abnormal patterns and analysing the effect they are having on the child's development.

Abnormal postural reflex activity is more evident in the child than in the infant because as the child grows and develops, there is reinforcement of abnormal tone and abnormal patterns. It is important to note the child's basic resting tone and how it changes with stimulus, with effort, and on movement. If there are associated reactions, the physiotherapist observes whether these are present continuously or only under certain circumstances, such as on loss of balance.

Reactions and reflexes are tested in the young child according to his chronological and developmental age, and as a result of the observation of the physiotherapist as she handles the child. A full description of the tests is in Appendix 1. The following reactions in particular should always be tested:

Equilibrium reactions.
Galant reaction.
Amphibian reaction.
Parachute reaction.

Tests for hand function and oral function

These are described on pp. 91–95 and in Carr (1979). Hand function is assessed in more detail in the child because of the greater range of activities normally possible. Some other functions to be assessed include the ability to discriminate the compressibility of objects, grasping and releasing of objects of different sizes and shapes, with arms close to the body and out in front. Hand function assessment suitable for children is described in Carr and Shepherd (1980).

Tests for sensation

Sensory testing is performed once the child is old enough to cooperate with simple test procedures. Sensation should be tested, particularly in hemiplegic children, as the problems of movement that many of these children experience can be traced to poor interpretation of sensory feedback. The aspects of sensation particularly relevant to the disorders of movement in these cerebral palsied children are:

Touch
Light touch.

Stereognosis.
Two point discrimination.

Joint position sense
The methods of testing these sensations are described below.

Touch
Light touch is tested by stroking the skin lightly with a piece of cottonwool. The child's eyes are closed or vision is obstructed and he is asked to say 'yes' each time he feels the cottonwool touch him.

Stereognosis is the ability to recognize common objects on touching and handling them without visual assistance. It involves elements of light and deep touch plus the ability to recognize the various aspects which make up the nature of the object. It is tested with the child's eyes closed, by placing in his hand objects which he should easily recognize. This will depend to some extent on his age, but a key, a marble, a block and a coin can be used.

Stereognosis also involves the ability to differentiate between different textures, and this can be tested in the older child with strips of material, such as silk, wool and sandpaper. Loss of stereognosis is called astereognosis.

Two point discrimination is the ability to appreciate fine pressure applied to two separate points simultaneously. This is tested by using a pair of dividers, the two points of which are applied simultaneously to an area such as the palm of the hand. The child, with eyes shut, is asked to say 'two' if he feels two separate points. The two points are moved progressively nearer to each other until the child can feel only one point. A normal 5 year old child will discriminate two points until they are approximately half an inch apart on the palm of the dominant hand and one inch apart on the palm of the non-dominant hand. This test is relatively complicated and can only be done with a child who is able to understand it.

Joint position sense
Presence of this sense indicates awareness of the position of a limb

or a part of a limb in space. It is tested, with the child's eyes closed, by placing a limb or an element of a limb, in a position of flexion or extension, then asking the child if the part is 'bent' or 'straight', or 'up' or 'down', using whatever words give the simplest explanation. If, for example, the terminal phalanx of the thumb is the part being moved, care must be taken to hold the thumb on its lateral surface in order to minimize touch sensation which may give the clue to the position of the thumb. Alternatively, the child's arm or leg may be placed in a particular position and the child instructed to place the opposite limb in the same position.

Most children find it either impossible to keep their eyes closed for a period of time, or the temptation to peep irresistible, so it is usually necessary to obstruct vision by placing a screen or curtain between the child's face and the limb being tested.

As well as astereognosis and the loss of two point discrimination and position sense, there are other problems of sensory perception which must be watched for in children with Cerebral Palsy, as they are not uncommon and may be the cause of problems of movement and function where the physiotherapist can find no motor cause. Perception has been defined as the organization of sensation for use, relating to the function of the sensory association areas in the parietal and occipital lobes of the cerebral cortex which turn the raw sensory data into a useful guide for controlling function. Problems such as visual agnosia and apraxia are described briefly in Appendix 4.

Disturbance of Body Image. This will occur where there is a lesion of the parietal lobe. It is seen sometimes in hemiplegic and quadriplegic children, who may ignore one limb, or one side of the body, or confuse the right and left sides of the body. These defects will affect movement also, and a child's refusal to use a limb may be due, not to motor dysfunction, or to deliberate naughtiness, but to unawareness or rejection of the limb itself. Such a disturbance may be recognized when the child draws a picture of himself, hemiplegic children, for example, sometimes drawing only one arm and leg attached to the body.

Other tests:

It will frequently be necessary for a child to have further assessments of such aspects of comprehension as space and form appreciation, appreciation of size, depth, distance, time, and ability to concentrate, as well as more specific tests of intellectual function. These may be performed by a psychologist in conjunction with an occupational therapist and a physiotherapist.

Note on Assessing Mildly Handicapped Children:

It is the mildly handicapped child who probably presents the most problems in assessment. He is the child whom parents and schoolteacher consider to be lazy, disobedient, or even mentally retarded. He may be referred for assessment because he is clumsy, poor at ball games, or lacking in concentration.

Assessment of gross motor development may show no abnormalities beyond a poor development of equilibrium reactions, demonstrated by an inability to stand on one leg, or walk along a plank. Assessment of manipulation may show a mildly spastic grasp, imprecise pincer grasp, or poor eye-hand control. An observant physiotherapist, if she watches the child as he moves about and plays, may detect signs of spastic hemiplegia or diplegia or general clumsiness in a child previously thought to be normal but lazy.

A boy of seven years was seen by the author prior to a psychiatric consultation, with the aim of eliminating abnormal motor development as a cause of his poor and worsening behaviour at school. He refused to play games with the other children, was bad-tempered and tearful. His mother reported that he refused to use both hands for a task, preferring to use the left. After a short assessment he was found to have associated reactions on the right side, made more obvious on effort, and abnormal patterns of movement. He reached out with his arm in internal rotation and pronation, and he had a typical, although mild, spastic grasp. When jumping he took most of his weight on the left leg. He ran asymmetrically with his right side slightly behind his left. When sensory interpretation was tested, he demonstrated astereognosis and poor two-point discrimination. A more detailed test by a psychologist indicated specific learning defects. His I.Q. was in the normal range. The child was classified as a mild spastic hemiplegic, yet he had passed as 'normal' in his family and amongst his peers.

An awkward clumsy child may be found on assessment to be mildly diplegic, with poor weight-bearing and slow automatic reactions in standing, inability or slowness to oppose thumb and forefinger being evident on assessment of manipulation. Mild ataxia or athetosis may make the child appear slow and clumsy in movement.

It must be noted that not all clumsy children have Cerebral Palsy, although they will benefit from treatment aimed at improving their co-ordination. In assessing the motor development of a child the therapist is assessing whether he has developed as far as the 'average' child of his age, rather than comparing him to some hypothetical 'normal'. As Illingworth (1970) has pointed out, it is impossible to say what is 'normal', although there is no difficulty in defining the 'average'.

It may be necessary for this child to have further tests of functions such as space and form appreciation, body image understanding, appreciation of size, depth, distance, time, and ability to concentrate. Abnormalities in these areas may be present in a child whose neurological assessment shows no abnormal signs although they may greatly interfere with his motor ability.

There is a further description of these children in Chapter 3.

PHYSICAL MANAGEMENT

The management of the cerebral palsied infant and child involves the interaction of the many aspects of treatment required by most of these children, in the areas of speech and communication, emotional, intellectual, and functional independence, and motor development.

The Concept of Neurodevelopmental Treatment

The term 'neurodevelopmental treatment' has been suggested by Bobath and Bobath (1967) to describe treatment directed towards the developing central nervous system of the infant and young child, and to distinguish this method of treatment from the more peripherally orientated approaches of Phelps and Collis. Temple

Fay devised a method of treatment which stressed the development of essential patterns of movement, and Bobath has developed this idea still further.

For treatment to be effective it must begin early (Bobath 1967, Köng 1970), preferably before the child is six months old. It can still be effective when the child is older, but abnormality is more established in the older child and carryover of treatment into daily life is more difficult to achieve.

The involvement of the child's parents is essential if there is to be any carryover of treatment. Great emphasis must be laid on teaching parents how to give treatment at home, and on showing them how to 'treat' their child by handling correctly in order to get a more normal response.

Similarly, there must be a complete link-up between the various people responsible for the child's treatment, physician, speech, occupational and physical therapist, and this link-up should extend to the school-teacher and psychologist. It has been suggested that the best approach is one in which all therapists are trained, not only to have a similar approach to treatment, but also to have an understanding of each other's work, so there can be some carryover in a practical sense. For example, the physiotherapist may prepare the child for speech therapy by normalizing tone and movement in the oro-facial region, by improving his respiratory co-ordination, and by inhibiting abnormal oral reflexes.

In order that the occupational therapist may improve the child's manipulative ability in play and self-care activities, the physiotherapist may prepare the child by facilitating more effective equilibrium reactions and by improving trunk and shoulder girdle control so he will be better able to use his hands. The speech therapist and occupational therapist will both need to know what the physiotherapist is aiming for in her treatment so there may be a carryover into their sessions with the child. At times it is preferable for two therapists to work together with a child. The speech therapist, for example, may encourage vocalization and stimulate more normal oral function during those times when the physiotherapist has facilitated more stable head control (figure 40).

Finally, it must be remembered that treatment is a preparation for function, and that function in the case of a young child is made up of play, of pulling himself to standing, and of dressing and feeding himself. The therapist who forgets this will not allow the child she is treating to develop his potential ability, but will transfix him in a treatment situation, isolated from the real world.

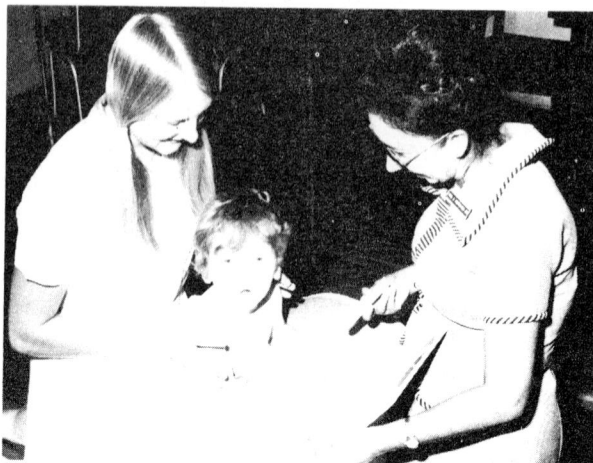

Fig. 40 Athetoid quadriplegia. Speech therapist encourages vocalisation while physiotherapist encourages a more stable position, with weightbearing on the forearms.

General Points in Treatment

In treatment an attempt is made to shunt nervous impulses from abnormal to normal patterns of activity as the child is handled by the physiotherapist and by his parents. This is termed *inhibition*, and the techniques used are called *reflex inhibiting patterns* (Bobath 1965). These are patterns in which the child is treated in order that his abnormal patterns of movement and posture may be changed. They constitute only one part of treatment but in the spastic patient are an essential part of the stimulation of functional movement.

A main aim of treatment with all cerebral palsied children is an active response to handling, but in order that this active response may be more normal in the hypertonic patient, and because a normal movement cannot be superimposed upon an abnormal posture, it is necessary for the abnormal postures to be inhibited. Sherrington stated that a reflex can be changed by changing the body position and this is the basis of reflex inhibiting patterns.

The term *key points* is used (Bobath & Bobath 1964) to describe those parts of the body, usually proximal, at which abnormal tone is inhibited and more normal movement is facilitated, and also those parts of the body from which the child's active movements can be guided.

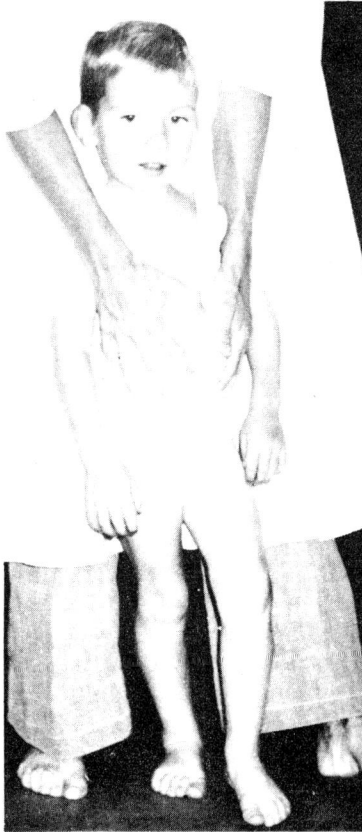

Fig. 41 Spastic diplegia. Facilitated walking, combining weight transference laterally and forward, with rotation of the trunk.

To *facilitate* a movement in this context means to make a particular movement happen automatically in response to the therapist's handling of the child. He may be facilitated from such key points as the head, shoulders, trunk or pelvis (figures 41, 42, 43, 44, 45). Where tone is too low to sustain a posture or a movement, stimulating techniques are used at the same time.

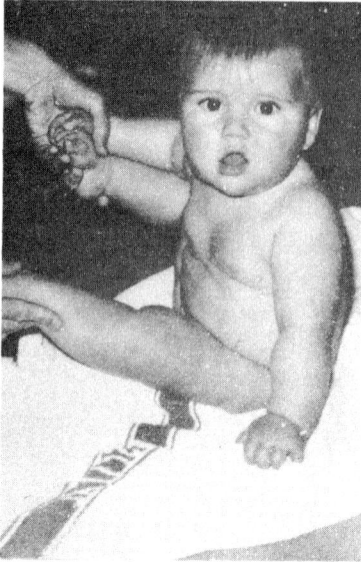

Fig. 42 Delayed motor development. Facilitation of lateral support on the hand.

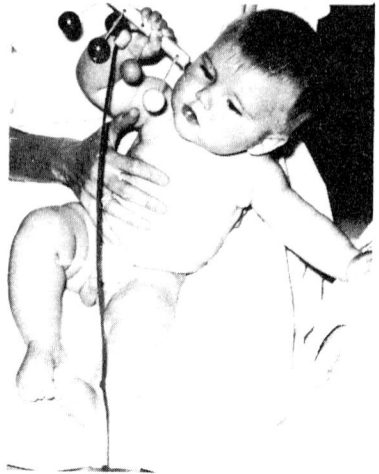

Fig. 43 Delayed motor development. Another method of facilitating lateral support on the hand.

The physiological mechanism of these techniques is not understood. However, in the spastic patient it appears that it is the changing of the movement from abnormal to normal as the child moves which results in the change in tone. The main problem in treatment of the older child is how to maintain this more normal tone as the child moves without guidance from the therapist. It is often movement, combined with several other factors, which brings the child back to his spastic state. These other factors are associated reactions which occur on effort plus the sensory feedback the child is receiving of the altered state of his tone. His brain has only been aware of abnormal tone and movement and therefore in a sense the child does not know how to move in this changed set of circumstances in which there is no longer such resistance to movement.

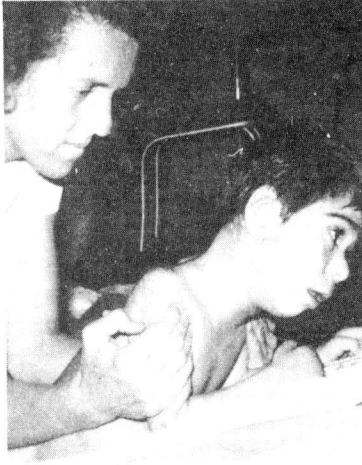

Fig. 44 Athetosis with marked hypotonia and intermittent tonic spasms. Facilitation of head righting and trunk extension with weightbearing on the arms. The shoulder girdle is used as the key point.

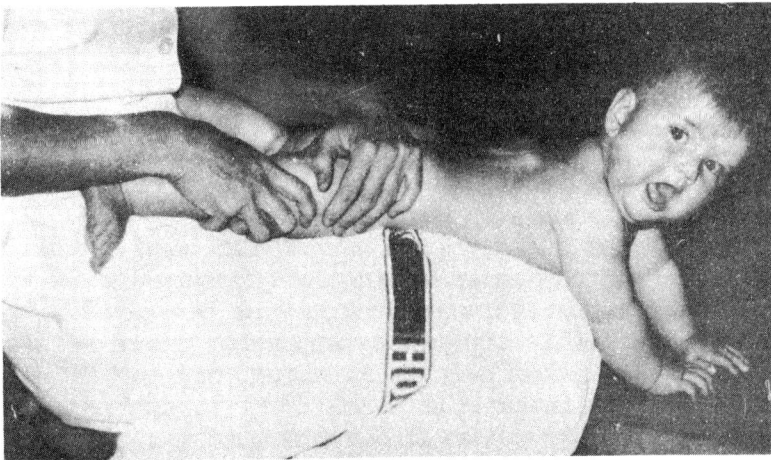

Fig. 45 Delayed motor development. Facilitation of head and trunk extension with protective support on the hands.

This poses a great problem in the carryover of treatment into function. The therapist must be able by her guidance to facilitate more normal movements, but the child may revert to his old abnormal method of moving because this seems more familiar. This is why it is so important to begin treatment in infancy while the brain is still developing and before there is a strong continuous feedback of abnormality which will cause the brain to be conditioned to respond abnormally. This is also why it is so important, both in the infant and the young child, that the physiotherapist ensures as complete a carryover as possible into the child's daily activities. There must be repetition of normal movements, or rather, repetition of the feedback from normal movements, in order that these may be *learned*.

Facilitation of automatic postural activity is an essential part of treatment. Movement cannot be effective until the child has developed some ability to make postural adjustments. Postural adjustments are those movements or tonus changes which are made in order to balance against gravity, as a preparation for movement and throughout movement. These adjustments are initiated in the brain as a result of feedback from the vestibular apparatus and the cerebellum and more peripherally from the proprioceptive mechanism. Facilitation techniques will therefore in particular be directed toward the development of head control (labyrinthine righting reactions), equilibrium reactions, and the basic movements necessary for such activities as rolling over, sitting up, propping on the hands, standing up, walking, dressing and feeding.

Symmetry of posture and movement are essential as it is difficult to function effectively against a background of an asymmetrical trunk or limbs. Abnormal body alignment interferes with movement and postural adjustment.

Techniques of facilitation and inhibition are used in order to enable the child to be active. He is encouraged to move about with the physiotherapist gradually relinquishing her guidance but always ready to inhibit abnormal or unnecessary movements when the child loses control over the movement, that is, when tone becomes either unstable or increased. The eventual goal for the child is independent movement, therefore it is important that the therapist can assess at what stage she can take her hands away (figure 46) and at what stage she should resume her guidance. The child should learn to use his newly-acquired movements in order to do things for himself, and the physiotherapist will be guided in her choice of movements to be stimulated by each child's functional requirements.

An understanding of how a child learns motor skills is very helpful for the physiotherapist. Unfortunately, the literature on the acquisition of motor skills is not always readily available to therapists as it is usually associated with other disciplines, such as psychology and physical education. Physical treatment designed to help the child to attain motor skill is considerably enriched if the therapist understands such factors as motivation, goal

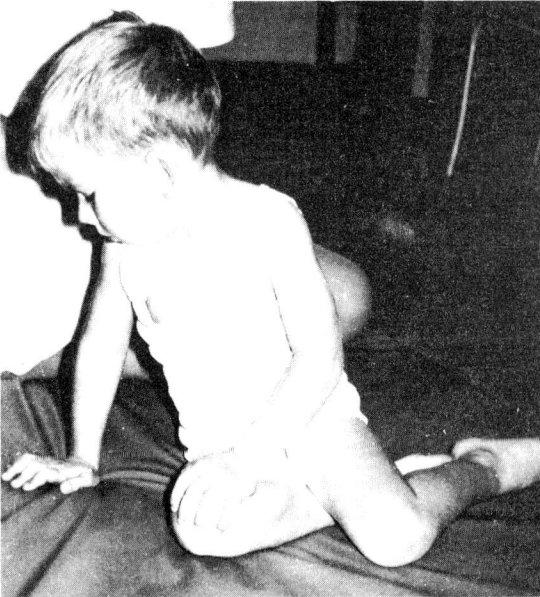

Fig. 46 Spastic diplegia. The therapist must know when to let the child try to maintain a posture or perform a movement on his own.

direction and practice, and the importance of auditory and visual feedback. Some introductory reading in this field is included at the end of Chapter 2 in Section 1.

119

Relationship between Development & Treatment

A detailed knowledge of normal child development is necessary as a guide for the physiotherapist assessing and treating the cerebral palsied child. However, it is not necessary, nor is it probably wise to attempt to follow too closely in treatment the various milestones, as there are many variations in normal development. Some children, for example, never crawl, preferring instead to walk on hands and feet, and later cruising around the furniture in an upright position.

It is important to recognise the overlap that occurs in normal development, the preparation for each new stage that a child gives himself, and the repetition of new movements until they are learned. Development must not be thought of only in terms of physical development, but as physical development progressing concurrently with the development of speech, intelligence, perception, and emotional and social behaviour. To some extent these aspects of the child develop as a result of motor development. Piaget (1952), for example, suggests that early motor experiences are essential for the development of cognitive behaviour. The cerebral palsied child may be slower to develop emotional maturity, for example, because of his greater dependence on those around him. His intelligence may develop inadequately if he cannot move around and learn about his surroundings, and if he cannot express himself effectively, either to others or to himself.

Treatment methods that stress the importance of understanding development are sometimes misunderstood. It is not necessary to wait until a child attains one stage in development before progressing on to the next. It is not necessary to treat the child in a particular sequence. He does not have to perfect rolling over, for example, before he tries to stand (Shepherd 1975). This is not what occurs in normal development. It is not necessary in treatment to fill in every gap in the child's development as this may hold the child back rather than allowing him to progress.

The approach to treatment should involve a realistic understanding of development aiming at useful function. The therapist will use this understanding to help the child *prepare* himself for each new skill or function, making sure she facilitates the various elements which comprise this new function. She must know, for example, that unless the child can gain sitting balance, the ability to reach forward and grasp, and the ability to flex the hips and knee fully and individually, the child will not be able to learn how to put on and take off his socks.

Involvement of Parents in Treatment

An infant who has parents to love and look after him will progress in treatment more than a child in an institution, where there may be too many children to be looked after by too few staff, and where there can therefore be no mother-substitute. A child whose parents have been taught how to handle him and treat him in order to evoke the best and most normal response possible will progress more quickly than a child whose parents are inadequately taught.

The instruction of the parents should begin during their first few visits to the therapist, and consists of simple descriptions of handling to be used when bathing, dressing, feeding, pot-training and playing with the child.

Suggestions are made as to the best way of looking after the child during the day. He may need to sit in a plastic blow-up chair or astride a roller at a table. If he has insufficient head control to maintain the sitting position even though supported, he may lie in prone over a wedge (figure 47), or in side lying. An infant may be nursed in a hammock if he has tonic extensor spasms (figure 48). A symmetrical head position may be encouraged by a headpiece attached to his stroller (figure 49).

Gradually, simple explanations of the abnormalities are given, and the parents are taught how to recognize an abnormal response to stimulation. They watch the therapist while she treats the child, and carry out some of the treatment techniques themselves under her supervision. The parents should only be asked to do what they can reasonably be expected to do, and this will depend on their intelligence and on the practical circumstances of their lives. Care should be taken, however, not to overburden the intelligent and enthusiastic parent. The therapist must take care to keep her suggestions for the care of the child as practical as possible, remembering that the parents have a responsibility towards their other children and to each other, as well as to their handicapped child.

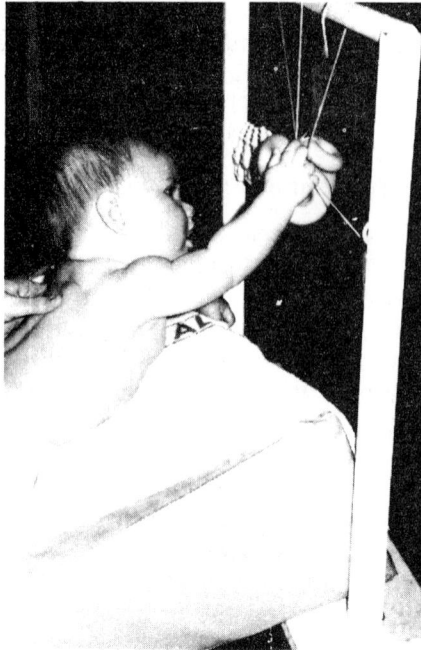

Fig. 47 Delayed motor development. Head
and trunk extension may be facilitated over a
wedge. The therapist helps the baby transfer
weight on to his left arm enabling him to reach
out with his right. He is encouraged to play in
this position at home.

Some Centres give parents a questionnaire to fill in. The answers give the therapists an idea of how much they have taught the
parents, and indicate the gaps left. The results of one such
questionnaire have been published (Bobath and Finnie 1970).

There is no place in this book for a detailed description of the
type of handling that must be done at home. The reader is referred
to Finnie (1974) for a guide to this aspect of treatment.

Specific Points in Treatment

In the treatment of a spastic child emphasis is on movement.
Spasticity will be inhibited by methods of handling which are
designed to inhibit the abnormal patterns (figure 50), and only

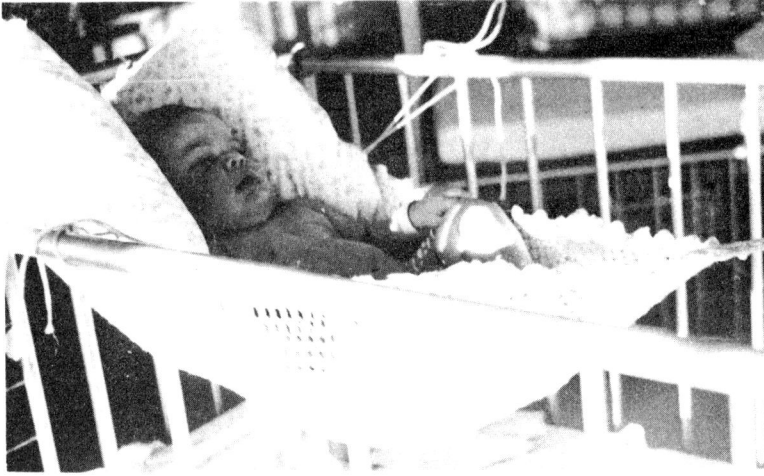

Fig. 48 The use of a hammock to inhibit intermittent extensor spasms or extensor spasticity in an infant. It also inhibits shoulder retraction and allows the baby to bring his hands to the midline.

then can more normal movement be expected. The therapist handles the child in such a way as to facilitate an active response and she does this from key points which are usually proximal, at the shoulder girdle or trunk for example (figure 51). By holding the child at these key points she can judge whether tone needs to be inhibited, whether she should facilitate an active response, or whether she should merely guide the child while he moves himself.

Emphasis is on movements involving rotation, this being an essential part of most functional movements, and also having the effect of inhibiting both flexor and extensor spasticity.

The child is discouraged from moving with effort, as this results in associated reactions, and consequent increase in tone makes normal movement very difficult or impossible. Associated reactions are inhibited by the therapist who can feel the built-up in tone as she handles the child and can therefore inhibit this at the appropriate key points.

In the treatment of an ataxic child the emphasis is on gaining stability. It may be necessary to use stimulating techniques in order to facilitate co-contraction, especially around the proximal joints. The child must develop stability if he is to maintain a

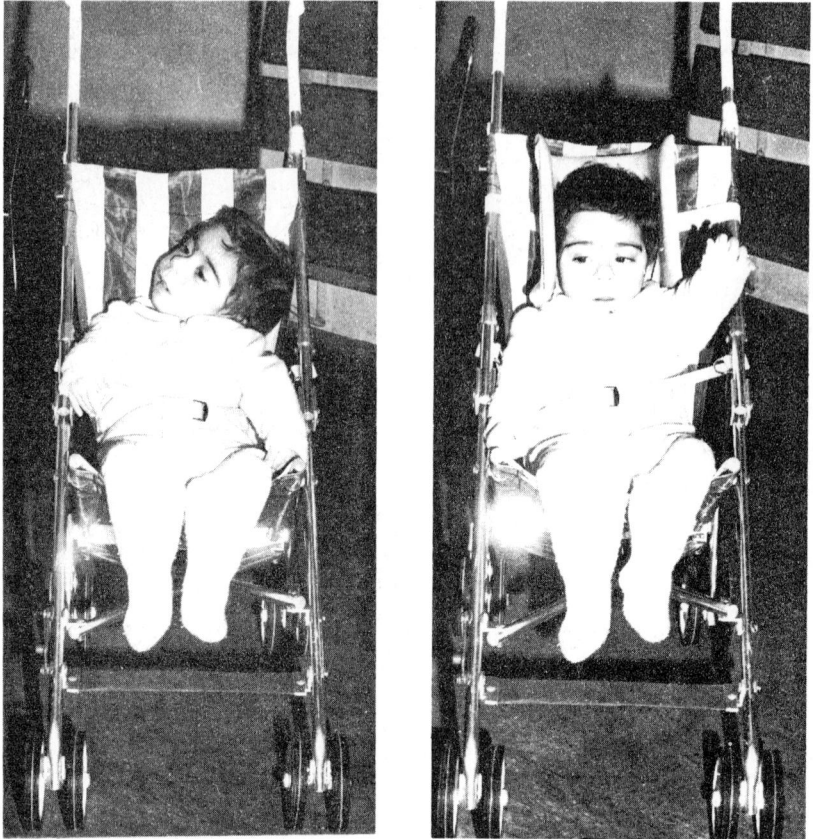

a   b

Fig. 49 (a) Athetoid baby with marked hypotonia and intermittent tonic spasms. Note asymmetrical head posture. (b) Same baby with head support. He can rotate his head a little but the support brings it back to the midline.

posture against gravity. Weight, pressure and resistance given as the child moves will stimulate stability by increasing co-contraction especially around proximal joints. The child is helped to gain control over the middle ranges of movement in particular, as it is in this area that control is most lacking.

When working for control over a posture or a movement of the upper limb, for example, the therapist may begin by holding

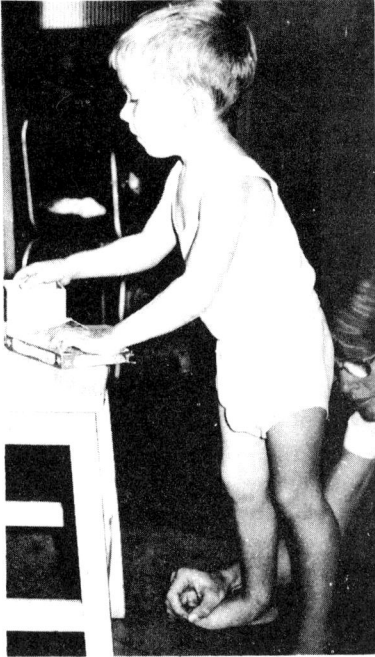

Fig. 50 Spastic diplegia. The spastic pattern of extension, internal rotation, adduction and plantarflexion is partly inhibited by the therapist. With his legs in external rotation and abduction, dorsiflexion of the toes maintains inhibition while the boy transfers his weight from side to side in play.

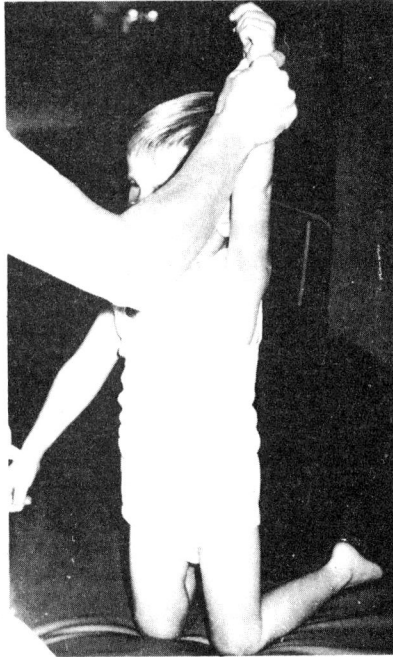

Fig. 51 Spastic diplegia. Facilitation of equilibrium reactions in kneeling. Flexion spasticity on the left side is inhibited by the therapist who holds his arm in elevation and external rotation while she facilitates the reaction.

proximally at the trunk or shoulder girdle, gradually allowing the child to gain control over movements of the hands while she maintains some control proximally.

The ataxic child must develop better balance especially in sitting and standing. Tapping to the trunk given alternately backward and forward helps the child learn the control necessary for balancing. The feet should be as close together as possible or one in front of the other in a small step. The child will use as wide a base as he can and this may have become an habitual posture. The therapist will have to watch carefully that he has a narrower base as she taps him, otherwise the technique can have little effect as it will not require any extra effort on the part of the child.

The wearing of a weighted belt may help give more stability in standing and walking, and may enable an ataxic child to walk where instability has made this difficult.

In the treatment of an athetoid child the methods used will depend upon whether the child has intermittent tonic spasms, dystonia, spasticity or a basically low tone with inability to maintain postures against gravity. It will also depend on his age, the older child being helped to control his own movements, the infant being guided and controlled more by the therapist. It is important to gain symmetry, head control and some coordination between eye and hand. Both athetoid and ataxic children frequently have poor eye-hand control, and learning to grasp with the eyes as well as with the hands is an important part of treatment.

In order that the child may gain some control over movement, intermittent tonic spasms (which are usually asymmetrical) and spasticity must be inhibited by guiding the patient from the key points already mentioned. The hypotonic athetoid child needs carefully graded stimulation to help him maintain postures against gravity and to move in a controlled manner against gravity. Techniques involving weight-bearing and compression will be useful with this child. Stimulation must be carefully graded to avoid the build-up of tone in abnormal patterns. The child with constant involuntary movements is encouraged to control these movements himself. Physical control by the therapist will usually result in an eventual increase in the extent of these movements and should not be used. However, verbal control from the therapist or from the child himself is often successful.

In the treatment of the flaccid patient the main problem is the extremely low tone and its potential changeability. Although emphasis must be on increasing tone in order to gain the ability to move and to hold a posture against gravity, care must be taken not to cause an increase in tone in abnormal patterns. The therapist must be able to recognize the development of intermittent spasms in an athetoid child, and the abnormal patterns of movement of the child developing spasticity, and should from the beginning attempt to inhibit them.

These children in particular have respiratory problems which result from lack of control over the respiratory muscles, which makes it difficult to breathe against the force of gravity, and impossible to cough effectively. Added to this the lack of tone in the oro-facial muscles makes the swallowing mechanism unreliable resulting in aspiration of feeds into the respiratory tract. The child's parents must be taught techniques of postural drainage and percussion in order to clear the airways when necessary.

In the treatment of the cerebral palsied child who is also hyperkinetic an attempt is made to organize the child and to help him to organize himself. Treatment must be very slow and relatively static. He is better treated in a quiet, darkened room, empty of objects which may prove too stimulating for him. Movements to counting or to precise commands may help him control his excess of movement. Primitive motor patterns must be inhibited in order to allow more mature patterns, particularly those of equilibrium, to develop. Smith and Phillips (1970) describe treatment of a particular hyperkinetic child.

All of these children will have defective automatic adjustment to changes in the centre of gravity, either through a failure of the equilibrium and righting reactions (Appendix 1) to develop or to abnormalities in these reactions. No matter into what category the child is classified, there must be considerable emphasis in treatment on development of these automatic reactions, as without them development of basic skills remains an impossibility. The body righting reaction may be facilitated in an infant by rolling him in a towel or by facilitating the movement from his legs. Equilibrium reactions may be facilitated with the infant lying on a ball, and with an older child in sitting and standing as well as on a ball. In attempting to gain any functional movement (sitting to standing, walking, dressing) the therapist makes sure to concentrate on the automatic adjustments which are necessary if the movement is to be more normal and effective.

Treatment of Oro-facial Dysfunction

Infants with abnormal oral function and consequent feeding problems require early treatment. In many cases it will be necessary to stimulate more normal muscular control, and in those infants with hypertonus or hypersensitivity to inhibit these.

Inhibition of such responses as a persistent strong bite reflex, a hypersensitive gag reflex, tongue thrust and immature swallowing must be gained before more normal oral function can occur. The therapist can desensitize the mouth of an infant with these abnormalities in the following ways.

To inhibit *hypersensitive lips and cheeks* a finger is rubbed gently around the lips, and as improvement occurs the finger is moved slowly into the infant's mouth and around his cheeks and gums. If there is a *persistent bite reflex* a finger is rubbed along the gums in an effort to desensitize them. Where there is a *tongue thrust* the finger is pressed firmly down and back on the blade of the tongue, then withdrawn and the lips and jaw quickly closed. Lateral vibration to the tongue with firm pressure downward may be more effective in some infants. If the tongue remains flat when the infant is sucking, the edges can be facilitated to elevate in the normal way if pressure is applied to the middle of the blade of the tongue, or if the lateral edges of the tongue are vibrated upwards by the finger. *Swallowing* is facilitated by lip and jaw closure and pressure applied externally to the base of the tongue.

Where the *gag reflex* is hypersensitive the infant may not be able to tolerate a finger touching his lips or the tip of his tongue. Inhibition of this hypersensitivity may be gained if the therapist begins by gently rubbing her finger around the infant's lips, gradually entering his mouth and rubbing along his gums. Only then does she approach his tongue, walking her finger along it in small stages until he can tolerate her finger pressing on the blade of the tongue.

The infant with a *hypotonic mouth* and a *flat atonic tongue* can be stimulated to suck and swallow more effectively if vibration is done as described above (Mueller 1977).

These procedures are done by the mother for a few minutes before she feeds the baby, where necessary during the feed and at intervals during the day. During feeding the mother will press the blade of the tongue down and back with the spoon as she puts the food in the baby's mouth, in order to inhibit a tongue thrust, then withdraw the spoon, closing the lips and jaw, and stimulating a swallow. *Chewing* may be stimulated by placing a strip of partially cooked steak between the child's gums or teeth and holding the jaw lightly closed (Mueller 1977). The child's head must not be allowed to extend as normal swallowing is impossible and lip and jaw closure unlikely in this position.

The physiotherapist will help the *development of speech mechanisms* if she encourages the baby to babble and vocalize. She can change the quality of the sound he makes by tapping over his lips or by giving vibrations to his chest. *Breathing control* is encouraged by vibrations on expiration, and manual pressure on the chest to encourage longer expiration. When the child is older, breathing control can be encouraged by games in which the child tries to bend but not extinguish a candle flame, blow a mobile or a ping-pong ball.

The initial assessment of the infant and child with oro-facial dysfunction may be done by a speech therapist and she will teach the child's mother how to carry out treatment at home. However, where the services of this therapist are not available, the assessment and treatment may have to be carried out by the physiotherapist or occupational therapist. When the time comes for speech itself to be trained, the child must be referred to a speech therapist for management of this aspect of his disability.

Splinting and Surgery

The use of splinting is not easily compatible with treatment directed at improving brain function. Apparatus which gives stability to the joints of the lower limb prevents the delicate interplay of postural adjustment in response to shifts in the centre of gravity which the therapist is trying to gain in these children. Treatment which aims to increase the scope of movement in a spastic patient will not be carried over into daily activities if the child is restricted in calipers. If bracing is applied to a young child his opportunities for learning basic motor patterns are limited. Some forms of splinting, if used temporarily, may help a child develop stability in the erect position; others such as serial weight-bearing leg plasters, may inhibit hypertonus (Hayes and Burns 1970). Benefit will only be seen, however, where such splinting is combined with physical treatment designed to normalize tone and gain more movement. Similarly, surgery will have limited effect unless it is followed by intensive physical treatment to gain movements which were impossible beforehand.

However, surgery is necessary for some of these children. It may enable physical treatment to proceed towards more independent activity in the older child by inhibiting hypertonus where conservative methods have failed, or by lengthening contracted soft tissues where these are preventing movement. It is hoped that physical treatment, if started sufficiently early, will successfully prevent these situations from occurring.

Other Methods of Treatment

There are other methods of physical treatment which must be briefly mentioned here. Cotton (1970) and Hari (1968) describe the method of *conductive education* devised in Hungary by Pëto. As its name implies, this method is an educative rather than a therapeutic approach to the problems of these children. The main principles behind the method are the relationship of speech to movement (Luria 1961) and recognition of the importance of a child developing in a total learning atmosphere. Rhythmic intention is used for training movement. The children state the intention, the movement is carried out to the rhythm of counting or of speech describing the movement. The child is placed in a situation in which he is taught the motor patterns essential for function, reinforcing his attempts at movement by vocalizing his actions as he performs them.

Biofeedback or sensory feedback therapy involves the use of a device which feeds back to the child an objective assessment of muscle activity and position in space. This can be done in a number of different ways. Harris, Spelman and Hyman (1974) describe the use of head position trainers to aid athetoid children gain head control. Halpern *et al* (1970) and Wolpert and Wooldridge (1975) also describe biofeedback training for children with cerebral palsy. Biofeedback may with some children be an effective adjunct to physical treatment by giving the child the opportunity to practise certain skills on his own with feedback as to his accuracy, and by providing a novel motivating factor.

Vibration. Stimulation of the tonic vibration reflex (Hagbarth and Eklund 1969) may be used to encourage activity in the muscle groups required for a particular function. A mechanical vibrator oscillating at between 100 and 200 Hz with an amplitude of 1 to 2 mm is applied directly to the muscle required to contract. Where spasticity is present, the vibrator is applied to the muscle groups antagonistic to the spastic muscles in order to have an inhibiting effect. Eklund and Steen (1969) describe its use with a group of children with cerebral palsy.

There are several contraindications to the use of vibration which should be considered. If applied directly to a spastic muscle it will cause a further increase in tone. It may cause an exaggeration in ataxic and athetoid movements and initiate spasms in athetoid and dystonic patients. Patients with rigidity may also be adversely affected.

THE DEVELOPMENTALLY DELAYED OR AT-RISK INFANT

The developmentally delayed infant may be an infant with brain damage or with mental retardation. He may, however, be developmentally delayed because he has a congenital heart defect or spina bifida, or because he was born premature, suffered infant respiratory distress syndrome or neonatal infection. He may catch up eventually with his peers or he may, at school age, show signs of minimal brain dysfunction.

He will be seen by the physiotherapist because of his developmental delay or because he is considered to be 'at-risk' and hopefully this will be early in his life, in the neonatal period if possible, as this is the best time to help him. It is also a time when his parents will most need help and guidance in rearing him. It has been suggested that by three months of age, a great deal of important interaction between infants and their parents has already occurred and that future patterns may already be set (Brazelton 1973).

The developmentally delayed infant poses problems for his parents, especially if he is first born and the parents are inexperienced in child rearing. If he is quiet and unresponsive they may worry about disturbing him, if he cries a lot they will feel guilty and uncertain as to how to act.

The objectives of the physiotherapist in his early weeks are to enable the parents to understand their infant, to appreciate their own skills in handling him, whether by stimulating him or quieting him, and to guide the parents in ways of getting the best out of him, behaviourally and socially as well as motorically. In this way the therapist helps the parents cement their relationship with the infant, while ensuring that his environment will be as enriching as it can be.

The Brazelton Neonatal Behavioural Assessment Scale (Brazelton 1973) is an effective method of both evaluating the performance of an infant in the first 30 days and of helping the parents understand their baby and how to handle him. This assessment, in conjunction with relevant parts of the assessment described earlier in this chapter, will give the therapist an understanding both of the infant's weaknesses and his strengths. The parents' handling of their developmentally delayed infant can then be concentrated on overcoming his problems both by direct stimulation of certain movements and functions and by using his positive abilities as an aid.

Probably the most important areas of function to encourage in the very early period are the following — head control in various positions, hand to mouth, visual and auditory orientation (both animate and inanimate) and suckling, swallowing and feeding. As the infant matures, he is encouraged to take weight on his arms in prone, reach out for objects in all positions, roll over, balance during all movements and vocalise. Gradually his activities are progressed. To encourage the maturation of development in all areas of function the therapist needs a good understanding of normal infant development. Campbell (1974) describes an infant stimulation programme which integrates the facilitation of early cognitive and motor skills in premature infants.

THE BLIND INFANT

A number of infants and children who have cerebral palsy have other handicaps such as deafness, or mental retardation, or blindness. Infants may be born with congenital blindness or may become blind as a result of various causes such as injury to the eye.

Blindness interferes with development in such areas as perception (for example, spatial relationships and form identification), cognition, socialisation (in terms of facial expression and the acquisition of social skills such as eating and dressing), personality formation and motor skill acquisition. The blind infant will therefore be referred for physiotherapy designed to prevent developmental delay, enable him to attain his maximum functional capacity and to help his parents cope with his special needs.

Some specific problems found in blind infants are outlined below. A stimulation programme for a blind infant will begin as soon after birth as possible and will aim to anticipate and prevent or minimise these problems.

Perseverant or stereotypic behaviours

These consist of actions such as eye poking, rocking, head banging and finger movement. The reasons for such behaviours are not understood, however there have been several suggested causes including sensory deprivation and emotional disturbance. It has also been suggested that the child may use stereotypic actions as actions to which he can regress when he is in a situation of extreme stress.

Antigravity posture and balance

Many blind infants are slow to develop head and trunk control against gravity, perhaps demonstrating the importance of vision as a motivating force. Touch, hearing and the stimulating effect of gravity itself need to be substituted for vision in providing stimulation to lift the head and trunk. The development of the balance required to move from one position to another, to sit, to crawl and to walk is slow to develop in blind infants. As Fraiberg (1968) has pointed out, the blind infant demonstrates his readiness for crawling by supporting himself on his hands and knees and rocking backward and forward. However, he does not crawl at this point but perseverates on this rocking action for months. Similarly, he may stand for several months before he is able to walk.

This may be due to the absence of the optical righting reaction's contribution to balance, to poor body orientation in space, to difficulties internalising his position in space, or to the fact that he is unable to learn from the example of others.

Crawling can be encouraged by stimulating lateral weight transference which is essential. The infant can be encouraged to reach out one hand toward an audible toy which will require him to transfer his weight laterally on to the other hand. Crawling itself can be encouraged by placing a towel under the infant's body and giving him the feeling of the sideways and forward motion necessary for crawling. It is probable that the onset of crawling is related to the ability to reach toward the sound an object makes, which is achieved at around 10 months. Reaching on sound is a major developmental step, a point which should be discussed with the parents, in order that they will not become discouraged by expecting their infant to achieve this step earlier than 10 months.

Again, in standing, it is the lack of lateral movement, both in terms of the transference of weight laterally and the lateral flexion of the head and trunk, which is a basic reason for the blind infant's slowness to develop walking skills. Such lateral movement should be encouraged whenever the infant is stood by his parents in order to encourage an awareness of position in space, as well as to stimulate balance adjustment to loss of centre of gravity.

Standing unsupported should be encouraged as early as possible. There is a tendency for these infants to persist in cruising sideways around the furniture once they have learned to do this. Gentle tapping to the trunk in standing, sufficient to displace weight, may help the infant learn the necessary adjustment. He also needs early experience of walking from one surface to another, for example, from floorboards to carpet, as this can be an obstacle to the further development of walking skills.

Gross motor play needs to be stimulated as early as possible in many different ways. Activities such as somersaulting, jumping, using playground equipment, will all help develop an awareness of self in space, a feeling for the pleasure of movement, and confidence.

Prehension

Blind infants tend to keep their arms abducted at shoulder level and are slow to engage their hands in the midline, reach, grasp, release and transfer objects from hand to hand.

Early in infancy the baby is encouraged to bring his hands to the midline, reach forward to touch objects and, once he can reach for them on sound, to search for them when they are moved slightly. Tactile sensitivity should be encouraged from an early age as touch will be used in many ways (in Braille perception, for example) to substitute for vision.

Blind children have difficulty throwing a ball. An audible ball can be used to encourage catching and an audible target to encourage throwing. It should not be assumed that a blind child cannot play ball games. However, he does need to be taught to substitute other senses for sight. He should not be protected from making mistakes as this is part of the learning process, even in motor skill acquisition. His errors may need to be more clearly defined for him so he can make the necessary corrections.

Attitudes of others

It is possible that the attitudes of those around the infant are as much to blame for his inability to acquire certain skills as is his blindness. Certain sensory and educational experiences may be denied the blind child by parents, friends and teachers who have certain expectations of the blind. Parents need to understand their infant's behaviour as their responses influence his future actions (Dubose 1976). One of the tasks for the parents of a blind infant is to encourage behaviour which is acceptable to society. Infants normally depend largely upon visual cues for this aspect of learning.

SUMMARY

The child with cerebral palsy demonstrates the complex effects of injury to or maldevelopment of the brain, and he requires the care of individuals experienced in their various fields.

The physiotherapist must have a thorough understanding of normal movement and its development in order to assess and treat these infants and children. In assessment there are certain particular factors interfering with function which should be looked for:

Asymmetry or abnormal body alignment.
Abnormal postural and movement patterns.
Retention of primitive reflex behaviour.
Gaps in development.

Detailed speech, perceptual and psychological assessments may need to be done by staff especially trained in these fields in order to complete the picture of the child's sensori-motor function.

It is difficult in assessing young babies to differentiate between those with minor cerebral damage, whose transient neurological signs will disappear as the baby matures, and those with definite cerebral palsy. Although it undoubtedly means that some normal babies are given treatment, the importance of a very early start in the treatment of those babies in whom cerebral palsy is suspected cannot be stressed too much.

The motor assessment is primarily an aid to diagnosis and a guide to treatment. On its own it has little prognostic value in the infant. Although it may enable the physiotherapist to compare a particular infant's development with the 'average' development of an infant of similar age, there remains the impossibility of determining what is 'normal' for an infant of a certain age.

No method of treatment can hope to effect a 'cure' for a cerebral palsied child, although in an infant, the chances of lessening the effects of brain damage seem certain. It must be kept in mind that no child will be helped towards achieving his potential if the therapist treating him sets unrealistic goals both for herself and for her patient. The therapist must be aware that helping the child attain the maximal amount of effective function is the principal objective in the treatment of any brain-damaged child, and that the only effective treatment is treatment which fulfils this objective.

It has so far been impossible to determine statistically the results of treatment available for these children. No two cerebral palsied children present for treatment with the same set of problems. It is difficult to assess the relative effectiveness of different methods as so much depends on the individual therapist's understanding of the total situation. Effectiveness will depend partly on how severely the child's brain is damaged, and partly on how well the therapist understands the child's particular problems and how capable she is of giving treatment which is directed at the main areas of dysfunction.

In the fields of medicine, psychology, education and therapy there is controversy about the best method of approach to the varied problems seen in these children. It is hoped that the graduate physiotherapist will study in depth the effects of brain-damage on movement, the factors involved in motor skill acquisition in childhood, and the various methods, which are developing all the time in various countries, of treating these children. This will be necessary for any therapist who intends treating brain-damaged children, children with developmental delay and children who are blind.

References

André-Thomas, Chesni, Y., and Dargassies, S.S.-A. (1960) *The Neurological Examination of the Infant.* London: Heinemann.

Bishop, B. (1975) Vibratory stimulation. *Phys. Ther.* **55**, 2, 139–143.

Bobath, B. (1965) *Abnormal Postural Reflex Activity Caused by Brain Lesions.* London: Heinemann.

Bobath, B. (1967) The very early treatment of cerebral palsy. *Develop. Med. Child Neurol.* **9**, 4.

Bobath, K. (1966) *The Motor Deficit in Patients with Cerebral Palsy.* London: Heinemann.

Bobath, K. and Bobath, B. (1964) The facilitation of normal postural reactions and movements in the treatment of cerebral palsy. *Physiotherapy*, **50**, 8, 246.

Bobath, K. and Bobath, B. (1967) The neurodevelopmental treatment of cerebral palsy. *J. Amer. Phys. Ther. Assoc.* **47**, 11.

Bobath, B. and Finnie, N. (1970) Problems of communication between parents and staff in the treatment and management of children with cerebral palsy. *Develop. Med. Child Neurol.* **12**, 629.

Brazelton, T. B. (1973) *Neonatal Behavioral Assessment Scale.* London: Heinemann.

Campbell, S. K. (1974) Facilitation of cognitive and motor development in infants with central nervous system dysfunction. *Phys. Ther.* **54**, 4, 346.

Carr, J. H. (1979) Oral function in infancy. *Aust. J. Physiother.* In press.

Carr, J. H. and Shepherd, R. B. (1980) *Physiotherapy in Disorders of the Brain.* London: Heinemann. In press.

Clarke, J. and Evans, E. (1973) Rhythmical intention as a method of treatment for the cerebral palsied patient. *Aust. J. Physiother.*, **19**, 2, 57.

Cotton, E. (1970) Integration of treatment and re-education in cerebral palsy. *Physiotherapy*, **56**, 4, 143.

Dubose, R. F. (1976) Developmental needs in blind infants. *The New Outlook*, Feb., 49–52.

Dubowitz, V. (1969) *The Floppy Infant.* London: Heinemann.

Eklund, G. and Steen, M. (1969) Muscle vibration therapy in children with cerebral palsy. *Scand. J. Rehabil. Med.* **1**, 35–37.

Finnie, N. (1974) *Handling the Young Cerebral Palsied Child at Home.* 2nd Edition. London: Heinemann.

Fraiberg, S. (1968) Parallel and divergent patterns in blind and sighted infants. In *Psycho-analytical Study of the Child.* New York: International University Press.

Goff, B. (1969) Appropriate afferent stimulation. *Physiotherapy* **55**, 1, 9.

Hagbarth, K. E. and Eklund, G. (1969) The muscle vibrator — a useful tool in neurological therapeutic work. *Scand. J. Rehab. Med.*, **1**, 26–34.

Halpern, D. *et al* (1970) Training of control of head posture in children with cerebral palsy. *Dev. Med. Child Neurol.* **12**, 290–305.

Hari, M. (1968) Address given at Castle Priory College, Wallingford, Berks.

Harris, F. A., Spelman, F. A. and Hyman, J. W. (1974) Electronic sensory aids as treatment for cerebral palsied children. *Phys. Ther.* **54**, 4, 354–365.

Hayes, N. K. and Burns, Y. R. (1970) Discussion on the use of weight-bearing plaster in the reduction of hypertonicity. *Aust. J. Physiother.* **16**, 3.

Illingworth, R. S. (1970) *The Development of the Infant and Young Child.* London: Livingstone.

Ingram, T. T. S. (1955) The early manifestations and course of diplegia in childhood. *Arch. Dis. Child.* **30**, 85.

Kabat, H. (1952) Studies in neuromuscular dysfunction. The role of central facilitation in restoration of motor function in paralysis. *Arch. Phys. Med.* **33**, 532.

Kolderie, M. L. (1971) Behaviour modification in the treatment of children with cerebral palsy. *Phys. Ther.* **51**, 10, 1083–1091.

Köng, E. (1967) Early detection and diagnosis of cerebral palsy. *Arch. Ital. di Pediat. e Pueri Coltura*, **25**, 1.

Köng, E. (1971) Early treatment of the motor handicap. Lecture given to American Academy for Cerebral Palsy.

Kukulka, C. G. and Basmajian, J. V. An assessment of an audio-visual feedback devise for use in motor training. *Am. J. Phys. Med.* **54**.

Lance, J. W. (1971) *A Physiological Approach to Clinical Neurology.* London: Butterworth.

Luria, A. R. (1961) *The Role of Speech in the Regulation of*

Normal and Abnormal Behaviour. London: Pergamon.

Mueller, H. (1977) Personal communication.

Piaget, J. (1952) *The Origins of Intelligence in Children.* New York: International University Press.

Prechtl, H. (1977) *The Neurological Examination of the Full-term Newborn Infant.* Edition 2. London: Heinemann.

Riddoch, G. and Buzzard, E. F. (1921) Reflex movements and postural reactions in quadriplegia and hemiplegia with special reference to those of the upper limb. *Brain* **44**, 397.

Scrutton, B. and Gilbertson, M. (1975) *Physiotherapy in Paediatric Practice.* London: Butterworth.

Shepherd, R. B. (1968) The Bobath concept in the treatment of cerebral palsy. *Aust. J. Physiother.* **14**, 3, 79.

Shepherd, R. B. (1975) Abnormal growth and development resulting from disease, trauma and deformity. *Aust. J. Physiother.* **21**, 4, 143-150.

Smith, B. S. and Phillips, E. H. (1970) Treating a hyperactive child. *Phys. Ther.*, **50**, 4.

Stockmeyer, S. A. (1966) An interpretation of the approach of Rood to the treatment of neuromuscular dysfunction. *Amer. J. Phys. Med.* **46**, 1.

Tronick, E. and Brazelton, T. B. (1975) Clinical uses of the Brazelton Neonatal Behavioural Assessment. In *Exceptional Infant* 3, edited by B. Z. Friedlander *et al.* New York: Brunner/Mazel.

Twitchell, T. E. (1959) On the motor deficit in congenital bilateral athetosis. *J. Nerv. Ment. Dis.* **129**, 105.

Voss, D. E. (1966) Proprioceptive neuromuscular facilitation. *Amer. J. Phys. Med.* **46**, 1.

Wolpert, R. and Wooldridge, C. P. (1975) The use of electromyography as biofeedback therapy in the management of cerebral palsy. *Physio. Canada*, **27**, 1.

Further Reading

Abercrombie, M. L. J. (1964) *Perceptual and Visuomotor Disorders in Cerebral Palsy.* London: Heinemann.

Adelson, E. and Fraiberg, S. (1974) Gross motor development in infants blind from birth. *Child Develop.* **45**, 114-126.

Bax, M. C. O. and MacKeith, R. C. (1973) Treatment of

cerebral palsy. *Develop. Med. Child Neurol.* **15**, 1.

Bobath, B. and Bobath, K. (1975) *Motor Development in the Cerebral Palsied Child.* London: Heinemann.

Brereton, B. Le G. (1972) Sensorimotor handicaps and cerebral palsy. Proc. XIIth. World Congress Rehabilitation International.

Brereton, B. Le G. and Sattler, J. (1967) *Cerebral Palsy: Basic Abilities.* Sydney: Spastic Centre of NSW.

Burns, Y. and Walter, P. (1971) Developmental perceptual-motor disorders. *Aust. J. Physiother.*, **17**, 3, 85.

Cotton, E. and Parnwell, M. (1967) From Hungary: The Pëto Method. *Special Education*, **56**, 4.

Critchley, M. (1966) *The Parietal Lobes.* New York: Hafner.

Denhoff, E. (1968) Motor development as a function of perception. In *Perceptual Motor Foundations.* Washington: Amer. Assoc. for Health, Physical Education and Recreation.

Denhoff, E. and Robinault, I. P. (1960) *Cerebral Palsy and Related Disorders — A Developmental Approach to Dysfunction.* New York, Toronto and London: McGraw Hill.

Ellis, E. (1967) *The Physical Management of Developmental Disorders.* London: Heinemann.

Fraiberg, S., Smith, M. and Adelson, E. (1969) An educational program for blind infants. *J. Spec. Educ.* **3**, 2, 121–139.

Fraiberg, S. (1971) Intervention in infancy. *J. Amer. Acad. Child Psychiat.* **10**, 3, 382–404.

Illingworth, R. S. (1962) *An Introduction to Developmental Assessment in the First Year.* London: Heinemann.

Levitt, S. (1977) *Treatment of Cerebral Palsy and Motor Delay.* London: Blackwell.

Reynell, J. K. (1971) The significance of developmental assessment and management of handicapped children. *Physiotherapy*, **57**, 4, 163.

Robinault, I. P. (1973) *Functional Aids for the Multiply Handicapped.* Maryland: Harper and Row.

Scott, R. (1969) *Making of a Blindman.* New York: Russell Sage Foundation.

Semans, S. (1967) The Bobath concept in the treatment of neurological disorders. *Amer. J. Phys. Med.* **46**, 1.

Strauss, A. A. and Kephart, N. C. (1955) *Psychopathology and Education of the Brain-Injured Child.* New York: Grune and Stratton.

Twitchell, T. E. (1964) Variations and abnormalities of motor development. *J. Amer. Phys. Ther. Assoc.* 424.

Wender, P. H. (1971) *Minimal Brain Dysfunction in Children.* New York: Wiley.

Chapter 2

Head Injuries

As well as the injury which may occur as a result of birth trauma, head injuries are seen in children as the result of car accidents, falls and sporting injuries. Children are prone to accidents, partly because of their unawareness of danger, partly because of their immature nervous system, which makes them clumsy and poor at maintaining their balance.

Walton (1971) lists the immediate effects of head injury as *concussion* (temporary and reversible), *cerebral contusion or laceration* (direct bruising and tearing of tissue) and *intracranial haemorrhage* (from tearing of the middle meningeal artery or its branches), *subdural haematoma* (injury to veins in the subdural space) or *subarachnoid haemorrhage* (commonly accompanying contusion or laceration). The effects frequently show widespread involvement of the brain, which is due to the brain's mobility within the relatively rigid cranium. Thus the effects of a blow to one side of the head may be seen on the opposite side where the brain has hit against that side of the cranium, as well as in the brain stem due to the movement of this confined area against the adjacent bony structures.

The problems of head injuries in children are basically the same as in adults, but the effects of such injury show some differences. The infant and young child's brain is relatively immature, and although a child may show severe signs of brain injury such as decerebrate or decorticate rigidity and long periods of un-consciousness, he will frequently make a much better recovery than an adult with a similar injury (Lewin 1966).

The clinical features depend upon the severity of the trauma and the areas of the brain involved. The early features may in-clude vomiting, restlessness, drowsiness, developing into un-consciousness, coma or decerebrate rigidity, while the later features include spasticity, ataxia, problems of sensori-motor integration, oro-facial and visual disability, temper tantrums, distractibility and impairment of memory and concentration, emotional lability with sudden crying episodes, headaches, diplopia, vertigo or epilepsy.

TREATMENT

Physical treatment depends upon the clinical features found in each particular child. A thorough assessment similar to that described for the cerebral palsied child will make clear the presence of spasticity or ataxia and any other disorders of movement which the child may demonstrate.

Rehabilitation should commence as soon as the child is admitted to hospital. Forward-looking care can prevent many subsequent disabilities, and the therapist should keep in mind the *quality* of the child's future recovery.

Early treatment involves the management of respiratory function, prevention as far as possible, of marked hypertonus and contractures, and the stimulation of functional movement.

Some of these children will require a tracheostomy in order to maintain a patent airway, and physical management will be directed towards maintaining effective respiratory function by assisted breathing exercises and the drainage of secretions. Postural drainage will need to be modified in many cases as a position with head dependent will be contraindicated where there is raised intracranial pressure. Anoxia and excessive carbon-dioxide produce and aggravate oedema of the brain, hence the importance of maintaining a patent airway and effective ventilation.

Stimulation of movement and prevention of contractures is very difficult where the child is severely spastic. Therefore, from the earliest possible time, the therapist must attempt to minimise the development of hypertonus. Where possible, the supine position should be avoided in children with tonic labyrinthine activity whose extensor spasticity may become opisthotonic in supine. If the child is small enough he may be nursed in a hammock (figure 48) which will inhibit retraction of the head and neck. He should not, however, lie in this position all day, but should be changed regularly to prone in his cot to prevent flexion contractures at the hips and knees. The older child is more difficult to manage, but he may be turned from semi-prone to side lying at two hourly intervals, and if he is well positioned in side lying with his arm forward and his leg supported from falling into adduction and internal rotation by a pillow, it may be possible to control his spasticity to some extent. In some cases merely the alteration of the head position will lead to a decrease in spasticity. Passive movements of the limbs, if these are done frequently enough, may also help the prevention of contractures. The therapist should concentrate on movement of the shoulder girdle (particularly protraction) and of the trunk. Movements should have some relation to function. They should include movements of the hands to touch different parts of the body in the hope that some degree of sensory awareness may be maintained. Similarly, those attending the child should talk to him, describing the movements he is doing, so that during the times when his level of consciousness improves, he may be kept in touch with his surroundings.

Plaster splints are of little use in controlling spastic limbs, as they tend to elicit the hyperactive stretch reflex, increasing the degree of spasticity and making it impossible to keep the splints in position. If a plaster splint must be used to prevent severe flexion contracture of the knee, it should be in the form of a cylinder which will allow no movement at the joint and therefore will not cause further hyperactivity of the stretch receptors.

Care must be taken to watch out for the signs of ossification around joints in those patients with prolonged unconsciousness, and to stop mobilizing exercises while this situation remains acute. Increasing stiffness, warmth of the joint and swelling may be signs of developing calcification in the soft tissues, and vigorous physical treatment is thought to increase this tendency (Lewin 1966).

Later treatment. As soon as possible the child should be given the experience of sitting and standing. The stimulation of the ability to regain his balance in these positions will be a major part of treatment to regain effective function.

Assessment and treatment will depend upon the child's particular problems. The reader is referred to Chapter 1 and to Carr and Shepherd (1980) for further details.

SUMMARY

The problems resulting from head injuries are only briefly discussed. They depend on the area and extent of the brain involved, and will affect sensori-motor function in ways similar to those discussed in Chapter 1. Physical treatment depends upon an accurate assessment of the child, and is aimed at ensuring quality in the child's recovery and at stimulating effective function.

References

Carr, J. H. and Shepherd, R. B. (1980) *Physiotherapy in Disorders of the Brain.* London: Heinemann. In press.

Lewin, W. (1966) *The Management of Head Injuries.* London: Bailliére, Tindall and Cassell.

Walton, J. N. (1971) *Essentials of Neurology.* London: Pitman.

Further Reading

Critchley, M. (1966) *The Parietal Lobes.* New York: Hafner.

Dekaban, A. (1970) *Neurology in Early Childhood.* Baltimore: Williams and Wilkins.

Hayes, N. K. and Burns, Y. R. (1970) Discussion on the use of weight-bearing plaster in the reduction of hypertonicity. *Aust. J. Physiother.* **16**, 3.

Jennet, B. (1972) Head injuries in children. *Develop. Med. Child Neurol.* **14**, 137.

Lansky, L. L. and Wolcott, G. J. (1975) Trauma to the Brain and Spinal Cord. In *The Practice of Paediatric Neurology*, edited by K. F. Swaiman and F. S. Wright. St. Louis, Mosby.

Loew, F. (1971) Pathophysiological basis for the management of head injuries. In *Head Injuries. Proceedings of an International Symposium.* Edinburgh and London: Churchill-Livingstone.

Plum, F. (1972) Persistent vegetative state after brain damage. *Lancet* **1**, 734.

Robarts, F. H. (1971) Causes of head injury in infancy and childhood. In *Head Injuries. Proceedings of an International Symposium.* Edinburgh and London: Churchill-Livingstone.

Teuber, H. L. and Rudal, R. G. (1962) Behaviour after cerebral lesions in children and adults. *Develop. Med. Child Neurol.* **4**, 3.

Todorow, S. (1975) Recovery of children after severe head injury. *Scand. J. Rehab. Med.* **7**, 93–96.

Walker, A. E., Caveness, W. F. and Critchley, M. (1969) *The Late Effects of Head Injury*. Illinois: Thomas.

Chapter 3

Minimal Brain Dysfunction

Under the title of this chapter are grouped all the children who demonstrate problems in coping with the demands of their environment and with various aspects of their lives, but who cannot be called mentally retarded or obviously brain-damaged. For many different reasons the children in this group do not fit in, whether to family life, the school class or their peer group. A great deal has been said about these children over the past few years, and considerable confusion exists, to some extent due to the varying and confusing terminology used to describe them. It is also due in part to the difficulty physicians and therapists have in evaluating their problems. It is always more difficult to evaluate relatively minor impairment. Where the child's problems exist in an area of function such as balance, about which there is little normative data, the problem of the person who wishes to improve the child's function becomes even more difficult.

This chapter is an attempt to clarify briefly some of the problems of function which may be found and to suggest some ways of approaching these problems. The reader is advised to consult the reading list at the conclusion of the chapter, then to embark upon a more extensive reading programme if she is to undertake the care of these children.

AETIOLOGY

In the presence of such a variety of abnormalities it is understandable that the aetiology is unknown in the majority of children with minimal brain dysfunction. With such a varied picture it is probable that there is also a varied aetiology.

Illingworth (1968), Gubbay (1975), Wender (1971) and others have suggested the following causative factors: organic brain damage (such as caused by anoxia in the perinatal period), dysmaturity, prematurity, delayed maturation, genetic transmission and psychogenetic determinants.

DIAGNOSIS

There are often difficulties in recognising the full extent of minor impairments before the age of 6 or 7 years when the child's learning difficulty and/or clumsiness are becoming apparent.

Nevertheless, it is interesting to consider whether infants who demonstrate transient neurological signs in their first year may be seen at a later age (say 3 or 4 years) with the problems referred to as minimal brain dysfunction.

Drillien in 1972 made a study of 300 infants of low birth weight (less than 2000 gms) in an attempt to identify at an early age the infants who might present with minor impairment at school age. He describes a syndrome he calls 'transient abnormal neurological signs' in the first year of life and suggests that this syndrome may be indicative of the minimal brain dysfunction evident at a later age.

It is possible that tests will eventually be able to anticipate with reliability those infants whose failure to become suitably competent in various areas of function will become obvious as they grow older. The Brazelton Neonatal Behavioural Assessment Scale (Brazelton 1975, Tronick and Brazelton 1975) may be one such test, Prechtl's (1977) another. These authors stress the importance of very early infant evaluation because of the tendency for early abnormal signs or behaviour to disappear, sometimes to reappear months or years later. These assessments can be combined with an evaluation of the infant's maturity at birth (Saint-Anne Dargassies 1966) and of intrauterine conditions of nutrition and/or depletion (the dysmaturity scale of Dubowitz *et al* 1970).

It should then follow that programmes can be developed for these infants which will enable each to develop his potential, that is, to become more competent than he would without special guidance.

DESCRIPTION

At the moment, many children with minimal brain dysfunction are not seen by the physiotherapist until they are at least 3 or 4 years old, and often not until they have been at school for 2 or 3 years. The child may then be referred because of clumsiness, hyperactivity, educational incompetence or under-achievement and behaviour disorders. He may be found to be suffering from a specific learning difficulty, such as difficulty reading (dyslexia), or writing (dysgraphia), difficulty with arithmetic, and poor comprehension and concentration. His clumsiness may be due to defects of sensory integration such as agnosia or dyspraxia or to disorders of motor function with mild athetosis, ataxia, spasticity or immature motor behaviour. Specific examples of clumsiness may include poor fine manual skills or poor balance. Speech defects and auditory imperception have been described as co-existing with clumsiness (Paine *et al* 1968). He may be unable to maintain antigravity control in prone or supine. He may be unable to cope with different kinds of movement, for example, swinging, spinning, motor car or boat movement.

The child with a cluster of the above problems will usually hold himself in low esteem and suffer considerable anxiety. He may not be popular with his peers or with others. Unfortunately, these children are often wrongly classified as mentally retarded, as behaviour problems or just as 'failures', without an attempt being made to find out the true nature of the problems.

Let us look at some of these problems in more detail.

Vestibular Dysfunction. Problems in vestibular function have been attributed to brain-damaged children (Bobath & Bobath 1972) as well as to children with minimal brain dysfunction (Ayres 1972). Abnormal responses to vestibular stimulation have been reported also in autistic children (Ritvo *et al* 1969) and in Down's syndrome children (Kantner *et al* 1976).

Stimulation of the semicircular canals normally produces nystagmus, although it can be inhibited in states of dreaminess (reverie), where the reticular activating system is unstimulated, and by fixation of the eyes. Responses to stimulation of the semicircular canals in children with minimal brain dysfunction are reported to be either hypo or hyperactive, and may vary in quality. In addition to changes in nystagmus, some children demonstrate considerable fear during or following the post-rotatory nystagmus tests, others become dizzy and vomit. Fear is a sign of postural insecurity, the other signs indicate an adversive reaction to movement.

149

The vestibular system affects tone through the connections between the labyrinths and the facilitatory reticular formation of the brain stem. It appears to exert an influence on gamma and alpha motoneurones (Pompeiano 1972, O'Connell and Gardner 1972, Ayres 1972).

The vestibular system together with the proprioceptive (kinaesthetic) system is responsible for our ability to respond to changes in our centre of gravity and body alignment. Many children with minimal brain dysfunction demonstrate an inability to use the head and/or trunk to respond to these changes. This results in difficulties with balance and with righting the head and trunk against gravity. For example, a child with this latter problem would be unable to push himself along the floor on a prone scooter (figure 88) because of inability to gain sufficient trunk and head extension. A child with balance difficulties, if carefully observed, will be seen to have poor or absent head and trunk movement, particularly in a lateral direction, and this will be a major reason for his inability to regain normal body alignment.

Steinberg and Rendle-Short (1977) found significant differences in post-rotatory nystagmus and head righting between a group of children with normal intelligence referred with minimal problems and a control group of randomly selected children without known problems. All the children were aged between 3 and 6 years.

They tested head righting in the horizontal and vertical positions. Poor head righting was greatest in the horizontal position with vision eliminated. 88% of their children showed complete lack of head correction. Even with vision head righting remained inefficient. Some of these children also demonstrated loss of postural tone in the horizontal and vertical positions.

Hyperactivity. Some degree of hyperactive behaviour is seen in the normal child between two and four years of age. This is a time when righting reactions are strongly developed and equilibrium reactions in the process of developing. The child is intensely mobile, mentally, emotionally and physically, and concentration is of a very short span. However, in the normal child, to the relief of the adult who must live with him, this is a passing phase. Unfortunately, some children with brain damage and many with minimal brain dysfunction demonstrate excessive hyperactivity and persist in this behaviour for a number of years.

Hyperactive behaviour is difficult to define. To some extent it is relative. A child may appear hyperactive in a family where all the other children are quiet. Nevertheless, this group of children with dysfunction demonstrate behaviour which differs markedly in both extent and quality from the behaviour seen in normal high-spirited children at certain ages.

Hyperactivity is characterised by excessive restlessness and inattentiveness. The child's activities and reactions are excessive. He hurls his toys instead of throwing them. He runs rather than walks, and he falls over a lot. He does not appear able to eliminate irrelevant stimuli around him, and in paying attention to everything, runs from one toy to the next, takes heed of all sounds without discriminating the most important. He appears a 'naughty' child, but his behaviour is really a manifestation of his inability to control himself or to inhibit unnecessary activity.

He cannot sit still in his seat or listen to stories for any length of time. He may be verbally hyperactive. In both speech and action he tends to perseverate and be compulsive.

In addition, the hyperactive child will demonstrate many of the other problems seen in children with minimal brain dysfunction. Perceptual-motor and cognitive disorders will add to his difficulties, particularly when he starts school. Problems of fine motor co-ordination result in clumsiness, inability to catch a ball or hold a pencil. Problems in balance will prevent him from learning to stand on one leg or walk along a balance beam. Visual-motor co-ordination is usually poor with difficulty in gaining eye-hand control. Tone may be rather low, although some of these children show signs of spasticity or athetosis.

The hyperactive child tends to be immature in both his development and behaviour. He is impulsive and throws temper tantrums. He may demonstrate emotional lability. He has difficulty with peer friendships. His movement ability often remains immature. Associated with his slowness in developing equilibrium reactions is the persistence of immature righting reactions.

Specific Sensory and Motor Problems. These vary greatly from child to child, but there are some particularly common problems which should be considered.

Fine-motor control fails to develop in some of these children and can be seen in the following examples:-

- An inability to appreciate the compressibility of objects. The child may be unable to control his grasp finely enough for it to be appropriate for a particular object even when he knows it is fragile. He will shatter fine glass, Christmas tree decorations and fresh eggs, or drop a glass of milk because he cannot make the necessary adjustment in his motor control.
- Difficulty maintaining the thumb in the abducted position required to oppose forefinger to thumb. The difficulty seems to be in stabilising the thumb at the carpo-metacarpal joint.
- A poor fine pincer grasp. He may be able to pick up a pen but not a pin, because a pin requires precise opposition of the tips of the thumb and forefinger.
- Difficulty using the hands effectively when his arms are stretched out in front of his body.
- Difficulty with rapid repetitive movements such as writing, tapping with the fingers.

These difficulties may be seen in combination with poor sensory discrimination or involuntary movements.

Inadequate sensory discrimination may be seen in poor tactile localisation, problems in stereognosis, in joint position sense and in two point discrimination.

Difficulty in eliminating unwanted activity is almost always seen in these children and probably best illustrates their motor immaturity. They persist in such immature associated movements as moving the fingers of both hands when one hand picks up an object.

Sensory Integrative Dysfunction. Ayres (1972) has been instrumental in pointing out disorders of sensory integrative function in these children. Following her studies of children with cognitive, perceptual and/or motor dysfunction, she has suggested that perceptual-motor dysfunction may be classified into a number of syndromes:- 1) Vestibular and bilateral integration dysfunction, which she considers is a dysfunction in brain stem processing. 2) Developmental apraxia, with either a vestibular or a somatosensory basis. 3) Generalised dysfunction. The reader should refer to Ayres (1972) for this author's description of the problems associated with sensory integrative dysfunction and her approach to treatment.

ASSESSMENT

Evaluation of groups of school children in various countries have discovered large numbers of children with supposed disability in perceptual-motor, cognitive and behavioural function. The wisdom of such evaluation programmes is to be questioned. Perhaps a child should not be assessed for a problem unless he or his parents or his school teacher thinks he has one. This is not to say that studies aimed at picking out infants at risk of joining this group should not be vigorously pursued, since this evaluation has a preventative function.

There is an ever-increasing number of assessments being developed and it is possible that there is a certain amount of over-assessment and under-treatment. A careful history from the parents, supplemented by a history from the school teacher when the child is having difficulties at school, together with careful and casual observation of the child as he moves about, handles toys and talks with the examiner, will indicate to the therapist, if she is familiar with normal children, what areas of function should be assessed. As time passes and the therapist gets to know the child and family better, other problems may become obvious or previously recognised problems clarified.

The tests to be performed for a particular child will develop out of the therapist's understanding of the apparent problems for which the child has been referred. In general, assessment may be performed in the areas of motor ability (including prehension, orientation and balance reactions, motor planning, ability to learn motor skills), significant neurological signs and primitive reflexes (see Chapter 1), tactile, proprioceptive, vestibular and spatial functioning, visual and auditory function.

Assessment should also be directed at the coping mechanisms present within the family. The therapist should aim to find out the strengths and not just the weaknesses of the child and his parents, and of their relationships with one another. Assessment must include behaviour as well as function.

Assessment may involve the skills of paediatrician, psychologist, audiologist, speech pathologist, paediatric neurologist and school teacher as well as occupational and physical therapist.

Ayres (1976) has designed tests for *sensory-integrative functions* the results of which can be measured against normative data.

153

Frostig (1963) has designed tests for *visual perceptual function.*

Balance is often tested by timing the child's ability to stand on one leg. This should, however, be widened to include tests of equilibrium reactions (page 491) with specific regard to the amount of head and trunk movement in response to alterations in centre of gravity.

The various aspects of *sensation* should be tested only if necessary (see Chapter 1), as should tests for *oral function* (see Chapter 1).

Significant neurological signs such as clonus should be observed for, but not necessarily tested. The therapist should look out for evidence of the abnormal patterns (synergies) of spasticity, for athetoid or choreic movements, tremor or ataxia (see Chapter 1).

In the absence of normative data, undue emphasis should probably not be placed on tests for dominance. Mixed dominance may be as common in the normal population as in the population with dysfunction. However, tests for foot, ear, eye and hand dominance may be considered of interest in adding to the therapist's understanding of the child's motor behaviour. The child may require other tests, such as the Bender-Gestalt visual motor test (Bender 1938) or a test for auditory memory skill. Touwen and Prechtl (1970) and Bergès and Lézine (1965) describe various tests appropriate to these children and the reader should consult these references.

MANAGEMENT

Not all children with minimal brain dysfunction require physiotherapy. Those who *do* may require individual treatment of particular problems for a period and/or group activities. These group activities may be organised and run by a physiotherapist or occupational therapist, where specific problems requiring the specialised care of a therapist are needed, or they may be performed in the school gymnastic group under the direct supervision of the physical education teacher with indirect guidance from the therapist. Some children will benefit from modern dance lessons.

Those children who also have behaviour and/or learning difficulties will require remedial teaching, psychiatric or psychologic counselling and behaviour control. Children with specific hearing and speech problems will receive treatment from the appropriate person.

There is evidence that improvement in motor skills and in schoolwork will affect behaviour when behavioural problems stem from these causes. Hence it seems reasonable to suggest that children with problems in motor function, learning and behaviour should have a trial period of physical and occupational therapy and remedial teaching before being referred for specific behaviour therapy.

The physiotherapist should be prepared to assess and deal with the child's problems away from a medical setting preferably in child care centres and in school. The child should not see movement training as 'treatment' because that suggests he is 'sick' but should see it as good fun, and an opportunity to acquire skill.

Group activity performs a useful social function. Some of the children will improve in social skills even if they remain relatively unskilled in motor function. As Abbie (1978) points out, a person can lead a fulfilled happy life without being particularly skilled in a motoric sense. This is not to say that these children should not be given the chance to develop skills which would not develop without guidance. Group treatment is described by Abbie, Douglas and Ross (1978).

Physiotherapy must be specific to each child's problems, which requires that assessment must be very accurate. It is not sufficient to say a child has poor balance. Poor balance must be analysed and training will then be specific to the particular problem. For example, if the head and trunk move ineffectively to restore balance when it is threatened in sitting, the appropriate response must be stimulated in sitting. Similarly, if a child has difficulty stabilising the metacarpo-phalangeal joint of his thumb in functions requiring controlled opposition of the thumb, he should practise this with whatever stimulation is necessary to enable him to be successful. If he has difficulty judging compressibility of objects, he can practise using compressible objects such as plastic foam cups. A child who has an aversive reaction to movements which stimulate the vestibular system will need therapy to improve his tolerance. This therapy may need to be combined with anti-motion sickness medication (Frank and Levinson 1973).

Parents may require advice on child rearing and on how to decrease the level of tension at home. They may need to appreciate how to anticipate routine restlessness and channel it into activity. They and the school teacher should know how to aim at the child's strengths so he can experience success.

Methods of treating hyperactivity are very controversial and include drug therapy, diet and behaviour control. Treatment which quietens the child may be good or bad depending upon whether the child's newly found control can be used to help him learn and socialise or not. There is also a considerable difference between treatment which controls the child and treatment which helps him control himself. Stewart and Olds (1973) give suggestions for parents on raising a hyperactive child.

Safer and Allen (1976) describe the medical (drug) and behavioural management of hyperactive children and the reader should refer to this work. Their studies showed that a group of children on stimulant medication (such as methyl-phenidate or dextroamphetamine) demonstrated a statistically significant improvement in their hyperactive behaviour, with less classroom restlessness, increased attention span, increased academic output and improved emotional and social behaviour. These children became happier, more motivated, more successful and therefore were better accepted into society.

Behavioural management may consist of biofeedback to increase self-control and desensitisation as well as other forms of behaviour therapy. The physiotherapy management of the hyperactive child is briefly described on page 127.

SUMMARY

In this chapter the author has attempted to introduce the reader to the variety of problems found in certain children who do not fit easily into family and school life. Evaluation tests should be appropriate to the child's presenting problems and follow on from the therapist's impressions of the child. In this way over-assessment will be avoided. Management of these children should, where possible, be in a non-medical setting, and parents, being responsible for the large part of management, should receive help and encouragement in rearing their child.

References

Abbie, M. (1978) Physical treatment for clumsy children — Not enough? *Physiotherapy*, **64**, 7, 198.

Abbie, M., Douglas, M. H. and Ross, K. E. (1978) The clumsy child: Observations in cases referred to the gymnasium of Adelaide Children's Hospital over a three year period. *Med. J. Aust.*, **1**, 65.

Ayres, A. J. (1972) *Sensory Integration and Learning Disorders.* Los Angeles: Western Psychological Services.

Ayres, A. J. (1976) *Interpreting the Southern California Sensory Integrative Tests.* Los Angeles: Western Psychological Services.

Bender, L. A. (1938) A visual motor Gestalt test and its clinical use. *Res. Monogr.*, 3, New York: Amer. Orthopsychiatric Assoc.

Bergès, J. and Lézine, I. (1965) *The Imitation of Gestures.* London: Heinemann.

Bobath, K. and Bobath, B. (1972) Cerebral Palsy. In *Therapy Services in Developmental Disabilities*, edited by P. H. Pearson and C. E. Williams. Springfield, Illinois: Charles C. Thomas.

Brazelton, T. B. (1975) *The Brazelton Neonatal Behavioural Assessment Scale.* London: Heinemann.

Drillien, C. M. (1972) Abnormal neurologic signs in the first year of life in low-birthweight infants: possible prognostic significance. *Develop. Med. Child Neurol.,* **14**, 575.

Dubowitz, L. M., Dubowitz, V., Goldberg, C. (1970) Clinical assessment of gestational age in the newborn infant. *Pediatrics*, 77, 1.

Frostig, M. (1963) *Developmental Test for Visual Perception.* Los Angeles: Consulting Psychologists' Press.

Frank, J. and Levinson, H. (1973) Dysmetric dyslexia and dyspraxia. Hypothesis and study. *J. Child Psych.* Oct. 690–701.

Gubbay, S. A. (1975) *The Clumsy Child: A Study of Developmental Apraxia and Agnostic Ataxia.* London: Saunders.

Illingworth, R. S. (1968) Delayed motor development. *Pediat. Clin. N. Amer.*, **15**, 569.

Kantner, R. M., Clark, D. L., Allen, L. C. and Chase, M. F. (1976) Effects of vestibular stimulation on nystagmus response and motor performance in the developmentally delayed infant. *Phys. Ther.*, **56**, 414.

O'Connell, A. L. and Gardner, E. B. (1972) *Understanding the*

Scientific Bases of Human Movement. Baltimore: Williams and Wilkins.

Paine, R. S., Werry, J. C. and Quay, H. C. (1968) A study of minimal cerebral dysfunction. *Develop. Med. Child Neurol.*, **10**, 505.

Pompeiano, O. (1972) Vestibulo-spinal relations: vestibular influences on gamma motoneurons and primary afferents. *Prog. in Brain Res.*, **37**, 197.

Prechtl, H. (1977) *The Neurological Examination of the Full-term Newborn Infant.* Edit 2. London: Heinemann.

Ritvo, E. R., Ornitz, E., Eviatar, A., Markham, C. H., Brown, M. B. and Mason, A., (1969) Decreased post-rotatory nystagmus in early infantile autism, *Neurol.*, **19**, 653.

Safer, D. J. and Allen, R. P. (1976) *Hyperactive Children. Diagnosis and Management.* Baltimore: University Park Press.

Saint-Anne Dargassies, S. (1966) Neurological maturation of the premature infant of 28 to 41 weeks gestational age. In *Human Development*, edited by F. Falkner. Philadelphia: W. B. Saunders.

Steinberg, M. and Rendle-Short, J. (1977) Vestibular dysfunction in young children with minor neurological impairment. *Develop. Med. Child. Neurol.*, **19**, 639.

Stewart, M. and Olds, S. (1973) *Raising a Hyperactive Child.* New York: Harper and Row.

Tronick, E. and Brazelton, T. B. (1975) Clinical uses of the Brazelton Neonatal Behavioural Assessment Scale. In *Except. Infant*, **3**, edited by B. Z. Friedlander et al. New York: Brunner/Mazel.

Touwen, B. C. L. and Prechtl, H. (1970) *The Neurological Examination of the Child with Minor Nervous Dysfunction.* London: Heinemann.

Wender, P. H. (1971) *Minimal Brain Dysfunction in Children.* New York: Wiley.

Further Reading

Arnheim, D. D. and Sinclair, W. A. (1975) *The Clumsy Child. A Program of Therapy.* St. Louis: Mosby.

Ayres, A. J. (1972) Improving academic scores through sensory integration. *J. Learn. Dis.*, **5**, 336–343.

Ayres, A. J. (1975) Sensori-motor foundations of academic ability. In *Perceptual and Learning Disabilities in Children*, **2**, edited by W. Cruickshank. Syracuse: University Press.

Cohen, H. J., Taft, L. T., Mahadeviah, M. S. and Birch, H. G. (1967) Developmental changes in overflow in normal and aberrantly functioning children. *J. Pediat.*, **71**, 39.

Connolly, K. and Stratton, P. (1968) Developmental changes in associated movements. *Develop. Med. Child. Neurol.*, **10**, 49.

de Quiros, J. B. (1976) Diagnosis of vestibular disorders in the learning disabled. *J. Learn. Dis.*, **9**, 39–47.

Fog, E. and Fog, M. (1963) Cerebral inhibition examined by associated movements. In *Minimal Cerebral Dysfunction*, edited by M. Bax and R. MacKeith, London: Heinemann.

Kephart, N. (1971) *The Slow Learner in the Classroom*. Columbus, Ohio: Merrill.

Wright, F. S., Schain, R. J., Weinberg, W. A. and Rapin, I. (1975) Learning disabilities and associated conditions. In *The Practice of Pediatric Neurology*, Vol. 2, edited by K. F. Swaiman and F. S. Wright. St. Louis: C. V. Mosby.

Chapter 4

Mental Retardation

The term mental retardation has been described as an intellectual deficit which is present from birth (Walton 1971), and as a state of arrested or incomplete development of the mind (Tredgold and Soddy 1963).

These children are classified as severely retarded (IQ below 25), moderately severely retarded (IQ between 25 and 50), mildly retarded (IQ between 50 and 75) and border-line normal (IQ between 75 and 95). Whether or not a child is regarded as subnormal in this borderline group will depend to some extent on where he is situated socio-economically. He may appear normal in many families, but should his parents be university educated he would, by comparison, appear retarded.

Generally speaking, the severely and moderately retarded are incapable of protecting or caring for themselves, the severely retarded being looked after in institutions, while the mildly retarded approach the lower limits of normal intelligence and manage to live and work in society. Illingworth (1970) has said that a child with an IQ over 50 will probably be able to earn his living in some capacity. Whether the child will be educable or not will depend on the presence and the degree of physical handicap. A very hyperkinetic child with an IQ in the borderline normal group may, for example, be ineducable because of his hyperkinesis.

AETIOLOGY

An aetiological classification of mentally retarded infants includes the following groups:

Metabolic and endocrine disorders (e.g. congenital hypothyroidism or cretinism, phenylketonuria, Wilson's disease)

Genetic or chromosomal abnormalities (e.g. Down's syndrome, Klinefelter's syndrome)

Malformations of the central nervous system (microcephaly, hydrocephaly, encephalocoele).

In addition, many syndromes have been described, including Noonan's, Möbius, Laurence-Moon, and Apert's syndromes.

Mental retardation occurs in some children with cerebral palsy, in some who are born dysmature or premature, or whose mothers were infected by rubella or herpes virus during pregnancy. It may also develop in children with epilepsy or following encephalitis, meningitis or head injury, and as a result of child abuse.

A degree of mental retardation has been found to be associated with muscular dystrophy (Dubowitz 1965) and spina bifida cystica. Deprived children are frequently found to have motor and mental retardation which disappears in most cases when their social situation improves. It is also possible for a child with a severe motor handicap from earliest infancy to suffer mental retardation which is secondary to his motor disability. This should, however, be preventable to some extent, with early treatment designed to overcome the motor handicap (Bobath 1963).

The importance of accurate assessment of children with developmental disorders cannot be too greatly stressed. Infants and children with developmental delay due to sensori-motor disability, to deprivation, or to specific learning difficulties (dyslexia, dysgraphia) must be distinguished from those whose developmental delay is due to mental retardation. There are many problems in assessing the intelligence of severely physically handicapped children and the tests are often of doubtful value as they require verbal or manual skills for their performance.

THE EFFECT OF MENTAL RETARDATION ON MOTOR
DEVELOPMENT AND MOVEMENT

Many mentally retarded infants are hypotonic for the first few months of life. Cowie (1970) suggests that this hypotonia may be due to delayed maturation of the cerebellum and cortical pathways.

The earliest signs of mental retardation may be *feeding* problems, with the infant unable to suck or swallow effectively, and apparently disinterested in feeding; *delay in social responses* such as smiling and recognition of his mother's face; an *excessive number of hours spent sleeping*; a *weak cry*; *apathy* and *little spontaneous activity*. He will be *slow to vocalise*, and when he does, he will lack the repertoire of sounds which a normal infant demonstrates. As he grows older he may develop *persistent hand regard*. *Mouthing* of toys and anything else he can hold will continue beyond the normal limit of twelve months of age. He may also develop *perseverent or stereotyped actions*, repetitive pointless movements such as hand flapping, head rolling, or rocking, which seem to occur at the stage when he is 'stuck' in a particular posture, lacking the balance and therefore the variety of movement which would enable him to move out of that posture. In *playing*, he will not go after his toys if he drops them, appearing to forget about them, and he may not move to get a toy which is out of reach. *Speech* will be very slow to develop, and in the severely retarded may not develop at all.

The extent to which movement develops in a mentally retarded child depends to some extent on the severity of his mental defect, gross motor development being less interfered with in most cases than the development of speech, fine manipulation of the fingers, and social and intellectual behaviour. Generally in the mildly handicapped child motor development proceeds as in a normal child but at a slower rate. His movements may be relatively normal although many children do not achieve a fully extended posture, maintaining some flexion of the hips, knees and trunk in standing. As well as poor posture, many mentally retarded children have poor muscular strength. Asmussen & Heeboll-Nielsen (1956) consider that in general low intelligence is associated with less muscular strength and endurance. Movements are performed more slowly by these children, although not by those who are hyperkinetic.

Motor development may come to a halt at any stage. The severely retarded child may arrest at an early stage before he even learns to sit. In assessment, the difference between, for example, a cerebral palsied child and a mentally retarded child may show itself by the difference in the progress of development. The cerebral palsied child's development may be patchy, with particular milestones left out while others may have developed. On the other hand, the development of a mentally retarded child usually shows a generalised arrest. It is as if he has become fixed at this point and can go no further. He may learn how to pull himself to standing, but will not go on to cruise around the furniture and walk alone.

Head control is slow to develop, particularly in the hypotonic child. This may be partly due in some cases to the reluctance of his parents to handle the infant, and play with him. An unresponsive baby gives his parents little reward for their efforts at communicating with him, and he may as a consequence be relatively unstimulated. Similarly, an infant who cries little and does not demand attention may also suffer such unintentional neglect. It is often this infant, appearing to his parents as good, docile and such little trouble, who spends his day lying in supine, a position from which he is unlikely to achieve head control and which will accentuate his disinterest in his surroundings and his general apathy. If he is picked up only rarely, he will lack this stimulus to gaining head control also.

Balance is always slow to develop, particularly if the child is lying down all day, or is propped securely in sitting, a position from which he has no stimulus to regain or maintain his balance.

As with normal children, there seem to be important periods in the child's progress at which the impetus toward a particular stage of development is strong. If this opportunity is missed in the retarded child it will be very difficult to recreate, and the child may never achieve that stage at all. For example, if he is not stood on his feet at an early age he may develop an aversion to having his feet on the ground and will pull his legs up or refuse to stand.

The mentally retarded baby may show little interest in his surroundings and in learning about them. He does not explore, as he seems unable to provide the stimulus for himself to do so. Eye-hand control is slow to develop, especially in a child who is late in getting his hands to the midline. If he is in an institution he will lack the stimulation he may have received at home, and because many of these institutions are over-crowded and shortstaffed he may be left to his own devices all day with no opportunity for developing whatever his potential abilities might have been.

His ultimate level of achievement and the rate at which he reaches it will depend upon the severity of his retardation, although it can be influenced to some extent by developmental stimulation if this is begun early enough. His ultimate motor development seems to be influenced to a very large extent by the amount of help, stimulation and guidance he receives from birth onward. If the child is referred for treatment for the first time when he is already two years old, he may derive some benefit but it will be impossible to help him reach the potential he would have reached had treatment started when he was a few months old.

Some children who were originally apathetic and inactive become hyperkinetic later. These children are over-active, noisy and difficult to control, causing considerable distress to their parents. Their problems have been considered in Chapter 3.

MANAGEMENT

Mentally retarded infants and children who are also brain-damaged, with spasticity or athetosis for example, will demonstrate problems described in Chapter 1, as well as the problems described here. Their treatment will, broadly speaking, follow along the lines described in Chapter 1.

Below is a discussion of some points in management of the mentally retarded infant and child.

The infant requires assessment at all levels of function, motor development, oral function and feeding, sensori-motor integration, sight, hearing and intelligence. The assessment may be done by a physiotherapist along the lines described in Chapter 1.

In analysing the motor assessment, the physician and physiotherapist must take care not to confuse the infant whose developmental retardation is due to delayed maturation of the central nervous system, with the infant whose retardation is due to mental deficiency (Illingworth 1970). The infant with delayed maturation will eventually catch up with his peers, and may demonstrate no apparent physical or mental abnormality in later months, but the mentally retarded child will become more obviously backward as he grows older.

There is general acceptance now of the need for stimulation of sensori-motor development in Down's syndrome infants. Several studies indicate the benefits (Connolly & Russell 1976, Montgomery and Richter 1977, Wolpert *et al* 1978).

Without stimulation the mentally retarded infant demonstrates certain predictable delays, all of which have an effect upon his relationship with people, his ability to go from one place to another and his ability to develop his potential learning capacity, no matter at what level that may be. Where parents are willing and able to stimulate their infant, as in the author's opinion most of them are, it seems a pity that more infants are not sent to therapists within the first few weeks of birth.

Stimulation of development, enrichment of the environment, whatever it is called, is always the parents' prerogative and often their pleasure. The therapist's role therefore involves helping the parents understand their infant, his needs, which are different from the needs of their other children, and the ways of bringing out the best in him. Parents need to understand not only what has to be done but also what problems need to be anticipated and avoided. For example, an infant left to his own devices tends to develop the habit of backward leaning in standing. Hence he may get as far as standing but no further since to walk he will need to transfer his weight forward. Similarly, he may get to sitting, develop sufficient balance to sit with his legs wide apart, and not ever be able to move out of the position. This would involve sufficient balance to be able to rotate the trunk in order to get into prone or four point kneeling. If the infant has habitually sat wide-based he will never develop the necessary balance, and added to this will be a fear of change, a fear of losing his balance, which will make him hold his breath then cry if the therapist places his legs closer together thereby narrowing his base of support.

Treatment which stimulates more normal tone and increases stability will be needed by the hypotonic infant as well as facilitation of motor development in those areas where it is lacking or where future difficulties can be predicted. The child's lack of intelligence or his inability to co-operate has in many cases little influence on treatment which depends upon facilitating an automatic rather than a voluntary response to stimulation. Of course, if an older infant is very obstructive and resents handling, then treatment cannot be so effective. Certain areas of treatment, such as the improvement of hand control, are made difficult by the inability to concentrate and the easy distractibility of many of these children.

Importance of parents
The birth of a mentally retarded infant brings a sense of loss and grief to his parents. Many authors have discussed these effects and the stresses facing parents of a mentally retarded infant. It is likely that they will have a very negative view of the infant's

future capabilities and this will, unfortunately, have an effect upon their developing relationship with the infant and upon the infant's immediate environment. It is important that they realise the help they and the infant can receive from the therapist and can understand the need for stimulation of feeding and motor function, of play and learning. This point can be discussed with parents without giving them unrealistic hopes for the infant's future. Discussions with the parents of children with Down's syndrome, for example, are usually helpful in giving new parents insight into the pleasures and difficulties involved in rearing a Down's syndrome child.

The parents of the young infant embark upon what will form a series of programmes. The first, and this should ideally start in the neonatal period, involves handling the infant, talking to him, encouraging him to follow his parent's face with his eyes, to follow sounds such as a bell or rattle. The objective here is not only to stimulate the baby's awareness of his environment but also to develop a close relationship between parents and baby. Other mini programmes will help the parents stimulate motor development, especially in the areas of head control, extension in prone, balance, manipulation, oral control, play and cognitive functioning.

Parents need to see all these areas of development as depending upon one another. The importance of picking the infant up and playing with him, and particularly of talking to him, to the development of his head control, eye-hand control, balance and intelligence needs to be explained. They may not understand unless it is pointed out to them that the child will need stimulus to explore his environment, and to develop balance and the other milestones in development that a normal child will achieve with minimum help. It is for these reasons that it is in the best interests of the mildly handicapped child to remain within the family if this is possible. However, the parents must not be left alone to cope with their problems, but must have support and advice, particularly throughout the child's early life.

Feeding

The Down's syndrome infant usually has a thick, hypotonic tongue which tends to protrude slightly between his lips. This flabby tongue is probably the major reason for his difficulty sucking and swallowing, and if nothing is done, the infant eventually has difficulty with solids and does not develop the ability to chew. Perhaps because of their low expectations of the child and the lack of help they so often receive with feeding, the parents tend to keep the infant on the bottle and on sloppy food for much longer than normal (Carr 1979). Lateral vibration to the tongue, done vigorously with the finger, with downward pressure on the tongue (Mueller 1977, Carr 1979) is most effective and when combined with treatment to desensitise the oral area if it is hyper-sensitive and to stimulate lip and jaw closure, the process of feeding the infant becomes much simpler.

Vibration to the tongue appears not only to make the tongue more active, it also causes it to contract to a more normal size. Presumably the stimulation to the small muscles of which it is made up causes this improved shape and function.

The infant should start on solid food at the normal time and should gradually be introduced to food which needs chewing. A most effective way to stimulate chewing is to place a strip of undercooked meat between the infant's gums or teeth (Mueller 1977) which is followed by stimulation of lip and jaw closure. The infant can chew on this without it falling to pieces, and for his efforts is rewarded by the flavourful juices of the meat. Parents should introduce the infant to foods of different flavours and textures early so as to avoid the development of an aversive reaction to different foods. Finger feeding should also be introduced as soon as possible, both as an early step toward independence and to enable the child to gain pleasure from eating.

Importance of the prone position

The mentally retarded infant is better lying in prone or sitting in a chair rather than lying in supine during the day. These positions will stimulate the development of extension of the head and trunk and control of head position. Extension of the trunk in prone and raising of the head, which are often difficult to elicit in the young hypotonic infant, may be stimulated on a ball by a fine shaking up and down, the hands holding the hips, and thumbs pressing downward firmly on the buttocks. When he is a little older he may lie in prone over a wedge (figure 47), which will enable him to look around the room, and to play with his toys. If he must lie in supine, mobiles of different shapes and sizes and colours may be hung in front of him and within reach. Shapes made from tinfoil will catch the light and attract his gaze. He may be similarly amused while lying on his side, a safer position than prone for the hypotonic infant.

Hughes (1971) has suggested that head rolling, a fairly common occupation of mentally retarded infants and children, may be prevented from developing if the supine position is avoided. It is certainly better to avoid if possible the development of this repetitive movement, as it is very difficult to stop once started. The development of many of the perseverent, repetitious movements of these children can probably be avoided if the child is given more variety of postures and movements with which to occupy his time.

Once he has developed some ability to bear weight through his forearms or hands, he should be stimulated to transfer his weight laterally and reach out with the other hand (figure 52). Otherwise, once he has achieved this position, he will become 'stuck' there.

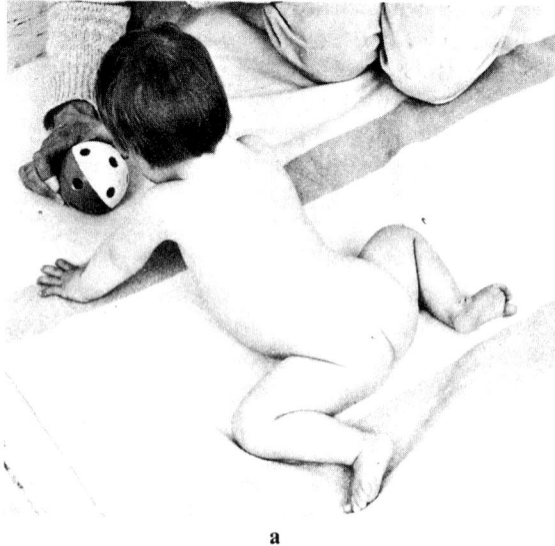

a

Fig. 52(a) This infant cannot get into four point kneeling, and cannot shift her weight laterally in order to reach out for a toy.

168

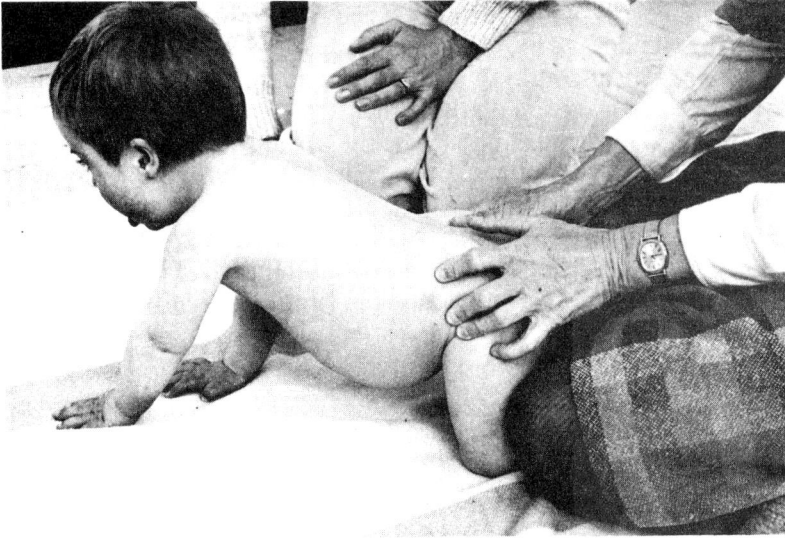

Fig. 52(b) Pressure is given downward through her hips and knees to give her the experience of four point kneeling.

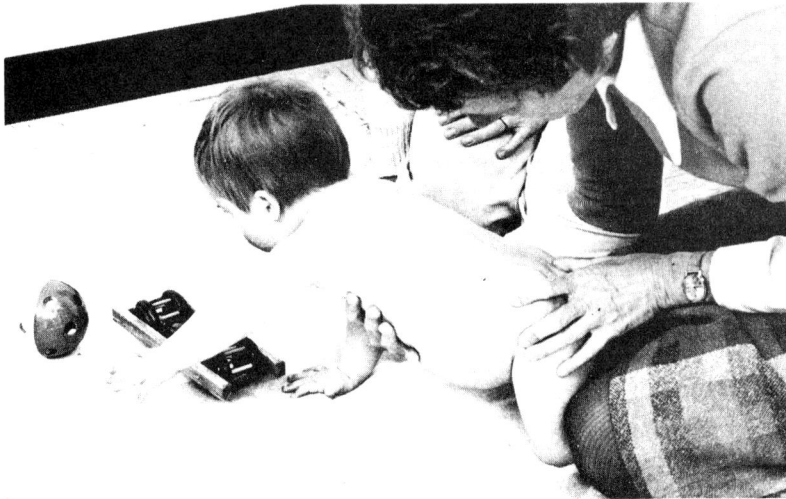

Fig. 52(c) The therapist shifts the infant's weight laterally and she is able to reach out with one hand.

169

The normal child, when he has reached the stage of bearing weight through extended arms, will usually descend on to one forearm while he practises reaching out, and the mentally retarded infant should be encouraged to do the same.

Figure 53 illustrates how quickly an infant can learn new movements if he is shown how. This 10 month old baby was photographed on the first day of a programme to stimulate his development. The speed with which success was achieved seems to indicate that external stimulation and guidance give the infant the chance to perform what his maturing brain is *already* capable of organising.

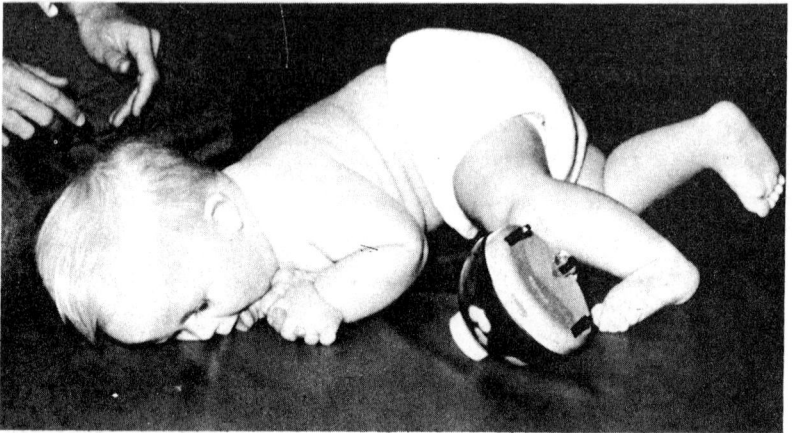

a

Fig. 53(a), (b), (c), (d) This infant was unable to lie in prone with weight through his hands. Extension of the head and trunk against gravity and weightbearing through the hands are stimulated. Within a few moments the infant is beginning to learn the components involved.

Importance of a variety of movements

Movement from one position to another is stimulated with the emphasis on gaining balance reactions throughout each movement and on gaining the ability to rotate about the body axis. Guidance ensures that body alignment is appropriate also throughout the movement.

The development of balance adjustments and of adequate

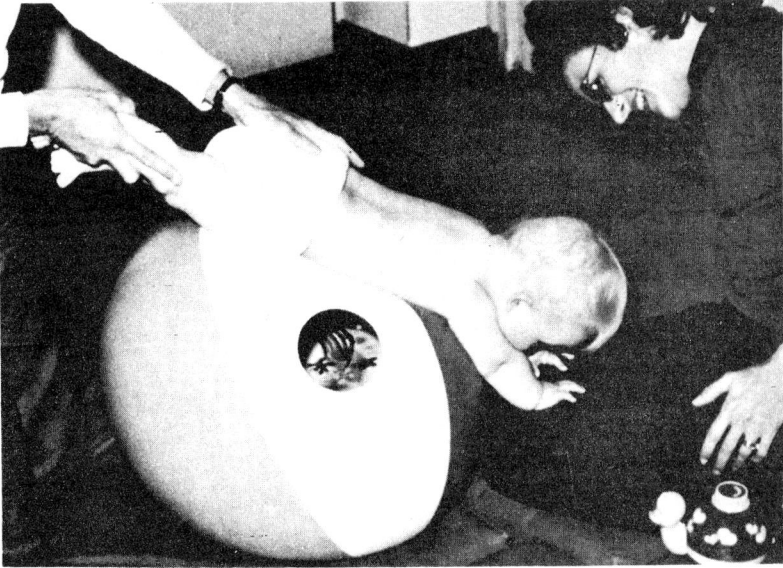

b

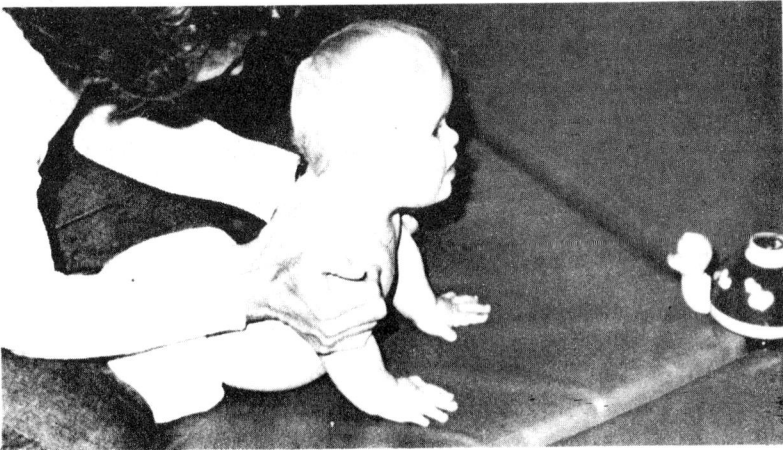

c

rotation within the body axis gives the child the ability to sit sideways from four point kneeling, pivot from side sitting to side sitting, stand up through half kneeling (figure 54) and eventually to walk. These movements can be facilitated from the head, shoulders, trunk or pelvis, the stimulus to move being applied by

171

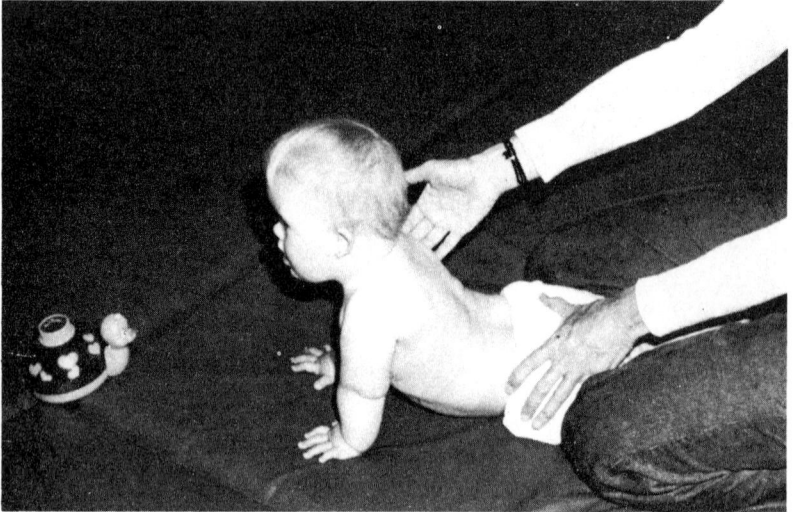

d

the physiotherapist at these points, the child responding automatically with the movement required. Care must be taken to avoid keeping the child in one position for too long. Although repetition is important for learning, the emphasis must be on a variety of movements. However, these movements must be important for function and not just movements for the sake of movement.

The infant needs early experience of standing. All parents stand their normal infants as soon as they can, so the infant very early in his life has experience of this upright posture long before he is able to balance in this position. The Down's syndrome infant is unlikely to be stood early because his hypotonia makes it very difficult for him to be held in this position. The development of antigravity extension, stimulated in prone, will gradually make this easier, but while his legs continue to give way beneath him, his parents will be reluctant to stand him. The provision of leggings made from canvas and firm light plastic struts (figure 55) will make it possible for the infant to be stood. One of the reasons for instituting a programme of early standing is to avoid the common tendency for the Down's syndrome infant to develop an aversion to standing. When this has occurred, the infant pulls his feet up

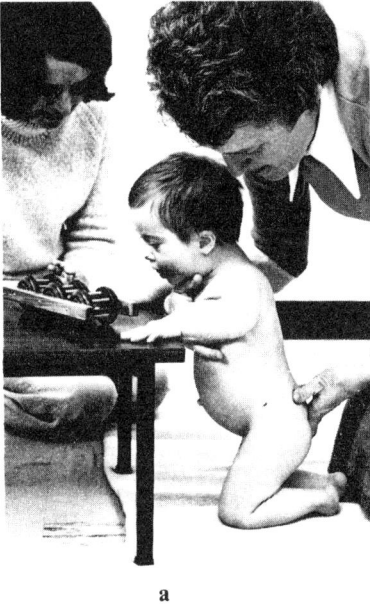

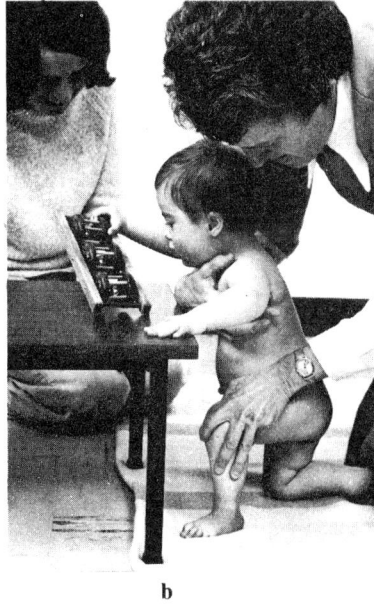

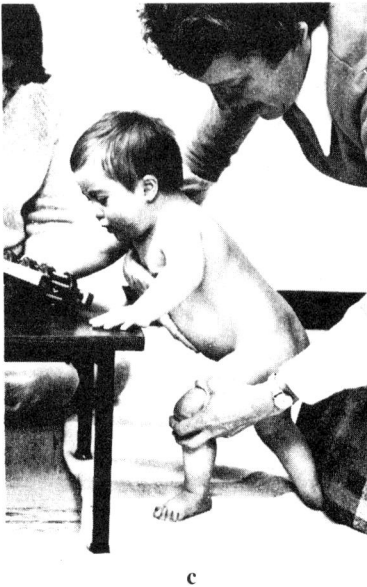

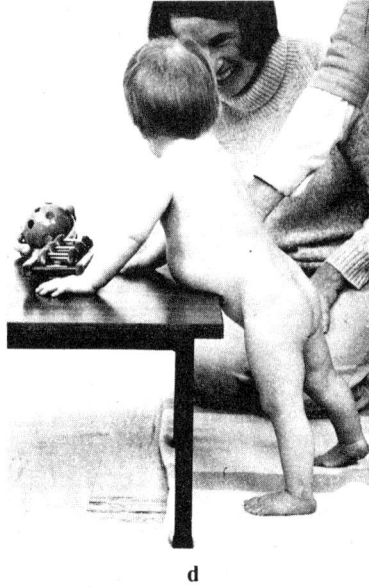

Fig. 54(a), (b), (c), (d) The infant is shown how to get from kneeling to standing. He is helped to practise the various movement components involved.

from the floor and will not allow the soles of his feet to be placed flat.

An aversion to having his feet on the floor is not the only negative response which the therapist should anticipate and avoid. Infants who are not accustomed early to taking weight through their hands seem to find difficulty in doing so, resent attempts to

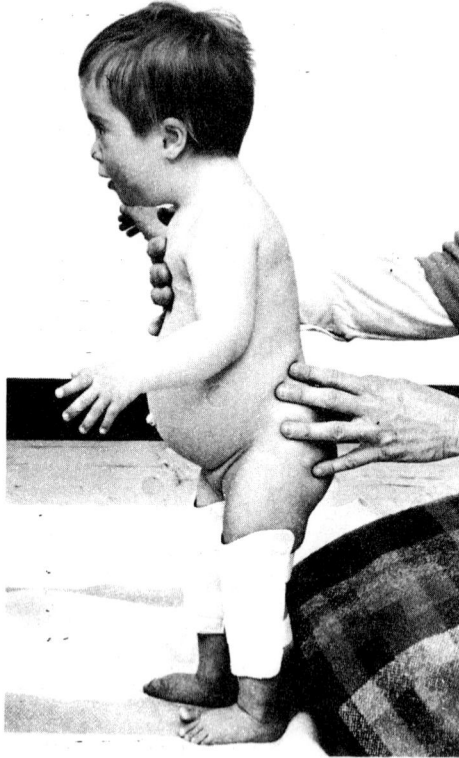

Fig. 55 The use of simple leggings makes it easier for this infant to remain in standing while his ability to shift weight laterally and to balance are stimulated.

gain this activity, and fall to sucking their fingers with renewed vigour. Perhaps this aversion stems from lack of opportunity — the untreated infant may never achieve enough extension in prone to weightbear through his hands, and if he is lifted into sitting and moved from one position to another by his parents he may never have the chance to develop this manual activity.

Once the infant has developed aversion responses, he must be gently desensitised. The use of various stimuli, starting from the most acceptable and working gradually toward the unacceptable is usually effective after a period of time. A mechanical vibrator placed on the arm or leg and gradually moved toward the dorsal then palmar or plantar surface of the hand or foot may also be effective as a desensitiser. The infant is encouraged to take weight as this becomes tolerated, and an enthusiastic response from his parents will reinforce his action.

As the child gets older activities are given which will increase endurance. Swimming instruction is important for safety as well as being a means of improving mobility. The child is taught how to float, encouraged to put his face in the water without inhaling, and how to move in the water. Two important points in teaching body control in water are the control of respiration which involves relaxation, plus the instinctive knowledge that movement of the head influences the position of the trunk and legs. That is, extension of the head in prone and flexion in supine cause the legs to sink to the bottom of the pool, while flexion of the head in prone and extension in supine cause the legs to float on the surface (Reid 1976).

Importance of stimulating balance

Balance is essential for effective movement. One of the major reasons for the infant's inability to move is poor balance development (Shepherd 1979). However, the problems of balance need to be analysed in detail. The important elements in regaining balance once it has been lost or almost lost is movement of the head and trunk and movement of the arms culminating in weight-bearing through the hands.

The infant tends to develop the ability to *maintain* a position, such as sitting, but only if he keeps a wide base of support and does not reach with his hands to that point where his balance is threatened (figure 56). At this point he may be assumed to have 'developed sitting balance'. However, he has not and this fact is illustrated by his inability to move out of the position (or into it), and his response when someone tries to narrow his base of support. At this point he may fall to one side with no lateral

175

movement of the head or trunk which indicates that he has no ability to regain his balance at all. The older child may sit on a chair with his legs wide apart. If they are placed together he will hold his breath, go red in the face, and tense his body, which are the manifestations of anxiety and fear which accompany very poor balance. In the author's experience these problems can be avoided, and the means are relatively simple. The infant should be given early experience of laterally oriented movement, with two objectives in mind, to accustom him to movement in this direc-

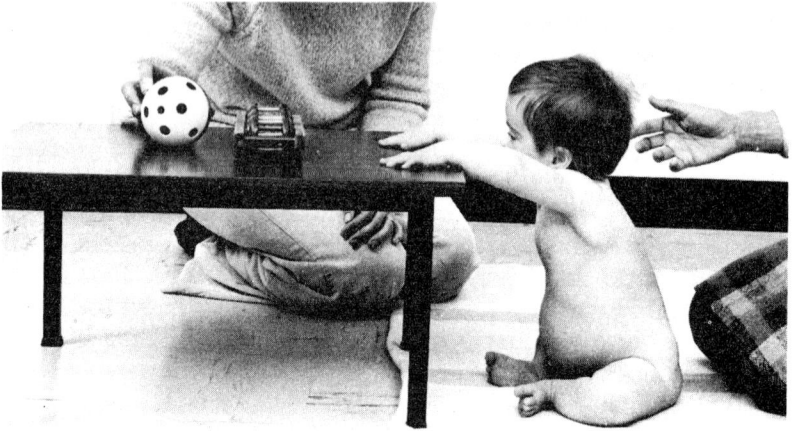

Fig. 56 This infant can maintain the sitting position but cannot move in or out of it as she has very little balance.

tion, and to stimulate the development of lateral movement of the head and trunk. This can be done in many different ways, for example, on a beach ball (figure 57) or on a parent's knee, in prone, supine, sitting, four point kneeling and standing. It is interesting that the usual development of the Down's syndrome baby and other mentally retarded babies seems to be concentrated in an antero-posterior direction with a tendency to avoid any lateral orientation. This is reinforced in many cases by continual experience of wide-based sitting and standing, and the antero-posterior orientation becomes habitual.

Importance of sensory and perceptual stimulation

Proprioceptive stimulation is given to encourage movement. Pressure may be applied to the sole of the foot or the palm of the hand to facilitate weight-bearing. Stimulation of a limb with a firm brush will stimulate movement in a particular direction. Tapping to the forehead in the direction of extension will stimulate head extension. Awareness of what constitutes a common object such as an orange will be stimulated if the child is helped to hold it in his hands, to feel its texture, and smell its strong perfume, and to compare it with some other object.

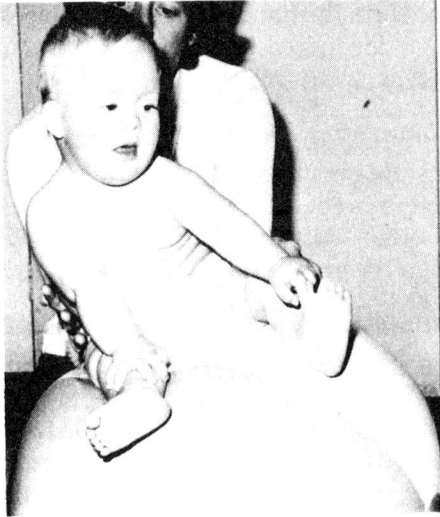

Fig. 57 Stimulation of lateral movement of the head and trunk, essential components of sitting balance.

Knowledge of parts of the body is an important part of training. The relationship of his body to objects in space is encouraged by activities that involve crawling under a table and through a tunnel, climbing over an obstacle, sitting on a chair. Eye control is usually slow to develop, and activities are designed to encourage control as the child moves about, although tracking with the eyes, both of animate (parent's face) and inanimate objects should have been stimulated since the first month after birth. The ability to distinguish between left and right is fully developed by seven years in the normal child, but the mentally retarded child will need considerable training in order to make this distinction.

Montgomery and Richter (1977) describe the effects of a

sensory integrative therapy programme on a group of mentally retarded children from age 5 to 12 years. They quote Ayres' (1973) hypothesis that improvement in sensori-motor integration will result in improvement in motor skills, academic achievement and language ability. The authors do not give details of their programme. However, in their study on the effects of vestibular stimulation on Down's syndrome children aged between 6 and 24 months, Kantner et al (1976) found that the stimulation resulted in improved motor performance which they suggested may reflect the acquisition of an increased level of central nervous system inhibitory control.

Importance of stimulating social development

When the child is old enough developmentally he may join a small group of children in order to play, and in this group he may learn to interact with other individuals, and may gain further stimulus to explore through the presence of these other personalities.

Importance of stimulating cognitive development

For the child to begin to learn even simple concepts, he must develop the ability to concentrate and to increase his attention span. Several programmes are being developed with the objective of improving the Down's syndrome infant's learning capacity.

Williams (1978) suggests that mentally retarded children are more handicapped by their overt behaviour than by their lack of development of internal concepts. He stresses that the child must be enabled to develop skills which will make him independent.

SUMMARY

Sensori-motor development is delayed in the mentally retarded child who tends to be hypotonic as an infant, lacking variety in movement, with little balance and a tendency to develop habitual responses which further hinder his progress. Sensori-motor development cannot be seen as separate from the development of social, emotional and cognitive functions.

Treatment must begin in early infancy in order to assist the infant to develop his potential, and to guide his parents in establishing a bond with the infant and in rearing him.

It requires patience and affection to treat these children, and also the conviction that something can be done to help them. It does seem certain that the mentally retarded infant will gain considerably from treatment designed to improve his motor function, and from parents trained to understand his needs.

References

Asmussen, E. and Heeboll-Neilsen, K. (1956) Physical performance and growth in children. Influence of sex, age and intelligence. *J. Appl. Physiol.* **8**, 4, 371.

Bobath, K. (1963) The prevention of mental retardation in patients with cerebral palsy. *Acta Paedopsychiat.* (Basel) **30**, 4, 141.

Carr. J. H. (1979) Oral function in infancy. *Aust. J. Physiother.* In press.

Connolly, B. and Russell, F. (1976) Interdisciplinary early intervention programme. *Phys. Ther.* **56**, 2, 155.

Cowie, V. A. (1970) *A Study of Early Development of Mongols.* London: Pergamon.

Dubowitz, V. (1965) Intellectual impairment in muscular dystrophy. *Arch. Dis. Child.* **40**.

Hughes, N. A. S. (1971) Developmental physiotherapy for mentally handicapped babies. *Physiotherapy*, **57**, 9, 399.

Illingworth, R. S. (1970) *The Development of the Infant and Young Child.* Edinburgh and London: Livingstone.

Kantner, R. M., Clark, D. L., Allen, L. C. and Chase, M. P. (1976) Effects of vestibular stimulation on nystagmus response and motor performance in the developmentally delayed infant. *Phys. Ther.* **56**, 4, 414.

Montgomery, P. and Richter, E. (1977) Effect of sensory integrative therapy on the neuromotor development of retarded children. *Phys. Ther.* **57**, 7, 799.

Mueller, H. (1977) Personal communication.

Reid, M. (1976) *Handling the Disabled Child in Water.* Assoc. of Paed. Chartered Physiotherapists, Birmingham.

Shepherd, R. B. (1979) Problem analysis with Down's syndrome children. *Aust. J. Physiother.* In press.

Tredgold, R. F. and Soddy, K. (1963) *Textbook of Mental Deficiency.* Baltimore: Williams and Wilkins.

Walton, J. (1971) *The Essentials of Neurology.* London: Pitman.

Williams, C. (1978) An introduction to behavioural principles in teaching the profoundly handicapped. *Child* **4**, 21.

Wolpert, R., Gouse-Sheese, J., Leuchter, S. L. and Sandmann, M. (1978) Stimulating developmentally delayed infants: evaluation of a short term project. *Physiother. Canada* **30**, 2, 78.

Further Reading

Bray, P. F. (1969) *Neurology in Paediatrics.* Chicago: Year Book Medical Publishers.

Brinkworth, R. and Collins, J. E. (1969) *Improving Mongol Babies.* London: National Society for Mentally Handicapped Children.

Clarke, A. M. and Clarke, A. D. B. (1974) *Mental Deficiency. The Changing Outlook.* London: Methuen.

Holmes, L. B., Moser, H. W., Halldorsson, S., Mack, C., Pant, S. S. and Matzilevich, B. (1972) *Mental Retardation. An Atlas of Diseases with Associated Physical Abnormalities.* New York: MacMillan.

Holt, K. S. (1958) The home care of severely retarded children. *Pediatrics*, **22**, 744.

Illingworth, R. S. (1961) Delayed maturation in development. *J. Pediat.* **58**, 761.

Illingworth, R. S. (1962) Some points about the guidance of parents of mentally subnormal children. *J. Ment. Subnormality*, **8**, 2.

Kiernan, C. C. (1974) Behaviour modification. In *Mental Deficiency. The Changing Outlook*, edited by A. M. and A. D. B. Clarke. London: Methuen.

La Frenais, M. (1971) *Language Stimulus with Retarded Children.* London: National Society for Mentally Handicapped Children.

Lawrence, K. M. and Weeks, M. R. (1963) Abnormalities of the central nervous system. In *Congenital Abnormalities in Infancy.* Oxford and Edinburgh: Blackwell.

Levy, J. (1973) *The Baby Exercise Book.* New York: Pantheon.

National Society for Mentally Handicapped Children (1967) *Stress in Families with a Mentally Handicapped Child. Report of a Working Party.* London: N.S.M.H.C.

Neumann-Neurode, D. (1967) *Baby Gymnastics*. London and Oxford: Pergamon.

Robinson, C. M., Harrison, J. and Gridley, J. (1970) *Physical Activity in the Education of Slow-Learning Children*. London: Arnold.

Robinson, H. B. and Robinson, N. M. (1965) *The Mentally Retarded Child. A Psychological Approach*. New York: McGraw-Hill.

Chapter 5

Infections of the Brain, Spinal Cord and Peripheral Nerves

ENCEPHALITIS, ENCEPHALOMYELITIS AND MENINGITIS

Inflammation of the central nervous system may result from many causative factors, and the clinical features will depend upon the severity of the infection and the specific area of the nervous system involved. The majority of infants and children who suffer from encephalitis, encephalomyelitis and meningitis recover without any apparent sequelae, but some are left with permanent evidence of neurological damage — mental retardation, behavioural abnormalities, speech disturbances, epilepsy and motor disability.

Neurological syndromes may complicate certain common childhood illnesses such as mumps, measles, chickenpox or pertussis, or may be the result of vaccination. Infants may be born with the evidence of congenital rubella encephalopathy due to maternal rubella, and will demonstrate cardiac defects, mental retardation, cataracts, deafness and skeletal deformities. Bacterial meningitis may be caused by *Haemophilus influenza*, *Escherichia Coli*, *meningococcus* or *pneumococcus*. The young infant may be particularly susceptible to bacterial meningeal infection during the period between his passively gained immunity and the development of active immunity. An encephalopathy may be caused by lead intoxication in children who chew on toys or furniture coated with paint containing lead. It is the accumulation of lead which causes damage to the brain and peripheral nerves as well as to other organs.

The neurological complications of encephalopathy are due to subdural effusion, hydrocephalus, brain abscess, to necrosis, or to haemorrhage, and the eventual clinical picture depends upon the area of the nervous system involved. There may be elements of ataxia, athetosis or spasticity in either a hemiplegic or a quadriplegic distribution. The signs evident during the acute stage include pyrexia, headache, vomiting, coma and convulsions, opisthotonus and irritability, and the cry may be high-pitched.

Management of these children in the early stages is supportive. Treatment of the unconscious child is described briefly in Section V, Chapter 4.

Physical therapy in the stage of recovery is directed towards the particular problems demonstrated by each child, and will be as described in Chapter 1 of this Section.

Viral encephalomyelitis may be caused by the poliomyelitis virus, and Guillain-Barré's syndrome is an encephalomyelitis of unknown origin. Management of children suffering from these diseases and their aftermath are described below.

ANTERIOR POLIOMYELITIS

This is an infectious disease caused principally by one of three strains of virus, the primary lesion of which is in the alimentary tract, and perhaps the nasopharynx. The infection is believed to be contracted through the ingestion of contaminated water and food. The virus travels via the circulatory system to the central nervous system, causing meningitic symptoms, and in a small percentage of cases, destroying the motor cells of the anterior horn of the spinal cord and brain stem causing a flaccid lower motor neurone type of paralysis. Physical effort or localised trauma during the period prior to the onset of paralysis apparently predisposes those particular cells to destruction (Sharrard 1971, Walton 1971). If the muscles of respiration are paralysed and if adequate ventilation cannot be maintained, or respiratory tract infection cannot be prevented or controlled, death will ensue.

The effects of the viral invasion can be prevented by oral vaccination, and consequently the disease is no longer common in countries in which large-scale inoculation programmes are practised. However, the disease still occurs in epidemic form in many underdeveloped countries, and in other countries is always likely to re-occur where parents may become careless about having their children inoculated.

Pathology

The neuronal lesions occur primarily in the anterior horn cells of the spinal cord. However, they may also occur in the motor cells of the medullary and pontine reticular formation, and in the cranial nerve cells of the medulla.

The cells are either destroyed, in which case no recovery of function will occur, or temporarily disabled. This disability is due either to inflammatory oedema occurring around the cells or to relatively minor damage being done to the cells. There is an inflammatory reaction in the region of the cells involved and the axons of these cells demonstrate Wallerian degeneration throughout the entire length of the nerve fibre. Cells concerned with the innervation of the abdominal organs including the bladder may be affected where there are areas of severe destruction. As a result of the inflammatory reaction and the destruction of the cells, the cerebrospinal fluid, when tested, shows an increase in cells which returns to normal 10 to 14 days after onset of the disease, as well as an increase in protein. The virus can be isolated in the stools and the child is said to be infectious while this situation continues.

Clinical features

These may be described as occurring in three stages. In the *preparalytic stage* the features are those of a febrile illness, with fever, malaise, vomiting, and, if there is meningeal involvement, pain in the neck, trunk and limbs. Symptoms may mimic a mild attack of influenza.

In a small percentage of those affected the disease progresses to a *paralytic stage* in which there is gradually developing weakness and paralysis with muscle tenderness. Reflexes are absent or diminished. The nerve cell involvement is haphazard in distribution and may cause paralysis of single muscles or almost total paralysis of trunk and limb muscles and the muscles of swallowing. Certain muscles have been found to be more susceptible to paralysis than others. Sharrard (1957) lists the following: tibialis anterior, tibialis posterior, the long toe flexors and extensors, the peronei, the calf muscles, and in the upper limbs, the intrinsic muscles of the hand, the deltoid and tricep brachii.

The degree of muscle weakness depends on the percentage of nerve cells destroyed. Sharrard (1955) states that more than 60 per cent of motor cells supplying a muscle have to be destroyed before weakness becomes clinically detectable.

Respiratory problems may arise in the presence of one or more factors. Paralysis of the diaphragm due to involvement of the phrenic nerve, paralysis of the intercostal muscles, paralysis of the abdominal muscles resulting in poor expiratory power and the resultant difficulty in clearing airways, or involvement of cranial nerves resulting in paralysis or weakness of the muscles of swallowing and the danger of aspiration of saliva, food, fluid or vomitus.

Pain and tenderness cause protective muscle spasm, and the child will resent handling while the disease is acute and will lie with the part protectively flexed. Apart from the pain and tenderness there are no other sensory changes. The child will be irritable and restless while the disease is in the acute stage.

The *stage of recovery* begins when the acute symptoms subside, leaving the child with weakness and paralysis of movement. The main period of recovery is in the few weeks following the acute phase of the disease, and this recovery is probably due to the resolution of inflammatory oedema which compresses but does not necessarily destroy the nerve cells. Further improvement takes place in the next twelve months. Damaged cells will not regenerate so the residual paralysis will be permanent. This further recovery will therefore be the result of treatment to hypertrophy those muscle fibres still normally innervated and to teach the child the use of trick movements.

Management

Preparalytic stage

During this stage the child must have complete bed rest, and he will be nursed in isolation as he is infectious. Analgesics may be prescribed to relieve pain.

Paralytic stage

This regime is continued during the active paralytic stage, and the child is disturbed as little as possible. Handling will increase his discomfort, and his muscles are often tender to touch. Management here consists largely of measures of prevention.

His respiratory condition must be assessed at frequent intervals day and night in case paralysis of the respiratory muscles or of the muscles of swallowing should suddenly develop. Should paralysis of the swallowing muscles occur the child may aspirate food or mucus and develop serious respiratory difficulty. He is therefore nursed from side to side or in prone with the foot of the bed elevated in order to minimise the risk of aspiration.

If paralysis or severe weakness of the respiratory muscles occurs the child may be nursed in a tank respirator which exerts a negative pressure upon the thorax. As air is pumped into the tank in which the child lies, the lungs deflate and air is expelled. As the air is removed from the tank, the lungs expand under the influence of the negative atmospheric pressure within the tank and air is drawn into the lungs. The advantage of this method of ventilation over intermittent positive pressure ventilation lies in the relative freedom from infection compared to the risk of infection present in positive pressure ventilation unless it is administered under scrupulously sterile conditions. The child is easily nursed in the tank respirator and can be given passive movements and warm packs through the portholes.

However, if the child also has paralysis of the swallowing muscles there is a definite risk of aspiration of mucus and food during the negative pressure phase of the cycle, as the negative pressure exerted by the machine will suck mucus and food from the oral cavity into the lungs. For this reason the child will be tracheostomized and ventilated on an intermittent positive pressure machine with a humidifier attached. Physical therapy for this child is briefly described in Section V, Chapter 4.

Where paralysis results in unopposed muscle action, and where it allows part of a limb to lose its ability to withstand the force of gravity, contractures will occur if steps are not taken to prevent this from the earliest possible moment. If positioning of the child is poor, it is the flexor groups which are most likely to become contracted in the limbs. A pillow placed under the knees will allow hip and knee flexor contractures to occur if the child cannot move his legs. A soft mattress may have a similar effect. Pain and protective muscle spasm may also result in flexion contractures, and the child should be nursed on a firm mattress, with a bed

186

cradle to prevent the bedclothes from pressing the feet into plantarflexion. If there is a need to prevent the knees from resting in a hyperextended position which is important if hamstring paralysis is present, it is better to apply a posterior plaster splint with the knee in 2 or 3 degrees of flexion, than run the risk of hip and knee flexor contractures by placing a pillow under the knee. Warm packs will effectively relieve pain and spasm in most cases, and will make it easier for the child to tolerate passive movements in the maximum painfree range. The child may also gain relief by lying on a ripple mattress.

Passive movements are done gently but in the fullest possible painfree range, and with as little handling of the tender muscle bellies as possible. To avoid distressing the child these may be done at intervals during the day for short periods only. Passive movements, provided they are frequently and effectively done, are probably more effective than splinting for the prevention of contractures in these early stages, as splinting may cause pain and further spasm. However, it is necessary to apply a posterior plaster splint to the lower limb to prevent contractures of the triceps surae and the long toe flexors. Similarly, for the forearm and hand, a plaster cock-up splint will help prevent contracture of the wrist and finger flexors. A long sandbag placed down the lateral side of the leg will prevent contracture of the hip external rotators while the child is lying in supine. Where splints are used they should not become substitutes for full-range passive movements done several times a day which are the most effective method of preserving the length of the soft tissues in this early stage.

Stage of Recovery

This stage usually begins some 3 weeks after the onset of the disease. While the disease is active the child is encouraged to lie as quietly as possible, since there is some evidence that activity increases the possibility of damage within the central nervous system. However, once the active stage is over, and this is signalled by a loss of the clinical features associated with the viral illness, the child may begin gentle active exercise.

If he has bulbar involvement or paralysis of the respiratory muscles, his recovery will depend very largely on the recovery of respiratory function. Artificial ventilation will continue until the muscular function is sufficiently improved. The child will gradually be weaned from the respirator, spending increasingly longer periods of time without it. He may progress to the stage where he can spend all day out of the respirator, going back into it at night, or he may be able to do without its assistance completely. An older child may be able to use glosso-pharyngeal breathing in order to spend periods of the day independent of the respirator. At this stage his physical treatment may be done during the periods when he is out of the respirator with the physiotherapist keeping a check on his respiratory rate. This child is always at risk of developing a respiratory tract infection and this should be prevented if possible and treated if it occurs by antibiotics and postural drainage.

Assessment

As soon as possible the extent of the child's disability must be assessed. A thorough assessment will not be done until the active stage is over, in order to avoid disturbing him and increasing the possibility of paralysis. A complete muscle chart is done in order to establish the range and extent of weakness and paralysis. The methods of testing the individual muscles are described by Kendall and Kendall (1949).

Unfortunately this method of assessment is very subjective although this effect can be minimized if the same therapist does subsequent reassessments. It does not give an accurate picture of, for example, spinal muscle involvement, as the small muscles of the spine cannot be charted. The chart may also be inaccurate because of the difficulty the therapist, particularly if she is inexperienced, has in discriminating between a trick movement which is effective and a movement in which the normal co-ordination of muscles is present.

The grade of a particular muscle will also depend on the degree of weakness of the muscles with a synergic or fixator action when the child performs a movement or holds a joint steady against resistance, as well as on the experience and skill of the therapist in assessing the relative strength of muscles. For example, if the hip abductors, adductors and rotators, and the abdominal muscles are weak, the hip flexors will appear weak because of the poor movement which results, even though these muscles may actually be grade 5 in strength. No group of muscles can perform a movement without the aid of normal synergist and fixator muscles, therefore in the absence of normal function in these groups it is very difficult to assess the real strength of the prime mover, and the therapist is really assessing the strength of the movement rather than of the muscle.

Despite the difficulties and inaccuracies it is hard to think of a more suitable physical method of establishing either the extent of paralysis or improvement in strength of muscles, and there are certain positive features of muscle charting to keep in mind. It enables the therapist to estimate potential deformities which may arise as a result of muscle imbalance, and to take steps to prevent these by suitable splinting and exercise.

An infant or small child too young to obey instructions can be tested relatively accurately although the procedure is more difficult and time-consuming. The testing involves watching for spontaneous movement and eliciting reactions to stimulation where possible. The therapist may stimulate reflex movements in the infant. Flexion of the toes, for example, may be tested by stimulating the tonic reaction of the toe flexors.

The usefulness of muscle charting may be explained by a look at the mechanism of nerve cell recovery. Singer and Rose-Innes (1963) have suggested that recovery occurs in some anterior horn cells during the stage of recovery in two ways. Those cells which have suffered a neurapraxia, probably due to inflammatory oedema, but which have suffered no actual histological change, will recover quickly. Those which have undergone some histological changes which stop short of complete chromotolysis will return to normal within a few months. The function of charting individual muscles does therefore given an indication of the rate of improvement in nerve cells, as well as an indication of the degree of hypertrophy of those muscle fibres which are still innervated. Once the chart shows improvement to be at a relative standstill, it may be of more use to change the form of assessment from this type of chart to one which gives a clearer picture of the child's function. This will serve as a guide for further management, for splinting, surgery or self-help apparatus.

Muscle length is tested during treatment, and does not require to be tested by special passive movements which waste time which would be more profitably spent in active exercise. It can instead be tested during active exercise, when any discrepancy in length should be obvious to an observant therapist.

Where there is respiratory involvement, function is tested regularly by the use of a machine which measures vital capacity and forced expiratory volume (Section V Chapter 4).

Physical treatment

As soon as the acute stage has passed, active movements are started within the limits of the child's comfort. Exercises must be begun gently and for the first few weeks any resistance given to a movement should be minimal to avoid strain to the soft tissues, and should progress slowly to maximal effort.

Exercises are given to encourage both specific movements, that is, those movements performed by using the weak muscle as prime mover, as synergist or as fixator, and general activities in which the weak muscle is encouraged to work in conjunction with other muscles in performing a function. For example, if the quadriceps femoris is weak, it will be strengthened specifically by exercises involving knee extension, and generally by resisted walking and other activities in which the muscle contracts as part of the particular synergy for performing a function.

Some techniques for the re-education of muscles are described below, demonstrating the methods used at various stages of the muscle's recovery. When a muscle appears paralysed, various methods may be employed to elicit a minimum contraction, if this is a possibility. For example, if tibialis anterior is charted as grade 1, a contraction may be elicited in whichever muscle fibres are still innervated in one of the following ways:

Sitting up from supine with the feet held.
Manual stimulation (by tapping, for example) to the belly of the muscle plus pressure on the dorsum of the foot while the child attempts to dorsiflex his foot.
Sitting on a stool with the feet on the floor, manual stimulation under the toes will facilitate contraction of the dorsiflexor muscles and toe extensors.
Supine lying with the plantar surface of the heel in the therapist's hand, pushing the heel down into the hand as though to elongate the leg.
Supine lying, resisting hip and knee flexion with resistance given at the thigh, and the other hand at the dorsum of the foot.

Standing, the child is pushed gently backwards and to each side in order to make him begin to lose his balance. Any technique which causes the child to try to regain his balance will elicit a contraction from tibialis anterior if there are any fibres capable of contracting.

As can be seen, due to recruitment of impulses, a weak muscle will be stimulated to contract if maximum resistance is given to another group in the same synergy.

When the muscle recovers to the stage where it is able to perform a movement, and as it becomes progressively stronger, so it is re-educated progressively by a variety of techniques, their variety being limited only by the physiotherapist's imagination. Some techniques will be more effective with a particular child than others, and it is as well to have the choice of a number of techniques in order to use those which are the most effective. Some of those mentioned below depend on the child's ability to co-operate with simple commands, some do not.

Assistance to a movement is gained by using the buoyancy of the water, manually, or by using springs and pulleys. Resistance to a movement can be applied by water, slings, springs, weights, pulleys with weights, and manual resistance using techniques such as repeated contractions and slow reversals (Appendix 5). The muscle is made to contract both isometrically and isotonically. The use of a short sharp stretch to the muscle's stretch receptors may help stimulate a contraction.

Whatever techniques are used, it is important to wait for a response, to give the child a chance to react. A muscle may respond in one part of a range, an inner range for example, but not in another. In many of the techniques mentioned above an attempt is being made to facilitate the muscle to contract at an automatic level. One of the most important functions of a muscle is its ability to contract automatically in response to a demand placed upon it, and this can be seen, for example, in tibialis anterior, which, in conjunction with other muscles in the limbs and trunk, works automatically to preserve balance in most activities. Thus, when a muscle is being re-educated, it should be exercised not only at a voluntary level but also at an automatic level.

Muscles are not only re-educated by specific exercises directed mainly at the particular muscle group involved, but also by more general activities involving the maintenance and regaining of balance, and the movement of the whole body. With children, these activities may consist of games, but there is little to be gained if the child is allowed to play haphazardly. Games are structured to facilitate the best response from the muscles to be re-educated. For example, a child with weak elbow extensors will use these muscles when he plays pat-ball with a balloon, and later with a light rubber ball. He can be encouraged to extend his elbow in different parts of its range if the ball is returned to him at different heights. Walking while pushing a weighted pram will strengthen weak hip extensors. Trunk and head extensors will be strengthened if he tries to wriggle on his tummy through a cardboard tunnel.

Not only strength must be re-educated but also endurance and agility. Responding to the vagaries of a balance board while standing or kneeling on it will re-educate the muscles in the lower limbs by making them adjust quickly to the changes in direction. Increasing the number of times he stands up on a stool will increase the endurance of the knee and hip extensors. Throwing and catching a ball while lying in prone with a pillow under his chest will increase the endurance of his trunk and head extensors, if the time spent in this activity is increased each day. Riding a prone scooter (figure 88) will have a similar effect.

If a child is too young to co-operate or obey simple instructions, his movements are re-educated by stimulation of automatic reactions, by placing him in such a position that he must react in a certain way, and by activities suitable for his developmental age.

The child may be treated in a warm pool. If he is nervous when he is first allowed out of bed he may find it easier to move about in a pool than on dry land. If his disability is severe he will be encouraged when he finds he can move in the water with so little effort. The exercises he does in the water can again be divided into those which are specifically for the muscles involved, and those which are more general, in which the muscles work in conjunction with others in performing activities. The water is used both for assistance, in which case it is buoyancy which gives assistance, and for resistance, when it is the weight of the water which resists. Walking is practised, first in deeper water using its buoyancy to hold him upright. The water offers some resistance as he walks, and the faster he walks the more the resistance increases. Further resistance may be added manually by the physiotherapist, the buoyancy of the water keeping the child steady. Respiratory function is improved by techniques which encourage him to breathe deeply, hold his breath and breathe out effectively. The physiotherapist will think of many activities herself, but blowing a sailing boat across the surface of the pool, swimming with the face in the water, picking up toys from the bottom of the pool are all useful activities as well as being good fun (Reid 1976). The water temperature should be neither too warm, which will be enervating, nor too cold, which will inhibit muscle action. The best temperature is between 32°C. and 34°C. The child should not remain in the pool too long as he will be easily tired.

Once the child is discharged to his home his parents will take over as much of his treatment as possible, returning with him at regular intervals to be taught how to progress his exercises and activities. The parents are taught how to care for his limbs. A flail limb has poor circulation and this will inhibit growth if the child is young. The limb will also be subject to trophic changes, including osteoporosis, with the danger of fracture on minimal strain. Skin ulceration will occur if the skin is not carefully protected, and these lesions are slow to heal. In cold weather chilblains are common. Indeed paralysed limbs are colder than normal throughout the year, and the child should be kept as warm as possible in winter, wearing woollen socks or stockings, and gloves.

Splinting

Splinting is designed for the child as soon as it is found to be necessary. In the early stages this applies particularly to the lower limbs and trunk. The child will not be allowed to stand or walk unsplinted if he has instability in the lower limbs or weakness of the trunk muscles which may lead to a paralytic scoliosis if he is allowed to remain upright without support. The instability which results from weakness or paralysis of muscles surrounding the joint will result in trauma to the surrounding soft tissues and eventually to permanent deformity if he is allowed to bear weight without adequate support.

If weakness of the abdominal muscles is present a corset or abdominal binder is worn. If weakness of the spinal musculature is present a brace such as Thomas' posterior spinal support,

Taylor's brace, or Milwaukee brace may be necessary, the latter brace being particularly necessary in the prevention and treatment of structural scoliosis.

Splinting for the limbs is similarly designed according to the distribution of the paralysis, to prevent the deforming effects of muscle imbalance and gravity, to give stability, to allow activity where paralysis or weakness prevent it, and to prevent strain being thrown on other parts of the body.

Paralysis of the quadriceps makes it impossible for the child to take weight on that leg without fully extending the knee which will result in a genu recurvatum deformity. Paralysis of the hamstrings will also result in this deformity because of the lack of posterior support for the knee. A long leg caliper with a posterior knee piece as well as a knee pad will give stability in either case. If the muscles remain paralysed, a knee locking mechanism is added to the caliper to allow knee flexion when the child sits down.

Paralysis of the anterior tibial muscles prevents a heel-toe gait and causes the child to step high with that leg to prevent the toes from dragging on the ground. A drop-foot stop or similar apparatus attached to a double below-knee iron will allow the child to put his heel to the ground. Paralysis of the tibialis anterior will allow the foot to roll into pronation on weightbearing, and this may be prevented from becoming excessive by an inside T-strap attached to a short single or double below-knee iron.

Paralysis of the hip extensors will cause the child to jack-knife forwards from the hips, and he will need to wear a pelvic band hinged to one or both calipers (figure 96). Eventually he will develop trick movements if there is no recovery in his hip extensors, and these will allow him to walk and stand without a pelvic band, by thrusting his pelvis forwards, gaining stability for his hips anteriorly.

Upper limb splints are designed to allow maximum hand function by holding the wrist extended or the thumb abducted to allow better grasp. It should be remembered that these splints will be useless and soon discarded if they do not give the child improved hand function. It will be of more use to the patient to develop trick movements if these prove more effective for function.

The problem of deciding which is the most suitable splinting for the child is difficult. It is necessary to prevent deformity from developing if possible, but splinting to fulfil this aim may conflict with the aim of allowing the child to function with maximum effectiveness.

The progressive deformities following as a result of paralysis may be formidable. Their full extent in children is only seen several years after the illness. They result probably from several factors, one of the most important being the effect of growth. The child continues to grow, but a flail limb, or a limb severely affected by muscle paralysis, does not grow at the same rate as the normal one, and by the time the child's growth is completed the flail limb will be shorter, sometimes by several centimetres, than the other. Another factor in the progression of deformity is the increasing mechanical advantage of stronger muscles over their paralysed or weakened antagonists. These weakened antagonists may eventually be unable to contract at all, so great may the disadvantage become. This will occur because of the gradual lengthening of the paralysed muscles and their adjacent soft tissues as the pull of gravity and the abnormal posture of the joint gradually force the part further into the deformed position. One 12 year old boy known to the author, severely paralysed since the age of 18 months, demonstrates the effect of walking for several years in a long caliper with the hip held in full external rotation. The soft tissues on the medial side of the knee have gradually stretched and bone growth has been influenced by the effect of the boy's weight being borne laterally at the knee. This has resulted in a gross genu valgum deformity which the caliper has been unable to prevent. However, it was only by maintaining this position that the boy had taught himself to walk.

Exercises and splints cannot hope to prevent the development of such deformities against these mechanical factors. It may be possible to slow their development by treatment and splinting designed to minimize the effects of gravity and posture, and splinting is continued for as long as recovery is occurring in the hope that the limbs and trunk will be kept in as normal and symmetrical a position as possible. Once improvement has ceased, the orthopaedic surgeon will consider what reconstructive or stabilizing surgery may be necessary either to gain more effective function or to prevent future deformities. Where the child's bone growth is still immature, splinting will be continued until he is old enough for surgery, and beyond that if it helps him to be functionally independent. The severely disabled child, when old enough to decide for himself, may prefer to use a wheelchair rather than endure the effort of being ambulant in splints.

The surgical procedures used for these children are described in detail by Sharrard (1971).

PERIPHERAL NEUROPATHY

Peripheral neuropathy may arise from one of many different causative factors. The cause may be infectious (e.g. herpes zoster), toxic (e.g. post-immunization, heavy metal poisoning), traumatic, metabolic (e.g. diabetes, vitamin B1 deficiency), vascular (e.g. dermatomyositis, lupus erythematosus), or neoplastic (e.g. leukaemia, neurofibromatosis). It may also be idiopathic as in Guillain-Barré syndrome.

Symptoms are muscle weakness and sensory impairment, and depend upon whether the site of involvement is the anterior or posterior nerve root or a mixed peripheral nerve.

Guillain-Barré Syndrome

Guillain-Barré syndrome is a polyneuropathy of unknown origin, although it has been suggested that the cause may indicate a hypersensitivity phenomenon, as it frequently follows an acute infection.

In diagnosis it must be distinguished from poliomyelitis which it closely resembles symptomatically. A feverish illness with vomiting and pyrexia precedes the sudden development of paralysis. However, the polyneuritis is symmetrical in distribution and usually affects all the muscles in a limb, often spreading gradually from lower limbs to upper, and there is usually sensory involvement, the child complaining of pain, numbness and paraesthesia, and suffering loss of position sense. The peripheral nerves with their roots are involved and in some cases the cranial nerves, particularly the facial nerve (Markland and Riley 1967). There is muscle tenderness, absence or diminution of tendon reflexes and a varying degree of weakness or paralysis of muscle. The disease tends to resolve slowly, most children making a good recovery, but some suffering remissions and exacerbations of symptoms. A few, due to paralysis of respiratory muscles and uncontrolled respiratory infection, may die.

Pathology

Changes found in peripheral nerves and their roots include myelin and axis cylinder degeneration. Eventually in most cases regeneration of the nerve structure occurs, but recovery is seldom complete.

Management

Treatment is symptomatic. There is no specific drug therapy. Physical treatment is as described for poliomyelitis. However, due to the involvement of the sensory fibres of the peripheral nerves and the anaesthesia which may result, appropriate care must be taken to avoid damage to the skin from pressure of bedclothes and ill-fitting splints.

TRANSVERSE MYELITIS

Transverse myelitis is the term given to an inflammation involving several spinal cord segments. The inflammation may progress upward (ascending myelitis) or remain stationary. Transverse myelitis may be associated with childhood viral diseases such as mumps and rubella or with certain vaccinations.

Clinical manifestations depend upon the part of the cord involved. For example, anterior horn cell damage causes flaccidity. Involvement of sensory pathways results in sensory loss up to the level of the cord lesion. Involvement of autonomic pathways causes autonomic dysfunction such as lack of sweating. Flaccidity will give way to hyperreflexia if central control over intact anterior horn cells is interrupted. Prognosis is usually poor in terms of full recovery of function.

Physical treatment depends upon the problems with which the child presents. Emphasis must be on stimulating growth and development, which requires that soft tissue contractures must be prevented, mobility must be ensured and social and educational isolation avoided.

SUMMARY

The main infections of the brain, spinal cord and peripheral nerves seen in children are described, with anterior poliomyelitis and Guillain-Barré syndrome described in detail. Physical treatment is symptomatic and preventive, aiming at maintaining the child in a condition which will allow maximum recovery of function to occur, by maintaining efficient ventilation, and by preventing soft tissue contractions, and at encouraging weakened muscles to develop their maximum strength, endurance and co-ordination. The management of the residual paralysis is the province of the orthopaedic surgeon and those skilled in designing apparatus for self-help.

References

Kendall, H. O. and Kendall, F. M. P. (1949) *Muscles-Testing and Function.* Baltimore: Williams and Wilkins.

Markland, L. D. and Riley, H. D. (1967) The Guillain-Barré Syndrome in Childhood. *Clinic. Pediat.* **6**, 3, 162.

Reid, M. (1976) *Handling the Disabled Child in Water.* Assoc. of Paed. Chartered Physiotherapists, Birmingham.

Sharrard, W. J. W. (1955) The distribution of permanent paralysis in the lower limb in poliomyelitis. *J. Bone Jt. Surg.* **37B**, 540.

Ibid. (1957) Muscle paralysis in poliomyelitis. *Brit. J. Surg.* **44**, 471.

Ibid. (1971) *Paediatric Orthopaedics and Fractures.* Oxford and Edinburgh: Blackwell.

Singer, M. and Rose-Innes, T. (1963) *The Recovery from Poliomyelitis. A Study of the Convalescent Phase.* Edinburgh: Livingstone.

Walton, J. N. (1971) *Essentials of Neurology.* London: Pitman.

Further Reading

Barr, J. S. (1949) The management of poliomyelitis. In *Poliomyelitis: Papers and Discussions, Presented at First International Poliomyelitis Conference.* London: Lippincott.

Dekaban, A. (1970) *Neurology in Early Childhood.* Baltimore: Williams and Wilkins.

Eccles, J. C. (1953) *The Neurophysiological Basis of Mind.* London: Oxford University Press.

Edds, M. V. (1950) Hypertrophy of nerve fibres to functionally overloaded muscles. *J. Compar. Anat.* **93**, 259.

Elkington, H. J. (1971) The effective use of the pool. *Physiotherapy*, **57**, 10.

Kabat, H. (1952) The role of central facilitation in restoration of motor function in paralysis. *Arch. Phys. Med.* **33**, 521.

McFarland, H. R. and Heller, G. L. (1966) Guillain-Barré disease complex. *Arch. Neurol.* **14**, 196.

Miller, H. G., Stanton, S. B. and Gibbons, S. L. (1956) Parainfectious encephalomyelitis and related syndromes. *Quart. J. Med.* **25**, 428.

Seddon, H. G. (1954) Poliomyelitis. In *British Surgical Practice.* London: Butterworth.

Swaiman, K. F. and Wright, F. S. (1970) *Neuromuscular Diseases of Infancy and Childhood.* Illinois: Thomas.

Toussaint, D. (1956) Facilitation technics achieve self-care in poliomyelitis patient. *Phys. Ther. Review*, **37**, 590.

Chapter 6

Brachial Plexus Lesions in Infancy

The brachial plexus of an infant may be injured during a difficult birth when a traction force is applied to the head during delivery of the shoulder. Babies involved are frequently of high birth weight, and breech presentations with an after-coming head. The traction on the plexus may cause injury to the upper roots (C5 and 6) resulting in the upper arm paralysis known as Erb's Palsy, or to the lower roots (C7, 8, TI) resulting in paralysis of the muscles of the hand and known as Klumpke's paralysis. Rarely, all the nerve roots may be injured and the infant will have a completely flail arm, an Erb-Duchenne-Klumpke type paralysis. Erb's Palsy is described below as it is the commonest of the three lesions.

As Adler and Patterson (1967) point out, recognition by obstetricians of disproportion between the infant's head and the mother's pelvis, and improved means of managing this complication, have dramatically decreased the incidence of so-called 'obstetrical paralysis' of the upper limb.

DESCRIPTION

The baby, immediately after birth, is noticed to lie asymmetrically, with the affected arm limply at his side instead of maintained in the predominantly flexed posture of the neonate. He is found on examination to have paralysis of the shoulder abductors (deltoid and supraspinatus) and external rotators (teres minor and infraspinatus), and supinators and flexors of the forearm (biceps brachii and supinator). The nerves to the rhomboids and serratus anterior usually escape injury. Sensory loss may occur over the lateral aspect of the arm but this is usually less than the corresponding motor loss. Where there is complete sensory loss in a severe whole arm paralysis, there will be absence of all sensation — pain, temperature, touch and proprioception.

PROGNOSIS

Prognosis depends on the extent of injury to the plexus. Times for maximum recovery vary from 1 month to 18 months. If it is merely a neurapraxia due to oedema and haemorrhage around the nerve fibres but with no damage to the neurilemmal sheath, to the axis cylinder, or to the neurofibrils, the paralysis will probably recover spontaneously in approximately one month with no resultant disability. If there is an axonotmesis in which the axis cylinder is disrupted but the nerves have remained intact, recovery, although probably not complete, will occur within approximately 18 months. However, if the injury is a neurotmesis due to actual rupture of the nerve fibres including the neurilemmal sheath, little or no recovery can be expected. The upper arm type of paralysis usually makes a better recovery than the lower arm type (Sharrard 1971).

If there is complete division of the axon, muscle wasting will be noticeable after the first few weeks. If recovery does not occur, normal growth will not take place in the limb which will be noticeably smaller than the normal limb as the child grows. The child with a complete paralysis is left with a flail insensible arm which eventually dislocates at the shoulder and is totally useless. In the case of an upper arm paralysis which fails to recover, it is remarkable how well the child can adapt the use of his shoulder girdle and arm to compensate for the disability if it is not severe. However many of these children require surgery when they are older in order to improve function. Relevant surgery is described by Lloyd-Roberts (1971) and Sharrard (1971).

ASSESSMENT

The infant is sent for treatment as soon as the injury is recognized and diagnosed. Assessment is carried out with the infant un-dressed and in a warm room. The way in which he holds his arm is similar to the posture of an infant with hemiplegia due to brain injury, so the physiotherapist does her assessment with an awareness of the possibility of this alternate diagnosis, although she must take care not to alarm the parents by inferring other problems. If she suspects brain damage, a suspicion which may only arise several weeks after birth when the lower limb may also show abnormal patterns of both posture and movement, she will send her report directly to the infant's referring doctor.

Tone is assessed in supine by raising the baby's arms above his head, and by moving them across his chest. In comparison with the normal side tone will be considerably lower, depending on the extent of the injury and the normally predominantly flexor hyperactivity will be absent with consequently no resistance to movement. Tone may also be tested in prone. Normally in the neonate this is the position of maximum flexor tonus and the arms should strongly resist any attempt at extension.

Movement is tested by observation. It is better for the physiotherapist to see the baby about one hour after he has been fed when he will be alert and active. Movement is also observed while testing reflex behaviour. The Moro reflex will be asymmetrical, with insufficient arm abduction, although the elbow and fingers may extend. The tonic reaction of the finger flexors will be present in upper arm types of paralysis, but not in lower arm or total lesions. It is normally accompanied by flexion of the elbow. In Erb's Palsy the absence of this element of flexion due to paralysis of the biceps brachii will cause the grasp to be weaker on the affected side. The neck righting reflex is also tested. If it can be elicited it will demonstrate whether or not there is any ability to abduct and flex the shoulder.

Joint range is tested by moving the whole arm through abduction, elevation, flexion, extension and rotation, and each joint separately through its range of motion. Normally it is impossible to complete the range of elevation and extension in a neonate because of the excessive flexor activity. The muscles prone to contracture in Erb's Palsy, for example, are the shoulder internal rotators and adductors, particularly the subscapularis. Contractures will not be found in the neonate, but they may develop as time passes if treatment is not being correctly and thoroughly carried out. Unopposed muscles will shorten unnoticed unless the physiotherapist checks carefully when she does passive movements that the scapula is not pulled into an excessive degree of external rotation when the arm is abducted passively from the side.

Development. The baby's general motor development may be briefly assessed along the lines suggested in Section 2, Chapter 1 and if there is any suspicion of abnormality other than brachial plexus injury, the physiotherapist will report her findings to the baby's doctor without causing anxiety to the parents.

TREATMENT

The baby's arm is rested for a few days after birth to allow haemorrhage and oedema to resolve. From then on treatment consists of full-range passive movements given several times a day by the baby's mother, supervised at regular intervals by the physiotherapist. Emphasis is placed on achieving full-range external rotation, abduction and elevation of the shoulder, with the mother taught how to maintain the length of the shoulder adductors by holding the scapula immobile while abducting the arm to approximately 75 degrees. This is particularly necessary if rhomboids are paralysed as their inactivity will allow the scapula to be pulled into external rotation by the action of both passive abduction of the arm and active adduction. All passive movements must be done very gently with no strain put upon the soft tissues surrounding the joints. In the case of total arm paralysis care must be taken that the mother does not stretch the arm beyond the normal range, particularly into abduction, because of the risk of dislocation.

Prevention of deformity is most important in children with poor recovery of muscle function, as it allows them to take advantage of muscle transfer operations designed to improve function and appearance.

The baby's mother is shown how to stimulate active movement of the arm and hand as the baby develops and becomes more aware of his surroundings. As he continues to progress, so she can be taught how to encourage such activities as reaching out for a rattle, putting his hands to his face and to different parts of his body including his toes, weightbearing on his forearms and hands in prone, rolling over to reach a toy, following as far as possible those normal developmental milestones which will also stimulate use of the weak muscles. Attention should particularly be paid to stimulating hand function, as inability to use the upper arm effectively makes use of the hand difficult unless the infant receives help from his parent or therapist.

Splinting in an abduction splint has been used in the past but is little used now. The aim of the splint was to hold the arm in a position which would discourage contractures, but passive full-range movements if they are carefully done will also prevent these from occurring. The splint has certain disadvantages. It prevents the baby from moving his arm, and it is thought to predispose to dislocation of the head of the radius by holding the forearm in a supinated position (Lloyd-Roberts 1971), and to dislocation of the shoulder joint by holding the arm in abduction (Sharrard 1971). It is sometimes suggested that the baby's arm be splinted in elevation by fastening the sleeve of his jacket to his pillow, but as this prevents him from moving about, and predisposes his shoulder to injury if he does move about, it is hoped that this means of splinting will eventually be completely discarded.

Sever in 1925, following observation of 1100 children, stated that splinting actually delays recovery. External rotation/abduction contractures have been found to occur in infants who were splinted without access to physiotherapy.

SUMMARY

Brachial plexus lesions may involve the whole arm or part of the arm. In many cases of total or lower arm paralysis recovery will fail to occur or will be incomplete. Upper arm lesions have a more hopeful prognosis. The role of the physiotherapist lies in teaching the baby's mother how to maintain normal muscle length and to stimulate active movement of the arm and hand. As with all infants suffering motor disability, care must be taken to encourage as normal development as possible.

References

Adler, J. B. and Patterson R. L. (1967) Erb's Palsy. *J. Bone Jt. Surg.* **49A**, 6, 1052–1064.

Lloyd-Roberts, G. C. (1971) *Orthopaedics in Infancy and Childhood.* London: Butterworth.

Sever, J. W. (1925) Obstetric paralysis: Report of 1100 cases. *J. Amer. Med. Assn.* **85,** 1862–1865.

Sharrard, W. J. W. (1971) *Paediatric Orthopaedics and Fractures.* Oxford and Edinburgh: Blackwell.

Further Reading

Aitken, J. (1952) Deformity of the elbow in Erb's Palsy. *J. Bone Jt. Surg.* **34B**, 352.

Dekaban, A. (1970) *Neurology of Early Childhood.* Baltimore: Williams and Wilkins.

Nelson, W. E., Vaughan, V. C. and McKay, R. J. (1969) *Textbook of Paediatrics.* Philadelphia, London and Toronto: Saunders.

Swaiman, K. F. and Wright, F. S. (1970) *Neuromuscular Diseases of Infancy and Childhood.* Illinois: Thomas.

Wickstrom, J. (1962) Birth injuries of the brachial plexus. *Clin. Ortho.* **23**, 187.

Section III

Congenital Abnormalities

1. *TALIPES EQUINOVARUS*

2. *TALIPES CALCANEO-VALGUS*

3. *CONGENITAL DISLOCATION OF THE HIPS*

4. *ARTHROGRYPOSIS MULTIPLEX CONGENITA*

5. *SPINA BIFIDA*

6. *CONGENITAL LIMB DEFICIENCIES*

Chapter 1

Talipes Equinovarus

This is said to be the commonest congenital abnormality of the foot (Sharrard 1971). The foot is plantarflexed at the ankle, inverted and adducted at the subtaloid (talo-calcaneal) and mid-tarsal joints. In severe cases the deformities may be fixed and the foot almost immobile. Lloyd-Roberts (1971) notes that the degree of rigidity may be variable between the two feet and also between the different elements of the deformity in the same foot. In milder postural cases the foot may be relatively mobile but the infant has difficulty in actively everting and dorsiflexing it.

This deformity may occur in an otherwise normal infant, but it is also seen in association with other congenital deformities such as dislocation of the hip, or as one of the deformities associated with arthrogryposis multiplex congenita or myelomeningocele. It also occurs in infants with congenital absence of the tibia. The deformity is often bilateral, in which case one foot is always more deformed than the other, but it may also be unilateral.

The cause of the defect is unknown, although there have been various theories. Browne (1936) suggested increased intrauterine pressure, Wynne-Davies (1964) said the aetiological factors were probably genetic and environmental while others consider a congenital neuromuscular abnormality may be responsible. A similar equinovarus deformity will result from muscle imbalance in poliomyelitis or in muscular dystrophy, caused by paralysis of the anterior tibial and peroneal muscles.

TYPES

The deformity may be divided into two groups, those which are postural, in which there is at first no bony or arthrotic abnormality, and those in which there are abnormalities of the bones themselves, with malpositioning of the joints, and soft tissue abnormality.

DEFORMITY

Where the deformity is severe (figures 58, 59 and 60), the affected foot is smaller in appearance than the other. The heel is usually small and undeveloped, the calf thin with poor development of the gastrocnemius. The talus is prominent on the dorsum of the foot. The skin on the medial side is wrinkled and on the lateral side stretched. The great toe may be abducted away from the other toes. The foot may be so displaced that its medial border is

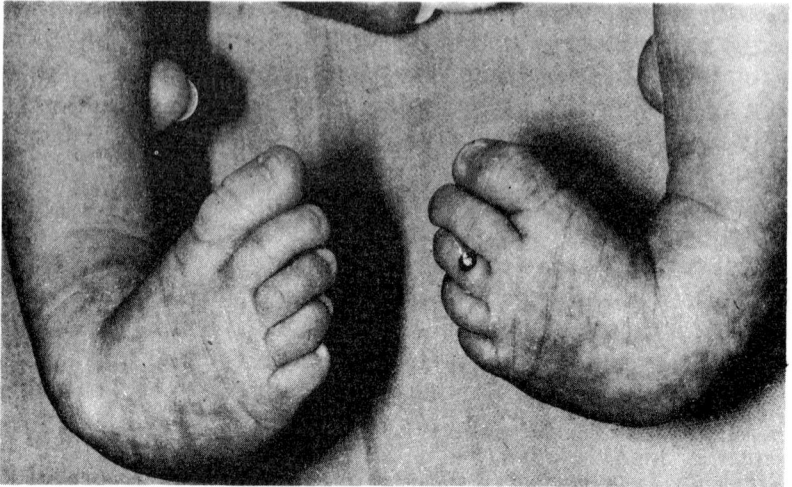

Fig. 58 A severe degree of talipes equinovarus. Note the extreme degree of inversion and metatarsus varus.

in contact with the medial side of the leg. If the foot is viewed from behind, the extreme degree of plantarflexion with contracture of the tendo Achilles is clearly seen (figure 59). The degree of inversion and adduction is noticed from the plantar aspect when the foot is seen to be curved in a banana shape. The foot with a postural equinovarus deformity may be of relatively normal size and shape, but will be held in an equinus and varus position (figure 61).

Pathological Anatomy

Schlicht (1963) reported a study he made of talipes equinovarus in stillborn babies and babies who died soon after birth. He performed dissections on the feet, all of which showed a severe degree of deformity. He did not, unfortunately, state whether the deformities were associated with myelomeningocele or arthrogryposis. He noted that the bones themselves showed distortion, particularly the talus, calcaneus, navicular, cuboid and metatarsals, the talus being the most affected. Not only were the bones themselves malformed, but their relationships with each other were also distorted (figure 62). In all the feet he dissected,

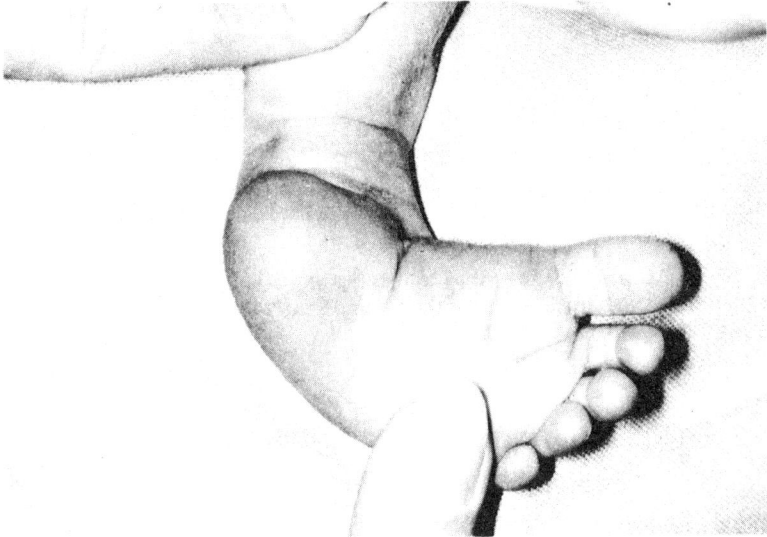

Fig. 59 A posterior view demonstrates the degree of plantarflexion and inversion. The contracted tendo Achilles is clearly visible.

the talus showed distortion of the facets on the superior surface and therefore the bone could not fit properly into the tibio-fibular mortice. He suggested that this bony block was an important cause of the persistence of the equinus deformity.

The talus and calcaneus in severely deformed feet are often smaller than normal, this factor contributing to the smallness of the affected foot in relation to the unaffected one. The convex shape of the outer border of the foot is due not only to the pull of the contracted muscles on the inner side of the foot and leg, but also to the subluxation of the calcaneo-cuboid joint, the ligaments and capsule of which are stretched.

211

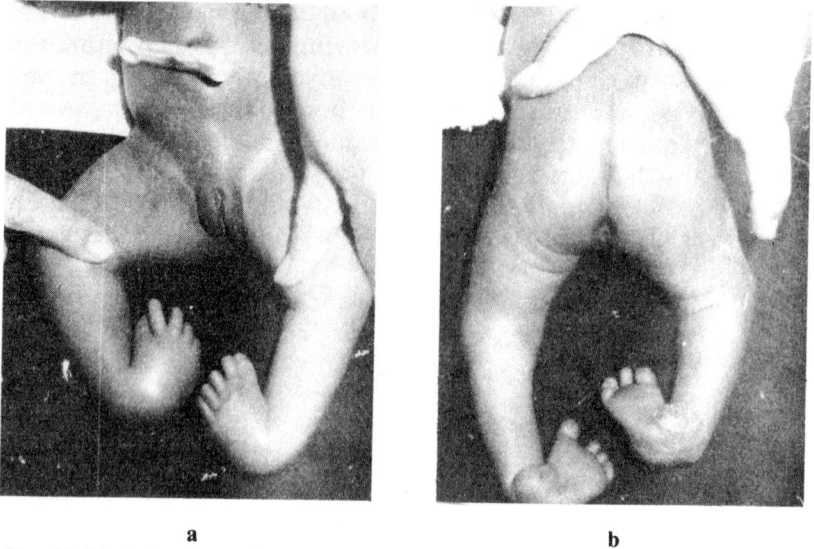

a   b

Fig. 60 (a) Arthrogrypotic type of talipes equinovarus. (b) Posterior view. Note the poor muscular development of the lower part of the legs.
(By permission of J. Harrison).

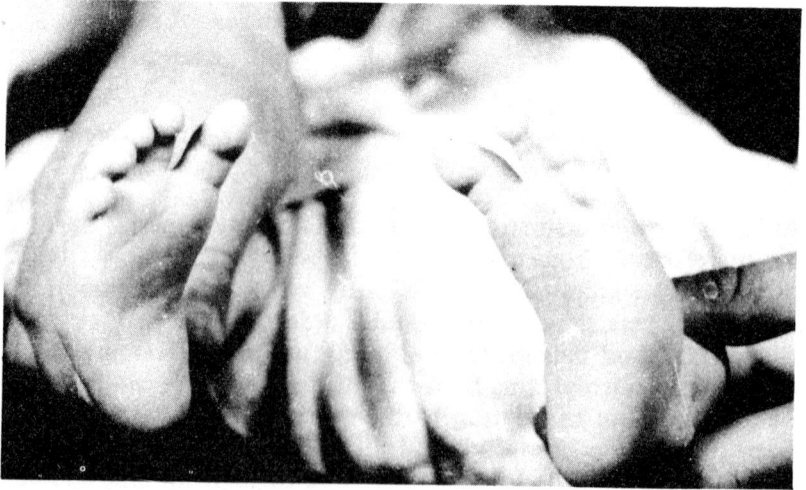

Fig. 61 Postural talipes equinovarus with metatarsus varus. Note the relatively normal shape of the foot compared to figures 58 and 60.

Schlicht found that the soft tissues were affected in all the feet he dissected and he considered the equinus and varus deformities to be maintained by tension in these tissues. Certainly contracture of gastrocnemius, soleus, tibialis posterior, flexor hallucis longus and flexor digitorum longus all appear to contribute to the equinus element, while contracture of tibialis anterior and posterior, flexor hallucis longus and flexor digitorum longus, of the deltoid and spring ligaments, and the small muscles along the

SKELETON OF FOOT

viewed from above

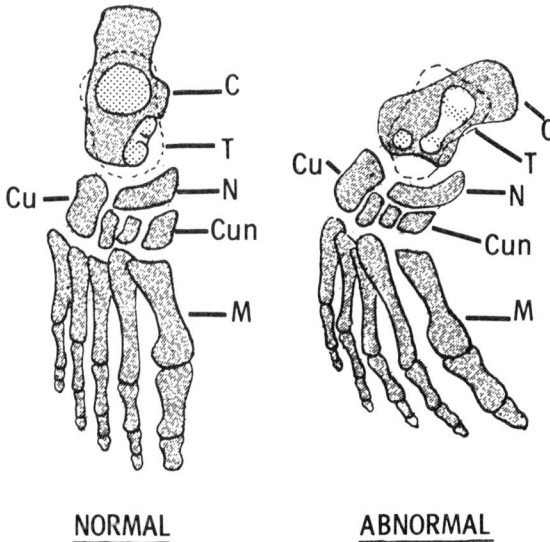

NORMAL   ABNORMAL

Fig. 62 Normal and abnormal skeletal structure. Note the distortion of the bones as well as their abnormal relationships to each other.
C = calcaneum. T = talus. N = navicular. Cu = cuboid. Cun = cuneiform. M = metatarsal.
(From Schlicht, D. (1963) The pathological anatomy of talipes equinovarus. *Aust. New Zeal. J. Surg.* 33,1.)

inner side of the foot contribute to the varus element. Surgeons have noticed the preponderance of fibres of the tendo Achilles inserted into the medial half of the posterior surface of the calcaneus, and this is probably also an important factor in the varus deformity.

PROGNOSIS

Most postural cases of talipes equinovarus correct with conservative treatment in an uncomplicated manner. However, many structural cases show a tendency to relapse despite treatment, although Sharrard (1971) suggests that this may not be a relapse in the sense of a loss of correction, but rather an indication that the deformities have not been completely corrected. These children will remain in the care of the orthopaedic surgeon for several years. If the deformity is either untreated or inadequately treated, secondary bony deformities will develop as the child grows. The relationship between the articular surfaces will alter, the subtaloid and calcaneo-cuboid joints in particular being altered in alignment (Lloyd-Roberts 1971). Eventually the child will be weight-bearing on the lateral border of his feet, with painful callosities forming under the cuboid and cuneiform bones (figure 63).

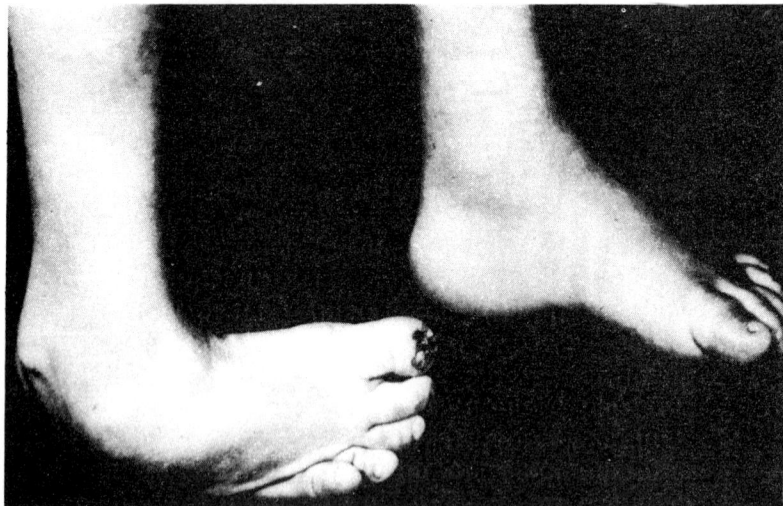

Fig. 63 Untreated talipes equinovarus with weightbearing on the lateral border of the foot.

MANAGEMENT

Treatment of this deformity has long been the subject of controversy. The methods of manipulating or mobilizing the joints of the foot into a corrected position, and the types of splinting used, vary from hospital to hospital. The author describes below one method of mobilizing the foot, and several methods of splinting. These methods of splinting have been found to be successful in the short term. Long-term results have not been adequately assessed. Until clinical trials on the various methods in use in different hospitals have been set up and their results made known, the student must expect to be confronted with a confusing number of alternatives. There is a disappointing tendency for many treated deformities of this type to relapse. The only effective methods of treatment will be those which prevent this tendency. This is an area of therapeutics in which the physiotherapist could well institute her own clinical trials in consultation with an orthopaedic surgeon.

ASSESSMENT

Details of family history and the infant's birth history are noted by the physiotherapist for her own records. It is sometimes found that similar deformities, talipes equinovarus or a contracted tendo Achilles, have been present in other members of the family. Note is made of any other congenital abnormalities which are also present, such as spina bifida occulta, dislocated hips, or the deformities associated with arthrogryposis.

The feet are examined and details of their shape, the extent of the deformity and the degree of mobility are noted, together with the degree of correction which can be obtained. The effectiveness of the evertors and dorsiflexors is tested by stroking the lateral border of the foot. The normal infant will respond immediately and strongly. In the infant with severe deformity, the response will indicate the deficiencies of the peroneal and anterior tibial muscles, or the degree to which they are inhibited by their contracted antagonists.

Photographs of the infant's feet are taken before treatment commences, and at frequent intervals until his eventual discharge. Periodic radiographs as the child grows will be useful in showing the true position of the joints.

PHYSICAL TREATMENT

Conservative treatment consisting of mobilizing and splinting must begin as early as possible after the infant's birth. It should be remembered that the deformity is present in an infant who will be subject to the mechanics of growth and development (Shepherd 1975). Mechanical structures (bone and soft tissue) develop according to the stresses put upon them. If the equinovarus foot is left untreated the bony structure of the foot and lower leg will be subject to unnatural stresses, the soft tissues will undergo further adaptive changes, and the actual deformity will be increased. The older the child is before treatment is commenced, the poorer the end result will probably be.

Mobilization

This technique takes into account the need to mobilize the foot as well as to correct the deformity, and in this way is probably more effective than the rigid forms of splinting sometimes used.

There is some controversy as to the order in which correction should be gained. There seems to be two conflicting views. In the first, emphasis is placed on the early correction of the hind foot equinus (Lloyd-Roberts 1971). Attenborough (1966) has made the observation that the infant's heel cannot be put in a valgus position, that is, everted, while the foot is in equinus. In the second view, the emphasis is on early correction of the midtarsal and subtaloid adduction and inversion before attempting correction of the equinus element (Browne 1936, Sharrard 1971). The technique described below allows for attempting correction of all three elements of plantarflexion, inversion and adduction in the same manoeuvre.

The mobilization of these feet should not be attempted by a physiotherapist unless she has detailed knowledge of the normal and pathological anatomy of the foot, plus an awareness of the plasticity of the infant foot. She should mobilize the foot always with due regard to the damage which may be caused to the undeveloped bones, to the epiphyseal areas of the tibia and fibula, and to the soft tissues around the foot. Forcible manipulation may result in further deformity of the talus (Sharrard 1971).

Technique

One hand holds the lower ends of the tibia and fibula and the calcaneus. This enables the therapist to protect the tibial and

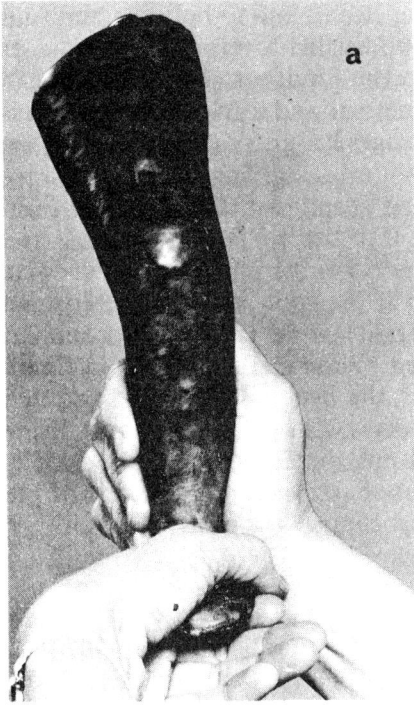

Fig. 64 Left talipes equinovarus. Mobilizing technique. (a) Mobilizing the forefoot in relation to the hindfoot. (b) Stretching the tendo Achilles.

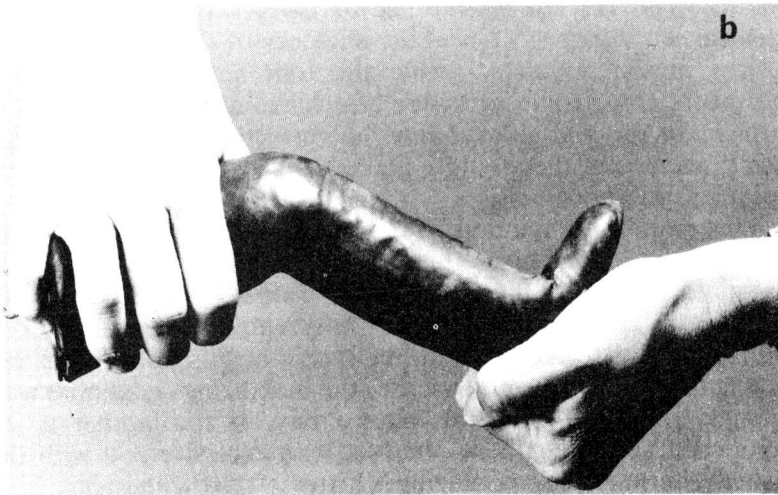

fibular epiphyses from a shearing strain, and to hold the hindfoot steady while the other hand mobilizes the forefoot away from its adducted position in relation to the hindfoot (figure 64). When this part of the foot (tarso-metatarsal and mid-tarsal joints) has been mobilized, the therapist changes her grip slightly, holding the foot with her thumb over the talus, giving gentle pressure downwards and backwards on the prominent talus, in an attempt to guide its articular facet back into the ankle joint mortice and gain as much dorsiflexion and eversion as possible. When some correction has been gained, and if the foot is severely deformed and immobile this may take several treatments, the tendo Achilles may be more effectively stretched by the method shown in figure 64. The foot is held in one hand, the heel pulled down to stretch the plantarflexors, and into eversion. Care is taken that it is the hindfoot that is corrected, and not the forefoot. If the foot is immobile as well as deformed, emphasis is on mobilization of the various joints rather than on maintenance of a passive stretch.

Precautions

The knee must be held flexed while the foot is being mobilized in order to avoid strain on the medial ligament of the knee. If the foot is everted on an extended leg it is possible to exert such strain on the medial ligament of the knee that a valgus deformity results. The risk in attempting to correct the plantarflexion element too vigorously lies in the tendency of the foot to 'break' at the midtarsal joints, giving the foot a rocker-shaped appearance. This pseudocorrection can be avoided if the therapist is content to proceed slowly with the correction of the hindfoot, gently increasing the mobility gained rather than attempting too great a degree of correction.

This mobilization is done by the therapist several times a day while the infant and his mother are in the maternity hospital, and the mother is taught the procedure, and does it herself under the therapist's supervision. When they return home the infant is seen by the therapist regularly, and emphasis at this point is on ensuring that his mother understands the mobilizing techniques well enough to do them several times a day. If the mother is incompetent or if she attacks the foot with excessive zeal with the risk of injuring it, the mobilizing is better left to the therapist.

Splinting

There are several methods of splinting in current use. Some are designed to allow active correction by the child as he kicks his legs, others are more rigid, holding the foot immobile in a position of some correction. Rigid splinting is avoided by some surgeons (Sharrard 1971) as it tends to leave a stiff immobile foot. Many prefer to correct the foot in an adjustable or removable splint which allows the joints to be mobilized regularly. The applications of three types of splinting are described below.

Strapping

This method of strapping holds the foot in a corrected position, the degree of correction being altered by adjusting the pull from the buckle (figure 65). Once the foot can be held in some eversion the infant will facilitate active contraction of the evertor and dorsiflexor muscles each time he thrusts with his leg into extension.

Materials

Zinc oxide strapping 3 inches wide.
Tincture benzoin compound.
Buckle.
Cotton wool.
Needle and cotton.

Method

The strapping is cut into pieces; the buckle is attached, and the strapping is sewn (figure 66). The therapist mobilizes the foot before applying the strapping. Tinc benz co is applied to the skin with cotton wool and allowed to dry before the strapping is applied. This will give some protection to the skin, but if the infant is allergic to this type of strapping it should not be used.

Step 1

Piece A is applied to the foot (figure 66-1). It should be wide enough to extend from the back of the heel to the web of the toes. The cut-out piece is deep enough to avoid cutting into the front of the ankle when the foot is dorsiflexed. The entire piece is long

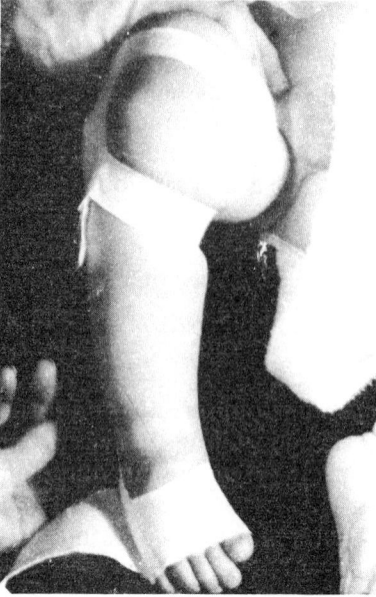

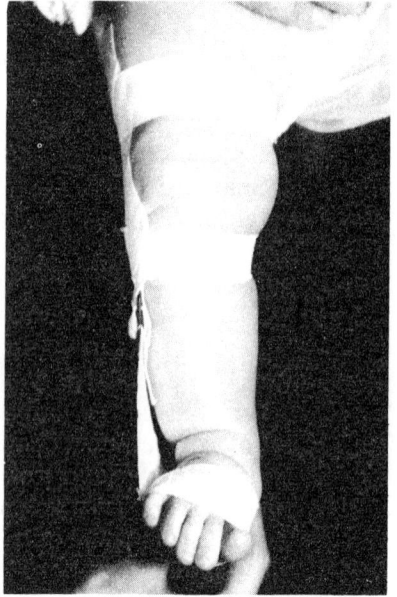

a   b

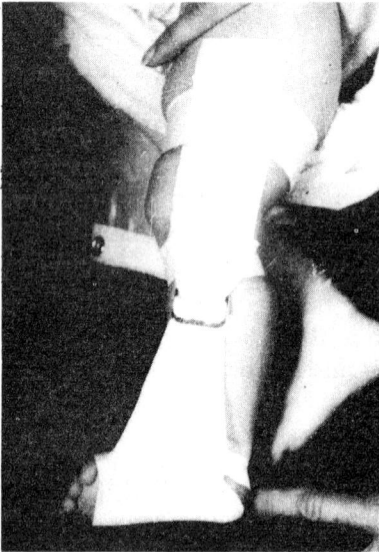

Fig. 65 Talipes equinovarus. Strap and buckle splinting. (a) Before being buckled up. (b) Anterior view of strap and buckle maintaining correction. (c) Lateral view.

c

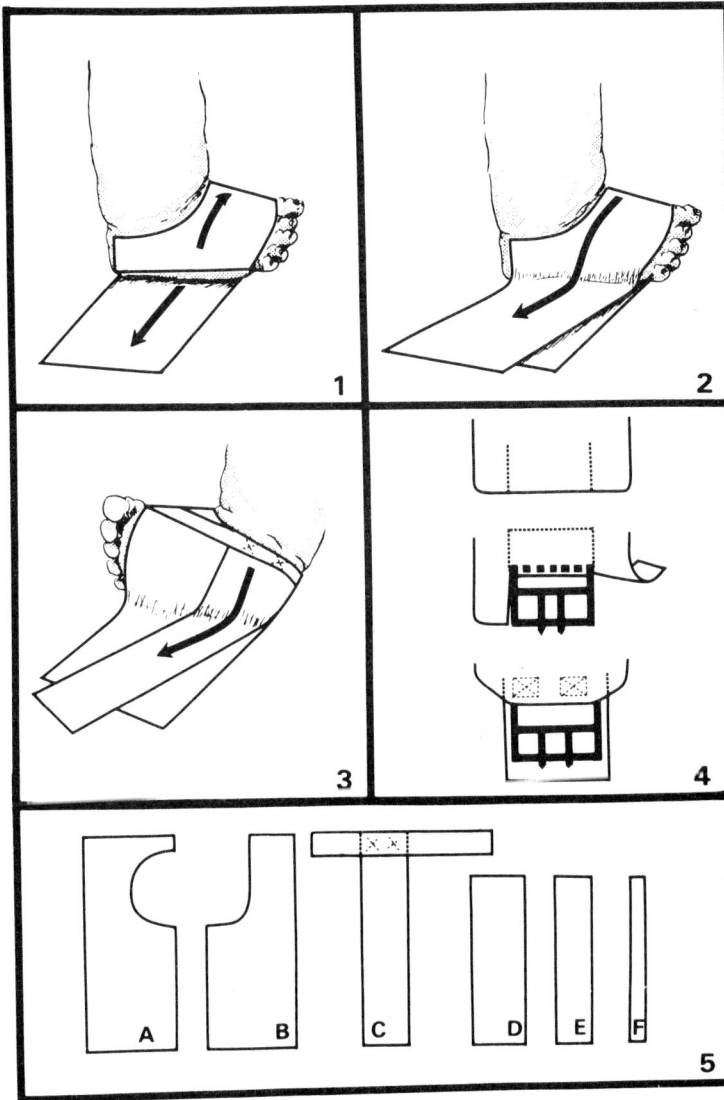

Fig. 66 Talipes equinovarus. Method of applying strap and buckle splinting to the right foot.

enough to extend from the lateral side of the dorsum of the foot, around the medial side, under the plantar aspect and up to the knee.

Step 2
Piece B is applied to the dorsum of the foot, extending from the medial side across the dorsum to join piece A laterally (figure 66-2). This piece is the lining for piece A, to which it is joined as near to the plantar surface as possible in order to pull the foot into dorsiflexion and eversion.

Step 3
Piece C is now applied (figure 66-3). The point at which the two pieces of strapping are sewn is placed at the medial side of the calcaneum with the horizontal piece passing from the great toe around the heel to the base of the fifth toe. The broader vertical strip is then taken under the heel and is attached to the combined pieces A and B. This piece reinforces the pull into dorsiflexion and eversion.

Step 4
With the foot pieces in place, piece D is applied to the lateral side of the thigh with the buckle just below the knee. Its exact position depends on the angle of pull required to correct the foot.

Step 5
Pieces E and F are applied around the top of the thigh and top of the leg in order to hold piece D in position. They are placed carefully, without tension, in order to avoid occlusion of the circulation. Piece F should not be placed over the popliteal fossa.

Step 6
The strapping is now too wide to pass through the buckle, so it is made narrower, being cut away anteriorly as far as necessary. As the pull is required particularly from the hindfoot, the strapping is not cut posteriorly.

Step 7
The combined pieces A, B and C are attached to the buckle after the foot has been pulled into the position of correction.

222

It has been suggested above that the foot be mobilized gently in order to avoid trauma to bones, joints and soft tissues, and this applies also to the splinting, which should not be applied too rigorously. A rocker foot may result if the strapping pulls the forefoot into dorsiflexion by 'breaking' the foot at the midtarsal joints instead of pulling the foot into dorsiflexion at the ankle joint.

The circulation of the foot is carefully checked by observing the capillary response to pressure on the toes. If the toes become dusky in colour, normal circulation can usually be restored by loosening the strapping at the buckle. Instructions are given to the baby's mother about caring for the strapping and the skin, and the purpose of the strapping is explained. She must avoid wetting the strapping when she bathes the baby, and must put his nappy on firmly and change it regularly in order to avoid soiling and soaking. She is shown how to undo the buckle in order to mobilize the foot during the day, and how to do it up again without applying too much force. If the infant's skin suffers an allergic reaction to the strapping other forms of splinting may have to be considered.

Modifications

If the foot is flexed at the midtarsal joints and the strapping does not correct this, a flat thin piece of aluminium shaped to the foot may be strapped to the plantar surface after the strapping has been applied. Similarly if the strapping does not correct a severe degree of metatarsus varus, a small metal splint is attached to the medial side of the foot from the calcaneus to the great toe.

Other forms of strapping, including that of Robert-Jones (Lloyd-Roberts 1971) may also be used.

Medial Plaster Splints

This splint is useful when a foot is so severely deformed and so immobile that strapping or Denis Browne splints cannot be put on effectively or safely, that is, when other splinting cannot be applied without a force which would damage the infant's foot. It is used for the first few days of treatment until some correction of the adduction and inversion element is obtained, and will be followed as soon as possible by a form of splinting which will encourage some active correction on the part of the child.

Materials

Plaster bandage 4 inches wide.
Piece of foam padding half inch thick.
Bandage 2 inches wide.
Scissors.
Bowl with warm water.

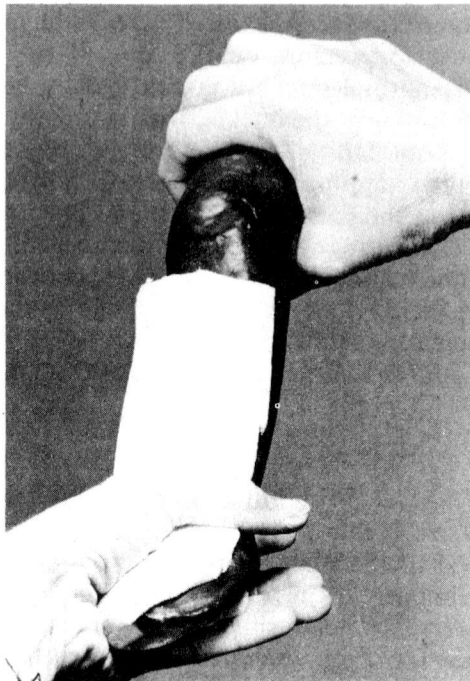

Fig. 67 Talipes equinovarus. Method of applying medial plaster splint to the left foot.

Method

A piece of plastic foam and a plaster slab of six thicknesses are cut to fit the anterior, medial and posterior surfaces of the foot and leg, from below the tibial tubercle to the tips of the toes. A narrow strip down the lateral side is left free. The foot is mobilized before the application of the plaster. The plaster slab is wet and is placed on the padding with any wrinkles smoothed out. This combined slab is applied (padding against the skin) to the leg and foot. The adduction and inversion element is corrected gently as in the mobilizing technique and held there until the plaster sets (figure 67). Indentations from finger pressure must be avoided. While the plaster is still wet, the bandage is soaked in water, then bandaged around the splint and foot leaving the toes free.

The capillary response is checked in the toes immediately after the plaster is applied, and at intervals for the next ten minutes. If the toes become dusky in colour, the splint is removed and reapplied.

This splint stays in position for two days, then is removed by

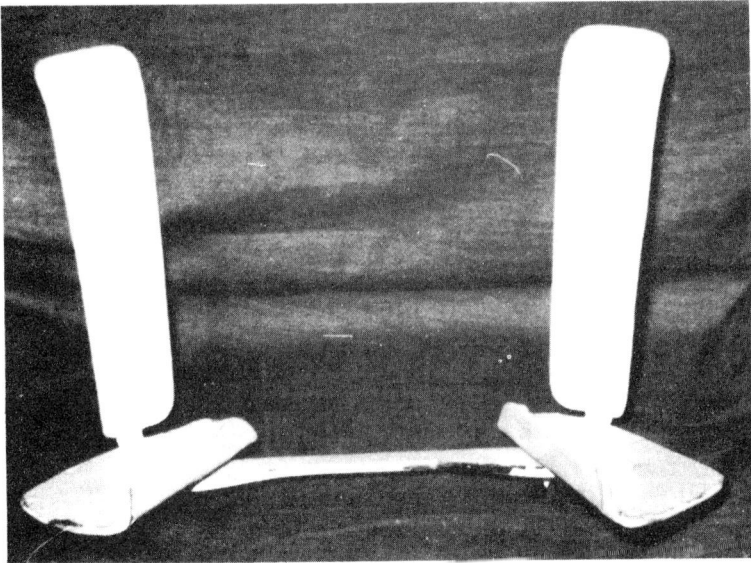

Fig. 68 Denis Browne splints.

cutting the bandage down the lateral side of the leg. The foot is mobilized again by the physiotherapist, and another splint applied. This routine is repeated three or four times, or until sufficient correction has been gained and a more active form of splinting can be applied. The mother is advised to check the circulation of the foot each day, and to remove the splint if the capillary response is not normal.

Denis Brown Type Metal Splints

This splint consists of two pieces of aluminium moulded into foot plates with extensions for the lateral side of the leg (figure 68). It is important that the foot pieces are the same size as the baby's feet. If they are too wide, the strapping will not be able to control the adduction element. The lateral extension should extend well up the leg. If it is too short it will eliminate the leverage required to hold the foot everted. In the case of a unilateral deformity the normal foot must be splinted as well. The splints are joined together by a removable crossbar which attaches by butterfly nuts to the footplates. The crossbar may be bent downwards to a small degree, and if the foot-plates are attached with the legs in some external rotation the position of the legs and feet probably helps facilitate eversion and dorsiflexion as the infant kicks into extension.

The effectiveness of this splint is questioned by some surgeons (Fripp and Shaw 1967) on the grounds that the feet are stiff and immobile after the splint is removed. The principal means by which correction of this deformity can be maintained, and the only way in which it can be relatively certain that the deformity will not relapse, is by facilitating active eversion and dorsiflexion of the foot. In the absence of efficient function of these muscles the deformity is bound to recur. If the Denis Browne splint really does, by the positioning of the feet on the splint, encourage contraction of these muscles, its effectiveness would be more obvious. This factor needs to be investigated thoroughly.

Materials

Denis Browne metal splints made to measure.
Adhesive felt ⅛ inch thick.
Strapping 1 inch wide.
Tincture benzoin compound.
Cotton wool.

Method

The splints are covered with felt which overlaps the edges a little. Small wedges of felt are cut out to pass from under the cuboid along the lateral border of the plantar surface of the foot. The number of pieces of felt in each wedge, that is, the height of the wedge, depends on the degree of correction obtainable (figure 69).

A narrow strip of felt is cut out which is long enough to pass along the medial side of the foot from the great toe to the calcaneus.

It is difficult to apply this splint without help, so assistance will be needed. One therapist, or the baby's mother, holds the foot firmly on the splint in order to gain the best correction, the other straps the foot on to the splint. At no time should force be used. The therapist holding the foot, holds with one hand at the toes and the other at the knee. The knee is flexed and gentle pressure downwards will keep the ankle in as much dorsiflexion as is obtainable. Tinc benz co is applied to the skin from the web of the toes to the knee, making sure to cover the skin thoroughly.

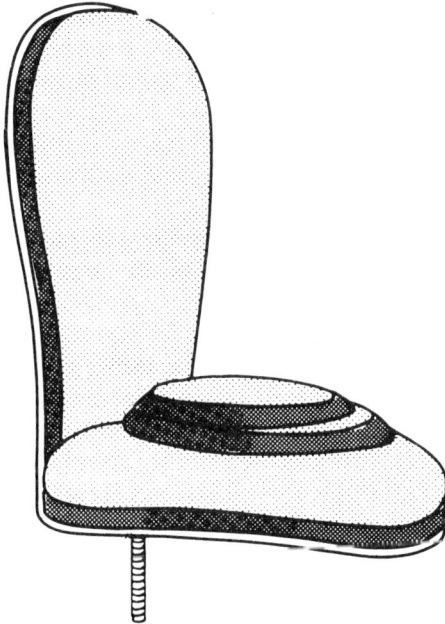

Fig. 69 Denis Browne splint for the left foot with felt and wedges attached.

The wedges are applied either to the splint or to the foot, extending laterally from the cuboid to the toes. These will hold the foot everted. The strapping is wound in circular fashion, leaving no gaps and starting from the web of the toes. Emphasis is placed on holding the ankle in as much dorsiflexion as possible by several turns around the ankle and under the heel, and the strapping is continued up the leg to the top of the splint. A narrow piece of felt is strapped on medially from the heel to the great toe to prevent the foot adducting from the splint. Alternatively, a small piece of padded aluminium may be applied in the same way.

The screws underneath the footplates must be free from strapping. The crossbar is attached (if it is curved the curve must be convex downwards) to the screws with the legs in as much external rotation as required. The butterfly nuts are then done up tightly (figure 70).

It is, unfortunately, easy to occlude the circulation during the application of the strapping, so the colour of the toes is checked carefully over a period of ten minutes, and the baby's mother is advised to continue these checks periodically for at least the next few hours. If the circulation does appear to be occluded and the obstruction cannot be relieved, the splint must be removed and reapplied.

Care must be taken when applying this splint that the dorsiflexion obtained is at the ankle joint and not at the midtarsal joints.

The normal foot is placed flat on the footplate with a piece of felt under the medial longitudinal arch, and is strapped on as described above.

If it is difficult to gain sufficient eversion by the above method, a strip of felt may be applied, with the sticky side against the skin, to pass from the medial side of the calcaneum and under the heel. At this point tension on the felt will pull the heel into some eversion. The felt is then attached to the lateral side of the leg, and acts as lining for the splint as well as a corrective force. The lateral wedges of felt are attached as before or on to the foot itself, and the splint is strapped on as described above.

Some advice to the baby's mother is necessary, and she is told how to look after the splint, and how to remove and reapply the crossbar which will have to be done when she is dressing and undressing the baby. The splint remains in place for one week. Ferguson (1968) suggests that the feet be suspended by a cord attached to the bar so the baby can kick more freely. At the end of this week the splint is removed by cutting the strapping along the lateral side. The baby may now be bathed and allowed to kick free for a few hours before the splint is reapplied. As the infant grows, so the splints will need to be remade in a larger size.

Other Forms of Splinting

Posterior plaster splint

A padded plaster splint is made to hold the foot either in the mid-position or in eversion and dorsiflexion. It is of no value in severe talipes equinovarus with its tendency to relapse, as even with firm bandaging it cannot control the tendency to return to an equinovarus position. However, the splint is useful in mild postural deformities to maintain correction until the infant can do so himself, and in infants with myelomeningocele where the leg is flaccid, with no muscle imbalance, and correction must be maintained until corrective stabilizing surgery can be performed.

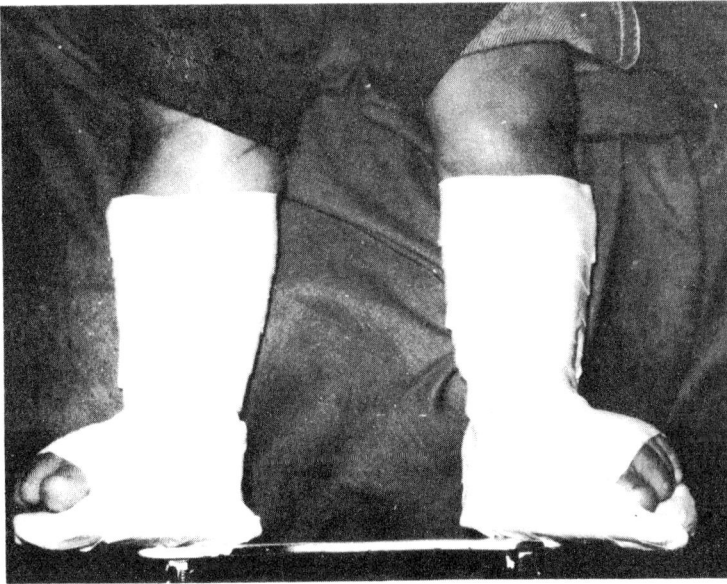

Fig. 70 Denis Browne splints, with strapping applied.

Denis Browne night splints

This splint is sometimes prescribed as a means of maintaining correction gained by strapping or by Denis Browne metal splints. It consists of a pair of boots attached to metal plates on a crossbar (figure 71). The principle is similar to that of the metal splint described above. The legs are held in external rotation and the feet

229

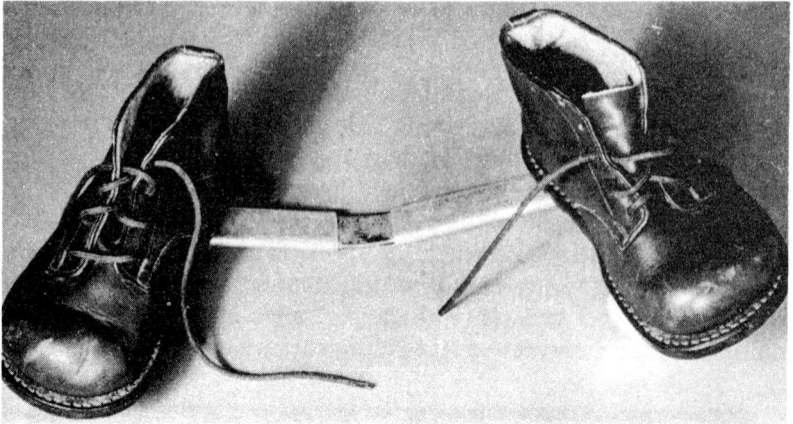

Fig. 71 Denis Browne night splint with boots and cross bar.

are everted and dorsiflexed. This splint is worn day and night, or at night only if the child is walking.

Active Correction

This is an important aspect of treatment. Mobilization of the infant's foot is followed by an attempt at stimulating active eversion and dorsiflexion by stroking the lateral border of the foot firmly with the tip of the finger in the direction of the heel.

When the foot is plantigrade the infant may be stood for a few moments with his weight on the affected foot and the heel well down, and moved gently from side to side and forwards and backwards to stimulate some active muscular control over eversion and dorsiflexion. At five months of age the normal infant in the supine position reaches up to grasp his toes and to play with them, and this should be encouraged by his mother as another way of gaining active correction. He should be encouraged to hold the lateral toes in order to stimulate eversion. Similarly, when he begins to sit at six or seven months he can be encouraged to play with his feet.

There are several ways of stimulating active eversion and dorsiflexion, and these include firm stroking of the antero-lateral aspect of the lower leg in an upward direction with a finger and mechanical vibration over the muscles required to contract

(Bishop 1975). Stimulation of the foot placing reaction (Appendix 1) will also facilitate active dorsiflexion. There are other methods of stimulating movement and these should be explored by the therapist.

Surgical Management

There are several surgical procedures involved at different stages of the management of this deformity, ranging from soft tissue release, and elongation of the tendo Achilles performed on the infant or young child, to the reconstructive procedures performed on older children with untreated or relapsed deformity. Most of these surgical procedures are followed by the application of long leg plaster casts for times which vary according to the nature of the structures required to heal or unite. It is beyond the scope of this book to describe such surgery, but details will be found in Lloyd-Roberts (1971) and Sharrard (1971).

SUMMARY

Talipes equinovarus is the commonest congenital deformity of the foot. The severe, rigid type is difficult to treat successfully and some show a tendency to relapse despite treatment. Methods of conservative treatment are still controversial. To some extent this is due to the lack of controlled trials on the various methods available. Mobilization of the joints of the foot is used to correct the deformity, and the physiotherapist must do this mobilizing with a thorough understanding of the anatomy of the foot, as well as with an awareness of the potential damage that may be caused by careless or forcible techniques.

References

Attenborough, C. G. (1966) Severe congenital talipes equinovarus. *J. Bone Jt. Surg.* **48B**, 1, 31.

Bishop, B. (1975) Vibratory Stimulation, Part 3. *Phys. Ther.* **55**, 2, 139-143.

Browne, D. (1936) Congenital deformities of mechanical origin. *Proc. Roy. Soc. Med.* **29**, 1, 409.

Ferguson, A. (1968) *Orthopaedic Surgery in Infancy and*

Childhood. Baltimore: Williams and Wilkins.

Fripp, A. T. and Shaw, N. R. (1967) *Clubfoot.* Edinburgh: Livingstone.

Lloyd-Roberts, G. C. (1971) *Orthopaedics in Infancy and Childhood.* London: Butterworth.

Schlicht, D. (1963) The pathological anatomy of talipes equinovarus. *Aust. New Zeal. J. Surg.* **33**, 1.

Sharrard, W. J. W. (1971) *Paediatric Orthopaedics and Fractures.* Oxford and Edinburgh: Blackwell.

Shepherd, R. B. (1975) Abnormal growth and development resulting from disease, trauma and deformity. *Aust. J. Physiother.* **21**, 4, 143–150.

Wynne-Davies, R. (1964) Family studies and the cause of congenital clubfoot. *J. Bone Jt. Surg.* **46B**, 445.

Further Reading

Blockley, N. J. and Smith, M. G. H. (1966) Treatment of congenital clubfoot. *J. Bone Jt. Surg.* **48B**, 660.

Böhm, M. (1929) The embryological origin of clubfoot. *J. Bone Jt. Surg.* **11**, 229.

Brockman, E. P. (1930) *Congenital Clubfoot.* Bristol: Wright.

Browne, D. (1956) Splinting for controlled movement. *Clinic. Orthop.* **8**, 91.

Clark, J. M. P. (1968) Treatment of clubfoot. *Proc. Roy. Soc. Med.* **61**, 779.

Dwyer, F. C. (1963) Treatment of relapse — calcaneal osteotomy. *J. Bone Jt. Surg.* **45B**, 67.

Kite, J. H. (1964) *The Clubfoot.* New York: Grune and Stratton.

Wynne-Davies, R. (1964) Review on completion of treatment. *J. Bone Jt. Surg.* **46B**, 464.

Chapter 2

Talipes Calcaneo-Valgus

In this congenital deformity (figure 72), the foot is held in dorsiflexion at the ankle joint and eversion at the subtaloid joint, and it cannot be moved passively into full inversion or plantarflexion. The soft tissues on the anterior surface of the ankle are tight. The deformity is thought to be a postural one if unaccompanied by spina bifida or bony abnormality of the foot. In children with spina bifida cystica, the deformity, although present at birth, will probably be the result of muscle imbalance.

The aetiology is unknown, although Jolly (1968) notes that it is seen in post-mature infants. Prognosis is good in the otherwise normal child, and with passive movements done daily by the parents, full range movement should be gained within a few weeks. However, in the child with muscle imbalance, although correction may be achieved, its maintenance is very difficult, and the effects of gravity and the pressure of bedclothes on the foot frequently results in a secondary deformity involving plantarflexion of the midtarsal joints with the ankle remaining in dorsiflexion.

MANAGEMENT

Physical treatment aims at mobilizing the foot by stretching the tight anterior structures and by stimulating the calf and posterior tibial muscles to plantarflex and invert the foot. The mobilization is done by the parents at home with regular supervision by the physiotherapist. Serial plaster splinting is useful for maintaining the correction gained. Surgery may be necessary eventually for the infant whose deformity is due to muscle imbalance.

Assessment

The physiotherapist takes note of the appearance of the foot, and tests the range of movement at the ankle and subtaloid joints. Photographs of the foot are a useful guide to progress.

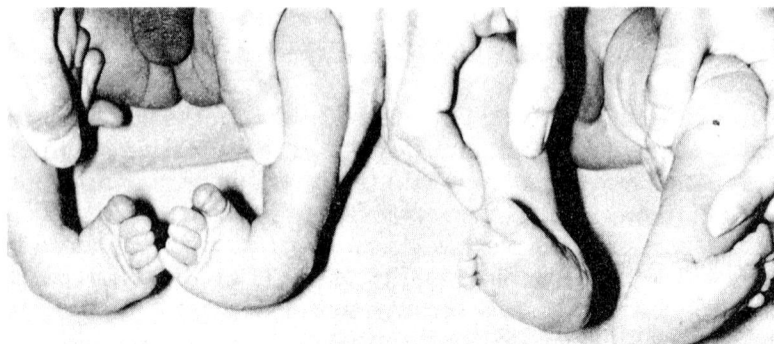

Fig. 72 Comparison of talipes equinovarus (on left) with talipes calcaneo-valgus (on right).
(By permission of W. Cumming.)

Physical Treatment

Mobilization

The foot is held in a handshake grasp with the lateral border of the foot in the palm. This grip enables the calcaneus to be inverted as the foot is plantarflexed. Care is taken to hold the foot near the ankle so plantarflexion will occur at this joint rather than at the midtarsal joints, otherwise a pseudocorrection will occur, with the ankle remaining in dorsiflexion while the forefoot is plantarflexed. This mobilization is done for five minutes at least three times a day.

Splinting

A plaster slab is made to fit the antero-lateral aspect of the foot and leg. It may be left unpadded provided it is made to fit smoothly, but must be padded in the case of the myelomeningocele infant with absent or abnormal sensation. The splint extends from below the knee to cover the toes. Laterally it covers the calcaneus in order to obtain maximum correction of the

234

eversion element. The wet plaster slab is applied using the same grip as in the mobilization technique, and the foot is gently corrected as much as possible, making sure it is true plantarflexion that is being gained. When the plaster has set, the splint is taken off and allowed to dry before being bandaged on with a 2 inch crepe bandage (figure 73).

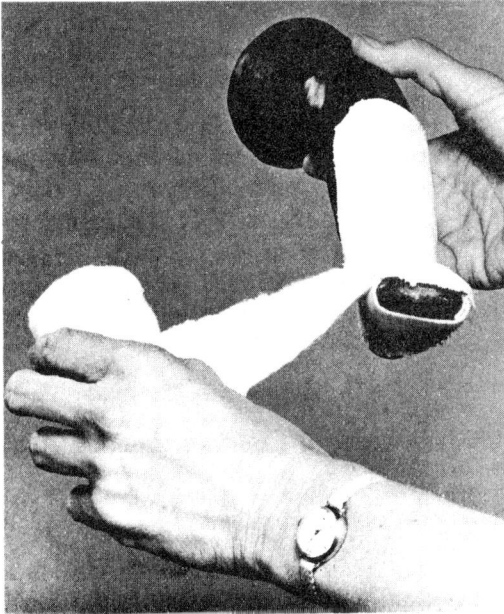

Fig. 73 Left talipes calcaneo-valgus. Antero-lateral plaster slab seen from the medial side. The heel must be bandaged up into the splint to gain as much plantarflexion as possible.

When the splint is being bandaged on, care is taken to hold the heel firmly enough to allow the anterior aspect of the ankle to fit well into the splint. If the splint is bandaged on with the heel sagging there will again be a tendency toward pseudocorrection. This must be carefully explained to the infant's parents. The circulation of the toes is checked after the splint is bandaged on.

A new splint is made every few days as the position of the foot improves. It may be worn day and night until correction is gained, with periods of the day spent in kicking freely without it, and eventually only at night until the baby can maintain active correction himself.

Active correction

The plantarflexors may be stimulated to contract by a variety of techniques. Pressure given upwards against the sole of the foot may stimulate plantarflexion, or the calf may be stimulated directly by fast brushing or vibration.

SUMMARY

In an otherwise normal baby talipes calcaneo-valgus poses no problems in management, the affected foot regaining full-range movement and a normal posture within a few weeks of treatment commencing. Where the deformity is the result of muscle imbalance, as may occur in a baby with myelomeningocele, maintenance of correction is difficult, and the infant may require surgery to correct the effects of the imbalance.

References

Jolly, H. (1968) *Diseases of Children*. London: Blackwell.

Further Reading

Giannestras, N. J. (1967) *Foot Disorders. Medical and Surgical Management*. London: Kimpton.

Lloyd-Roberts, G. C. (1971) *Orthopaedics in Infancy and Childhood*. London: Butterworth.

Sharrard, W. J. W. (1971) *Paediatric Orthopaedics and Fractures*. Oxford and Edinburgh: Blackwell.

Chapter 3

Congenital Dislocation of the Hips

The treatment of unstable hips in infants and of dislocated and subluxated hips in infants and older children, is the province of the orthopaedic surgeon. However, it is important for the physiotherapist to understand the methods of testing clinically for the presence of instability or dislocation, as this is frequently her responsibility. If she suspects hip instability or dislocation in a baby she is treating she must refer the baby to his doctor immediately as early treatment is essential. In many paediatric departments the physiotherapist is responsible for the application of splinting, and a description of the methods of application of the most commonly used forms of splinting is given below.

DESCRIPTION

In actual dislocation the head of the femur lies superior and posterior to the acetabulum (figure 74). It separates the gluteus medius from the ilium. The joint capsule is stretched and the ligamentum teres greatly elongated. The psoas, adductors and hamstrings become contracted. Sometimes the cartilaginous limbus which forms the rim of the acetabulum is inverted, and this may be a difficult obstacle to reduction. If the dislocation remains unreduced, the head of the femur changes shape and may become flattened.

AETIOLOGY

True dislocation of the hips is said to occur in a ratio of 6:1,000 of the population. It is more common in girls than in boys, and occurs more often unilaterally than bilaterally. Although it often occurs in otherwise normal children it is also seen associated with other congenital abnormalities such as spina bifida and arthrogryposis, and in babies with severe asymmetrical hypertonus associated with cerebral palsy. A number of infants demonstrate instability of their hips at birth. The majority appear spontaneously to become stable, others frankly subluxate or dislocate.

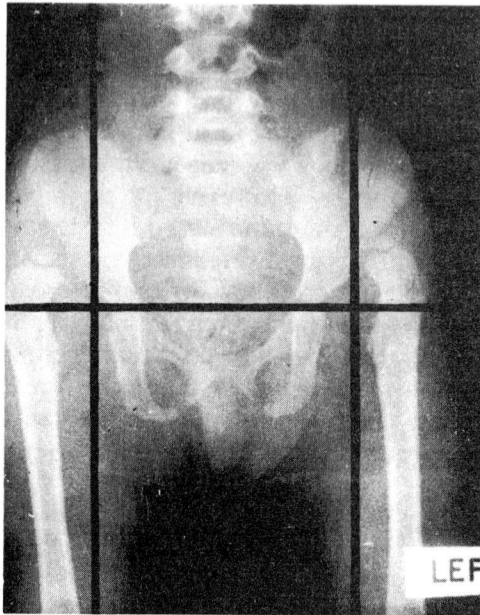

Fig. 74 Radiograph of bilaterally dislocated hips. Note the position of the head of the femur in relation to the acetabulum.

There are several factors which may be responsible for this congenital abnormality (Illingworth 1970, Lloyd-Roberts 1971, Sharrard 1971), and among them are:

Breech position *in utero*.
Severe hypotonia with generalized joint laxity.
Shallow acetabulum.
Family history, i.e. genetic factors.

DIAGNOSIS

Attempts are being made in many obstetric hospitals to detect hip instability or dislocation soon after birth. Infants are subjected to routine assessment in the hope that actual dislocation may be prevented in those infants with instability, and that early treatment of actual dislocation will be more effective than treatment begun when the infant is older.

Tests for Hip Instability in Infants

There are several tests for hip instability. One is described below.

Barlow's sign

With the baby in supine on an examination couch, his hips and knees are flexed to 90 degrees, and the hips abducted. Pressure is given by the operator against the greater trochanter towards the acetabulum (figure 75). If a jerk is felt the sign is said to be positive. It is caused by the head of the femur slipping over the posterior rim of the acetabulum into the socket. The absence of a jerk does not necessarily mean the baby's hips are normal, but could indicate that the dislocation is irreducible.

With the hips in the same position, pressure is then given with the operator's thumb on the medial side of the thigh over the hip, down towards the hip joint. Another jerk may be felt indicating that the head of the femur is being pushed out of the acetabulum again (figure 75).

Other signs to look for which may indicate *unilateral dislocation* in an infant may be:

Decreased abduction in one hip (figure 76).
Asymmetrical skin creases.
Apparent shortness of one leg (figure 77).
On palpation, one greater trochanter is felt to be higher than the other.

In the case of *bilateral dislocation* the signs may include:

Wide perineum.
Female shape of pelvis.
Increased lumbar lordosis.

Once the child begins to bear weight and walk the following signs will be evident:

239

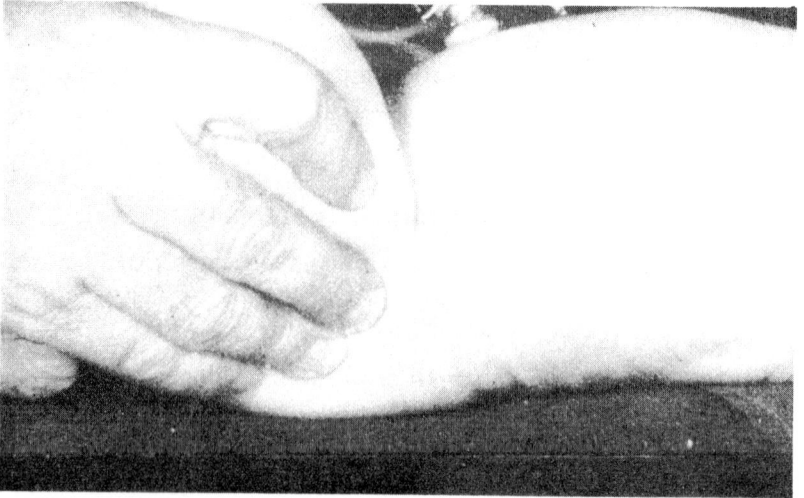

a

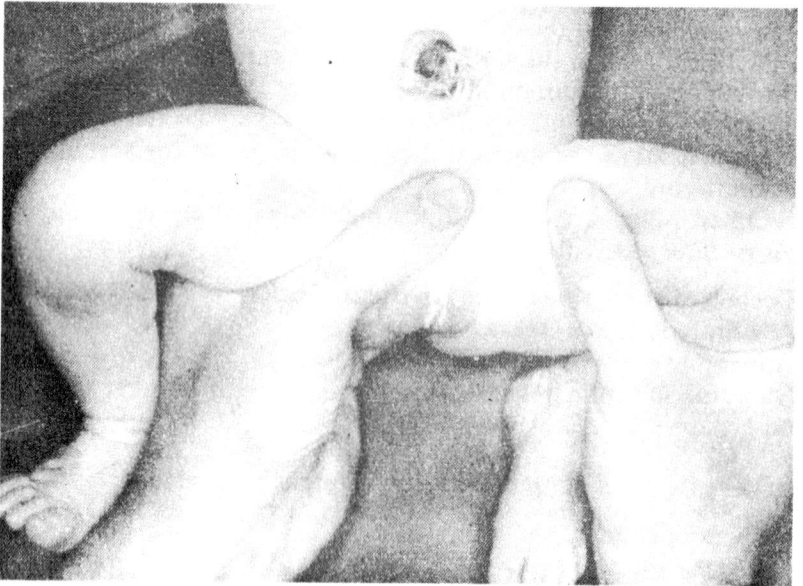

b

Fig. 75 Barlow's test for dislocation of the hips. (a) First manoeuvre. (b) Second manoeuvre. (By permission of W. Cumming.)

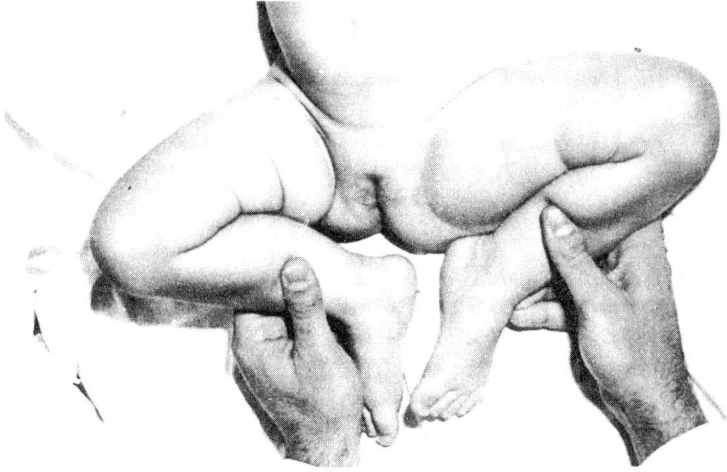

Fig. 76 Dislocation of the right hip. Note the limited abduction of this hip compared with the left.

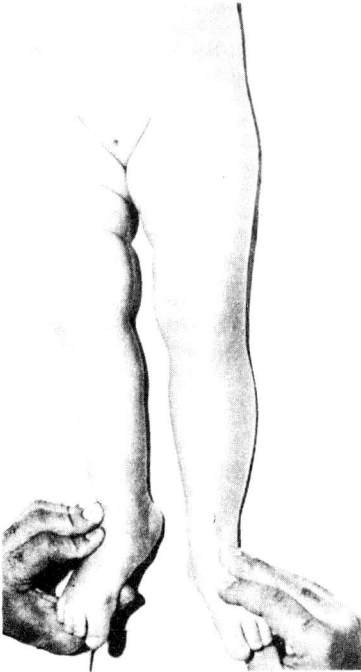

Fig. 77 Dislocation of the right hip. Note the apparent shortness of the right leg and the asymmetrical skin creases.

241

Trendelenburg sign.

Abnormal gait:

    Unilateral: Limp due to apparent shortness and lateral hip instability.

    Bilateral: Waddling gait due to lateral hip instability.

MANAGEMENT

Treatment is usually conservative. If this is unsuccessful surgery may be necessary. In both cases, the object is to reduce the dislocation and maintain its reduction with minimum trauma to the head of the femur and the soft tissues around the hip joint. Orthopaedic treatment varies from one paediatric centre to another, and is described in detail by Ferguson (1968), Lloyd-Roberts (1971) and Sharrard (1971). It may consist of one or more of the following modalities.

Traction

Weight traction with skin extensions may be employed to reduce the dislocation. The hips are gradually moved into a position of wide abduction in either flexion or extension.

Splinting

There are several forms of splinting in use: double nappies, Frejka pillow, Von Rosen splint, Pavlek harness, Denis Browne hip splint, plaster hip spica in Lorenz' position. Some of these are described in detail below.

Frejka pillow (figure 78)

This consists of a moulded piece of firm rubber or felt, covered with waterproof material. The pillow is enclosed in a jacket into which the child is fitted, the pillow fitting between his legs, holding them in abduction and flexion to 90 degrees. The pillow itself extends from the lumbar spine posteriorly to the umbilicus anteriorly. This splint is an alternative to double nappies and may be prescribed for a small infant with unstable or subluxated hips.

Von Rosen splint (figure 79)

This splint also holds the baby's legs in flexion and abduction to 90 degrees, and is used particularly for the young infant with either dislocation or instability of the hip. It allows movement in a small range at the hip with the joint always returning to the required position. The parents are taught to care for the baby's skin under the splint, making sure there are no pressure areas.

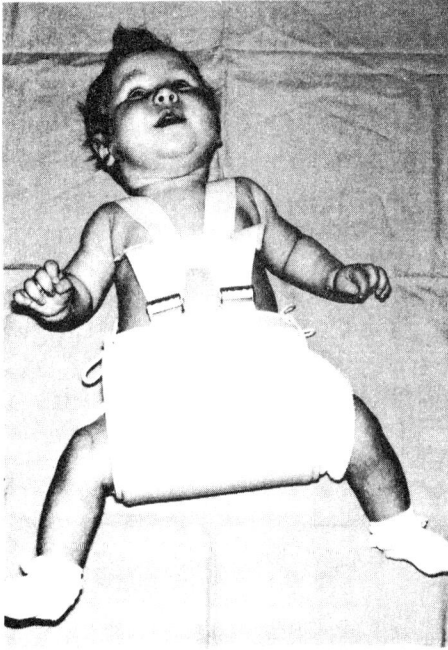

Fig. 78 Frejka pillow.
(By permission of W. Cumming).

Denis Browne hip splint (figures 80 and 81)

This splint also holds the hips in flexion and abduction, and permits a small amount of movement at the hips. When the child is old enough he can crawl and some children even learn to walk in their splints. The parents are taught how to care for the child's skin.

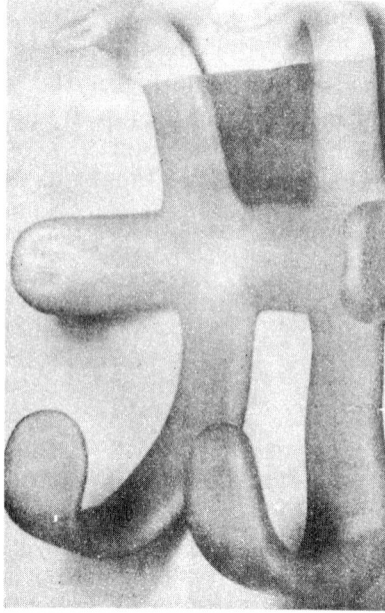

Fig. 79 Von Rosen splint.
(By permission of W. Cumming.)

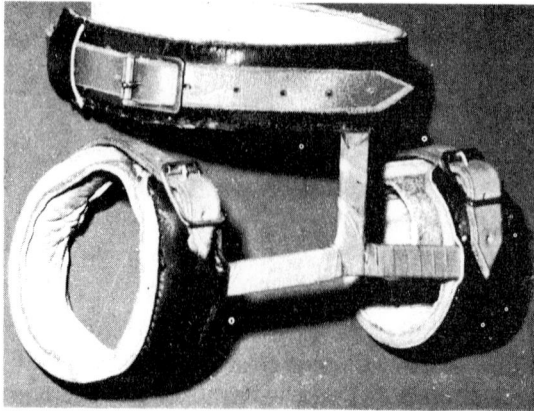

Fig. 80 Denis Browne hip splint.

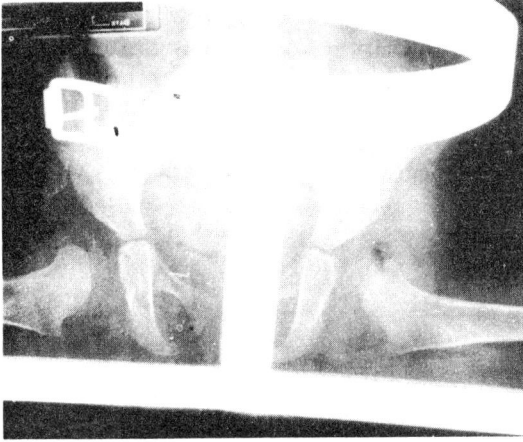

Fig. 81 Radiograph demonstrates the reduction of the dislocation gained in the Denis Browne hip splint.

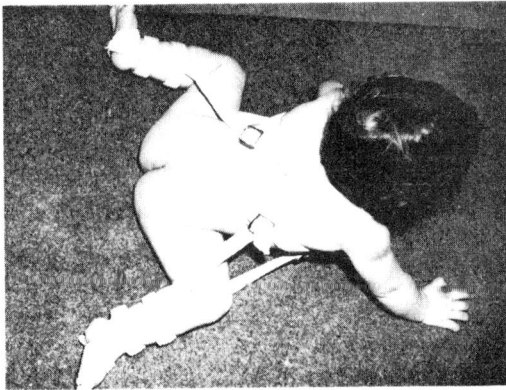

Fig. 82 Pavlek harness.
(By permission of W. Cumming.)

Pavlek harness (figure 82)

This webbing harness also holds the hips in flexion and abduction, and allows the child to crawl about.

Plaster hip spica (figure 83)

This is a frequently used method of splinting babies and young children with dislocated hips. It is usually applied under general anaesthesia and is preceded by a few weeks spent in weight traction in order that tight soft tissues around the hip may be stretched, and in order to avoid trauma to the blood supply of the femur by a forced manipulation. If the hip adductors are still contracted when the child is anaesthetized and ready for the plaster, a closed tenotomy is performed by the surgeon.

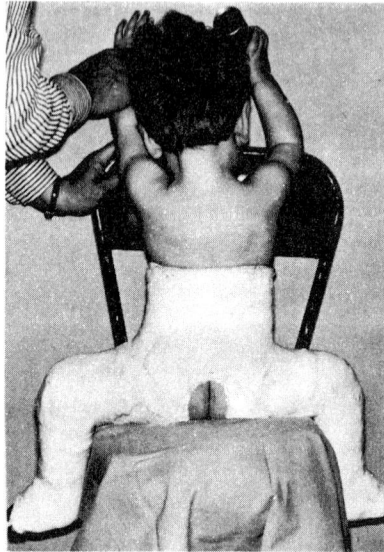

Fig. 83 Plaster spica ('frog' plaster).
(By permission of W. Cumming).

Materials

4 inch and 6 inch wide plaster bandages.
Wool bandages.
Sacral rest and box.
Knife or plaster shears.
Basins with warm water.

Method

Two people are required for the application of this plaster.

Step 1. The child is placed in supine on the box, his sacral area on the rest, his hips flexed and abducted to 90 degrees (Lorenz' position). Three plaster slabs are made of six thicknesses each from the 4 inch bandages. These slabs are to reinforce the anterior and posterior nursing holes and the areas which are most likely to take strain. Slab A must be long enough to pass from the middle of one knee to the middle of the other with the child's legs in the position described above. This slab has a semi-oval piece cut out which will form the anterior part of the nursing hole. Slabs B and C must be long enough to pass from the waist anteriorly down along the edge of the nursing area and up posteriorly to cross above the nursing area in the sacral region.

Step 2. While the slabs are being made, the wool bandage is placed around the child from as high as the nipple line down to the knee. The wool must not be too thick but must cover the skin completely in order to prevent pressure areas.

Step 3. Wet circular bandages are now applied from the nipple line to the knees, covering the trunk and thighs. Care must be taken not to crease or gather the bandages into folds as these may cause pressure areas, particularly in the popliteal fossae and on the lateral aspects of the hips.

Step 4. The slabs are now applied in order as above (figure 84).

Step 5. These slabs are held in place by more circular bandages. The plaster must be applied swiftly and the plaster cream well rubbed in to bind the bandages together and ensure a strong splint. The circulars are extended down to the malleoli. Some surgeons continue plaster to the webs of the toes.

Step 6. The nursing hole will have to be carefully trimmed with plaster shears or a knife. It must not be too large or the hip position will not be maintained. If it is too small the edges will become wet and soiled. Finally the wool may be turned down around the nursing area, the thorax and legs, and is held neatly in place with a plaster bandage or with waterproof adhesive strapping. This ensures that it is the wool which comes in contact with the patient's skin and not a sharp plaster edge.

Step 7. When the plaster is dry a waterproof plastic material may be applied which helps prevent disintegration of the plaster in the event of sometimes unavoidable wetting.

The child is nursed on a special wooden frame with a basin underneath the nursing area to collect urine. The head of the bed is slightly tilted to prevent urine from running backwards into the plaster. The older child needs a special chair for sitting in at home, and a stroller to make it easier for his mother to move him about.

247

His parents are taught correct lifting techniques for their own protection, as the weight of child plus plaster may be considerable. The child may also move himself about with the aid of a trolley on castors. Carpenter (1970) describes some suitable equipment.

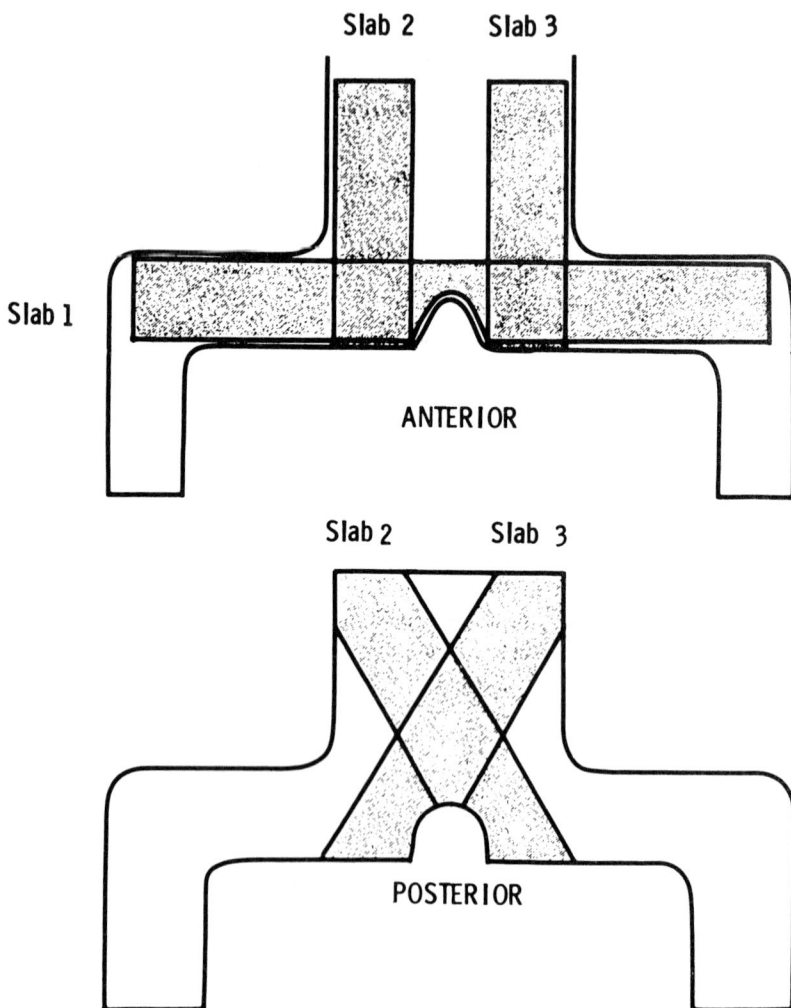

Fig. 84 Diagram showing the application of slabs for a hip spica plaster. (See figure 83.)

Precautions

The child is put on a plaster chart in the ward and his circulation is checked at regular intervals for the first 24 hours and then rechecked at 24-hour intervals. If the plaster inhibits respiration by being too tight or too high around the thorax it must be cut down a little to relieve the pressure.

Splinting is continued until the surgeon considers the hips will remain reduced. This decision is made with the aid of X-rays which show that the acetabulum is covering the femoral head sufficiently well to prevent it from redislocating. Plaster splinting may be followed by a period in a Denis Brown hip splint. If conservative measures such as those outlined above are unsuccessful, surgery may be necessary to realign the angle of weight-bearing or to reconstruct the superior aspect of the acetabulum. Surgery is described in detail by Salter (1961) and Sharrard (1971).

Physical treatment

It is unusual for a baby or small child to require extensive physiotherapy when splinting is removed. Small children do not suffer the stiffness and lack of function that follow long periods of splinting in adults. If a child is stiff or frightened of moving following a period spent in a plaster hip spica, mobilization can be encouraged in a warm pool, and full-range movement is more gently and safely achieved in this way than by vigorous exercise which may place an undue strain on the reduced hip.

SUMMARY

The physiotherapist should be able to test for hip dislocation whenever she finds suspicious signs, such as apparent shortening in one leg or limited abduction at the hip, in the babies she is treating. The place of physical treatment in the management of subluxation or dislocation lies in the application of splinting, and the explanation of care to the baby's parents, rather than in any specific exercise programme.

References

Carpenter, E. M. (1970) Equipment for children in plaster. *Occupational Therapy*, **35**, 10.

Ferguson, A. B. (1968) *Orthopaedic Surgery in Infancy and Childhood.* Baltimore: Williams and Wilkins.

Illingworth, R. S. (1970) *The Development of the Infant and Young Child.* London: Livingstone.

Lloyd-Roberts, G. C. (1971) *Orthopaedics in Infancy and Childhood.* London: Butterworth.

Salter, R. B. (1961) Innominate osteotomy in the treatment of congenital dislocation and subluxation of the hip. *J. Bone Jt. Surg.* **43B**, 518.

Sharrard, W. J. W. (1971) *Paediatric Orthopaedics and Fractures.* Oxford and Edinburgh: Blackwell.

Further Reading

Barlow, T. G. (1966) Congenital dislocation of the hip in the new-born. Early diagnosis and treatment of dislocation of the hip in the newborn. *Proc. Roy. Soc. Med.* **59**, 1, 103.

Hass, J. (1951) *Congenital Dislocation of the Hip.* Illinois: Thomas.

Lloyd-Roberts, G. C. (1967) The hip joint and pelvis. In *Clinical Surgery — Orthopaedics.* London: Butterworth.

Rosen, S. Von (1962) Diagnosis and treatment of congenital dislocation of the hip in the newborn. *J. Bone Jt. Surg.* **44B**, 284.

Chapter 4

Arthrogryposis Multiplex Congenita

DESCRIPTION

The infant is born with multiple and often grotesque deformities and contractures. The pattern will vary from child to child, but the infant may demonstrate talipes equinovarus, flexed or extended knees, flexed hips either abducted or adducted, clubbed and clawed hands, flexed or extended elbows, adducted shoulders. The joints are held rigidly in these positions. This is a non-progressive disorder, but the degree of deformity is frequently very severe. The joints appear at first sight to be involved, however there is no bony ankylosis although there are thickened inelastic joint capsules (Walton 1969). The deformities appear to be due to the absence of muscles, to their replacement by fibrous tissue, or to muscle imbalance *in utero*

AETIOLOGY

This is a relatively uncommon disorder, and its aetiology is unknown. Cases of congenital hypotonia and severe but non-progressive muscle weakness with histology typical of muscular dystrophy have been found to have associated arthrogryposis (Pearson and Fowler 1963). Other cases have been found at autopsy to lack anterior horn cells in spinal cord segments which correspond to the paralysed muscles. This has led to a classification in which these children with their congenital deformities are grouped under the two headings of neuropathic and myopathic arthrogryposis (Adams, Denny Brown & Pearson 1962).

MANAGEMENT

The deformities with which these children are born are extremely

251

difficult to correct as they tend to be rigid, and maintenance of correction is difficult because of lack of muscle power. However, if they are treated early enough with passive mobilizing and splinting, and if this is followed by mobilizing or reconstructive surgery, many of these children will make surprisingly good progress. It is very worthwhile for the phsyiotherapist to spend time in mobilizing these infants, although it does involve a great deal of time as so many deformities are involved. Many of these children are intelligent and have good personalities, and with help and encouragement may accomplish far more as they grow older than would have seemed possible when they were infants.

Physical Treatment

This aspect of treatment consists of stretching the tightened soft tissues, gentle mobilizing of joints, encouragement of active limb and trunk movements and assistance with the attaining of normal milestones, with progressive splinting to maintain the correction gained. This regime should be pursued as intensively as possible, especially during the child's first year, but it is likely that he will need treatment and support at least until he is employed, then assistance when necessary during the rest of his life.

His parents' help is enlisted in carrying out the above treatment at home. The mobilizing techniques and stretching should be done for short periods several times a day, although the physiotherapist must take care not to be too demanding of the parents' time. Care should be taken to teach them how to be gentle and effective in their treatment, and they will need encouragement to be patient, for results are slow to be gained.

Severe talipes equinovarus may be splinted with medial plaster splints, progressing as soon as possible to strapping which allows the physiotherapist and parents to mobilize the foot. Rigid splinting is avoided where possible, the emphasis being on mobility. Prone lying is encouraged as soon as practicable, to stretch the structures anterior to the hip, or to maintain hip extension after surgery to correct hip flexion deformity.

All splints and calipers should be as light and unencumbering as possible, so the child will be less likely to reject them, and will have as little extra weight to lift as possible without limiting effectiveness.

Where deformity makes it difficult for the child to play, and to explore both the environment and himself, he will need assistance, and this part of his management could be taken over by the occupational therapist. Toys may have to be altered or specially designed, self-feeding may be taught using adjusted tools, and time spent by both therapists in encouraging the child in his explorative activities.

Surgical Treatment

Reconstructive surgery will eventually be needed in the majority of cases, but probably not until as much movement as possible has been gained by conservative means. Capsulotomy of the structures posterior to the knee and elongation of the tendo Achilles are commonly done to release soft tissue tightness, while reconstructive surgery is often necessary to correct resistant talipes equinovarus and other limb deformities. Dislocated hips are treated by traction, adduction tenotomy, release of a tight psoas muscle, and splinting, or if necessary, open reduction of the hips with iliopsoas transplant, if hip extensors are nonfunctioning. Surgery for the upper limbs is usually not attempted until the child's future needs can be in some measure assessed, although self-feeding remains a major target, and the child with extended arms will need surgery to give him sufficient flexion to enable him to get his hands to his mouth.

SUMMARY

The infant with arthrogryposis demonstrates a picture of congenital abnormalities consistent with intrauterine neurological or muscular pathology. The role of the physiotherapist lies in the correction of the deformities by physical methods, frequently in conjunction with surgical correction, and in encouraging the most normal development possible for the child.

References

Adams, R. D., Denny Brown, D. and Pearson, C. M. (1962) *Diseases of Muscle; a Study in Pathology.* New York: Hoeber.
Pearson, C. M., and Fowler, W. G. (1963) Hereditary

non-progressive muscular dystrophy including arthrogryposis syndrome. *Brain*, **86**, 75.

Walton, J. N. (1969) *Disorders of Voluntary Muscles.* Baltimore: Williams and Wilkins.

Further Reading

Drachman, D. B. and Banker, B. Q. (1961) Arthrogryposis multiplex congenita. *Arch. Neurol.* **5**, 77.

Dubowitz, V. (1970) The myopathies. *Physiotherapy*, **56**, 4, 384.

Ferguson, A. B. (1968) *Orthopaedic Surgery in Infancy and Childhood.* Baltimore: Williams and Wilkins.

Friedlander, H. L., Westin, G. W. and Wood, W. L. (1968) Arthrogryposis multiplex congenita. *J. Bone Jt. Surg* **50A**, 89.

Lloyd-Roberts, G. C. (1971) *Orthopaedics in Infancy and Childhood.* London: Butterworth.

Lloyd-Roberts, G. C. and Lettin, A. W. F. (1970) Arthrogryposis multiplex congenita. *J. Bone Jt. Surg.* **52B**, 494.

Mead, N. G., Lithgow, W. C. and Sweeney, H. J. (1958) Arthrogryposis multiplex congenita. *J. Bone Jt. Surg.* **40A**, 1285.

Sharrard, W. J. W. (1971) *Paediatric Orthopaedics and Fractures.* Oxford and Edinburgh: Blackwell.

Chapter 5

Spina Bifida

DESCRIPTION

Spina bifida is a congenital abnormality in which there is a developmental defect in the spinal column with incomplete closure of the vertebral canal due to a failure of fusion of the vertebral arches. There may or may not be protrusion and dysplasia of the spinal cord or its membranes.

The primary developmental defect is thought to occur in the neural tube before its closure is complete (Patten 1953), with the vertebral malformation occurring secondarily. The defect must therefore arise within the first few weeks of gestation, but whether the cause is genetic or environmental is unknown.

Spina bifida is the commonest of the major congenital abnormalities, comprising between one and two per 1,000 liveborn babies (Durham Smith 1965, Lorber 1968). It is possible that there are other manifestations of this myelodysplasia, although without the vertebral abnormality. These may include some cases of talipes equinovarus, congenitally dislocated hips and arthrogryposis (Sharrard 1971).

CLASSIFICATION

A number of varieties of spina bifida have been described. The following classification is from Durham Smith (1965).

Spina Bifida Occulta

The vertebral arches are unfused, however there is no herniation or displacement of the meninges. Skin changes over the defect, pathological changes in the spinal cord, and therefore neurological signs, may or may not be present.

Spina Bifida Cystica

Meningocele. The vertebral arches are unfused and there is herniation of the meninges. Neither myelodysplasia of the spinal cord nor neurological signs are present. Part of the cord or nerve roots may be present in the sac but if so they conduct impulses normally (figure 85).

MENINGOCOELE

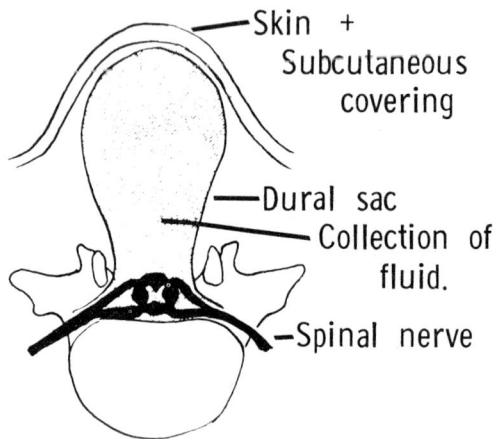

Fig. 85 Diagram of the defect in meningocele.

Myelomeningocele. There is herniation of the meninges as in meningocele, but there is also an associated abnormal development of the spinal cord and neurological signs (figure 86).

It is the child with myelomeningocele who most concerns the physiotherapist. However, occasionally a child with neurological signs arising from spina bifida occulta may be referred for treatment.

The commonest site of myelomeningocele is the lumbosacral region, although it may occur elsewhere in the spine, and as surgical skill improves increasing numbers of children with this defect are surviving. Durham Smith (1965) notes that 'with the declining incidence of poliomyelitis and tuberculous bone and joint diseases, myelomeningocele now stands second only in

256

importance to cerebral palsy as a cause of chronic locomotor disability in childhood.'

The discussion which follows is devoted to children suffering from myelomeningocele. The problems involved will be examined and suggestions made for the management of these children, who are increasingly to occupy the time and thoughts, not only of

MYELOMENINGOCOELE

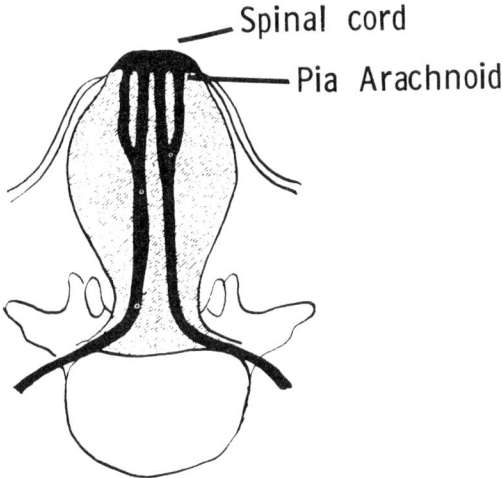

Fig. 86 Diagram of the defect in myelomeningocele.

physiotherapists in the field of paediatrics, but also of other physiotherapists who may play a part in the habilitation of these children and their eventual entry into an active adult world.

PATHOLOGY OF MYELOMENINGOCELE

The spinal cord

Evident in the myelomeningocele mass at birth is a neural plaque containing spinal cord tissue. Some anterior and posterior horn cells may be recognizable histologically and may have connections with muscles which can be shown by faradic stimulation. Nerve roots and posterior root ganglia are often well formed. The spinal cord may be tethered low in the vertebral canal and the nerve roots will then pass laterally to their foramina instead of caudally.

The spinal cord is abnormal in every case. The dysplasic changes usually extend below the level of the main myelomeningocele mass, which means that if the mass is in the lumbar or sacral region, the dysplasia may extend down to the conus medullaris. If the cord is dysplasic below the level of the main mass there will be no anterior horn cells intact. As the final common pathway is interrupted there will be no stretch reflex reaction and hence the lower motor neurone flaccidity usually found in these children. However, if part of the cord is intact below the level of the lesion there may be some anterior horn cells intact, and these children will show some signs of spasticity. This manifestation of an upper motor neurone lesion will be due to the interruption of descending inhibitory and facilitatory pathways which normally exercise control from the brain upon the anterior horn cells. Spasticity in these cases is usually isolated to particular muscle groups, such as the hip, and knee flexors.

The vertebrae

Lamina growth is apparently arrested at various stages, some vertebrae showing a failure of laminae and spines to fuse posteriorly, others showing a failure of the laminae to develop at all.

The skin

The skin is rarely intact over the lesion. The myelomeningocele mass shows itself as a raised mass on the back, covered laterally and at its base by normal skin, the summit of the mass being devoid of skin (figure 87). The surface may appear ulcerated and granulated. The dura mater is usually fused with the edges of the skin defect, the sac being covered by arachnoid membrane only.

The cerebrospinal fluid

Over 80 per cent of infants born with myelomeningocele are said to have an associated hydrocephalus. A common cause is the Arnold-Chiari malformation in which there is displacement of a tongue of cerebellar tissue comprising the inferior part of the cerebellar vermis and an elongated medulla oblongata into the cervical part of the spinal canal via the foramen magnum. This causes hydrocephalus by obstructing the flow of cerebrospinal fluid from the fourth ventricle into the cerebral subarachnoid space, so interfering with its absorption. Distension of the cerebral ventricles occurs leading to pressure on the bones of the skull which become thin. The cranial sutures separate, the anterior fontanelle enlarges and there is marked congestion of the veins of the scalp. However, signs of increased intracranial pressure are usually minor due to the expansibility of the skull in infancy. In uncontrolled hydrocephalus, neurological signs become evident as the child develops, and there will almost certainly be a degree of mental as well as motor retardation as a result.

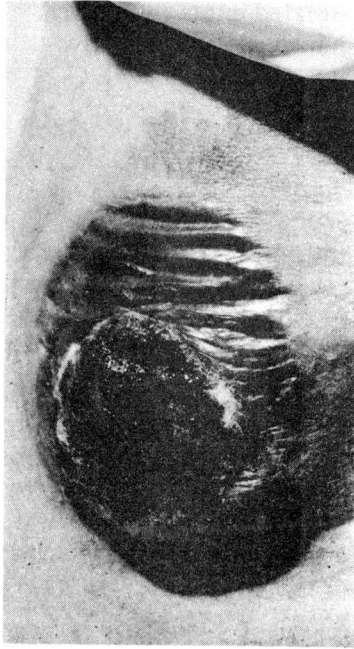

Fig. 87 Myelomeningocele mass in newborn baby. Note the central area devoid of skin.

CLINICAL FEATURES

The clinical features seen in these children vary according to the level of the lesion. The commonest site of myelomeningocele is the lumbosacral region. The clinical features evident in the infant and young child with a lumbosacral myelomeningocele are:

Flaccid paralysis.
Muscle weakness.
Muscle wasting.
Decreased or absent tendon reflexes.
Decreased or absent exteroceptive and proprioceptive sensation.
Rectal and bladder incontinence.
Paralytic and congenital deformities.
Hydrocephalus.

As well as the above features, children with lumbar or thoracic lesions may demonstrate spasticity in isolated muscle groups due to the influence of isolated intact reflex arcs.

Eventually secondary clinical features will almost certainly develop:

Pressure ulceration of the skin due to absent sensation and poor skin nutrition.
Severe vasomotor changes.
Osteoporosis with probability of fractures.
Retarded mental, physical and emotional development due to the child's inability to move about and explore his environment, to play normally and to inter-relate with other children.
Soft tissue contractures and eventual skeletal deformity, due to unopposed muscle action, gravity and posture.

Associated with the congenital malformation of the spine and spinal cord there may be other congenital abnormalities such as dislocated hips, talipes equinovarus, hemivertebrae with resultant scoliosis, local kyphosis due to the vertebral anomaly, hare lip, cleft palate, cardiac and urinary tract abnormalities.

THE PROBLEMS INVOLVED AND THEIR MANAGEMENT

The problems involved in this gross congenital disorder are extremely complex and cannot be considered in isolation. Their management requires the co-operation of a large team of people, the child and his parents, a neurosurgeon, urologist, psychiatrist, physiotherapist, social worker and orthopaedic surgeon. The problems will be described under the following headings:

The myelomeningocele mass.
Hydrocephalus.

Social and psychological factors.
Incontinence of bladder and bowel.
Deformity.
Absence of sensation.
Disorder of movement.

The myelomeningocele mass
Surgery to repair the defect is usually performed within the first few hours of birth, usually within the first 24 hours. This is thought (Sharrard, Zachary, and Lorber 1967) to minimize the risk of ascending meningitis and of further damage to the spinal cord with resultant paralysis. During the surgery as much of the neurological tissue as possible is conserved and the defect is covered with dura mater and sound skin.

Hydrocephalus
If the hydrocephalus is uncontrolled the infant will suffer eventual brain damage and will not survive. If he does survive for a few years he will be severely retarded mentally and physically. However, many of these children now have surgery to control the hydrocephalus, and there are many methods of draining the cerebrospinal fluid which are currently in use. Some involve drainage of the cerebrospinal fluid from a cerebral ventricle to the atrium of the heart by means of a silicone rubber tube. The tube passes down to the heart in one of the veins of the neck. A valve is incorporated into the system which will only open in one direction therefore allowing fluid to flow down to the heart but preventing blood from flowing back into the brain. The valves open only when pressure in the ventricles becomes elevated. This apparatus reduces the abnormally high pressure within the cranium to within more normal limits. As the child grows the tube will be replaced by a longer one. Surgery may also be necessary to revise the shunt should the tube become blocked by growing brain tissue. This blockage will cause the pressure within the cranium to rise and the child will become drowsy, develop a headache, vomit, fit or lose consciousness.

Even when the hydrocephalus is controlled the weight of the enlarged head will make head control slow to develop in the infant, and the child's general motor development will be correspondingly slowed. He will sit later than usual, balance may be slower to achieve, his mental and emotional development will also be slower than normal. Many of these children show some degree of mental subnormality despite control of their hydrocephalus. It appears that a major factor in influencing the intelligence of children with spina bifida is the development of hydrocephalus.

Social and Psychological Factors

The parents

After the child is born the immediate problem for the parents is one of acceptance of the child who is often the first born. There may be feelings of resentment or guilt, or a sense of inadequacy with regard to the problems ahead. There will be an atmosphere of sorrow around the birth of this child, where the parents had expected only joy. At this time the parents are seen by the social worker and by the doctor in charge of treatment, who will be able to give them some idea of what lies ahead, of the treatment required, and any other counselling that may be necessary in order to allay fear and anxiety.

Practical problems for the parents will include the expense of medical and hospital care, with apparatus by no means a small consideration. There is the problem of schooling and eventual habilitation. There is the fear of having further afflicted children. The other children in the family may be neglected by parents who feel the need to spend extra time with the disabled child. Parents will have to take care not to overfeed the disabled child, who, being relatively inactive, may become increasingly obese as he grows older.

There is a profound stress on all those who come in contact with this child, and it is one of the responsibilities of the physiotherapist to watch for signs of mounting anxiety in the family and to refer them where they will find help. The physiotherapist, because she spends so much time in the company of the child and his mother, has the opportunity of developing a close relationship with them, and she may herself allay some of the mother's anxiety, especially at the time when the child is learning to walk, by counselling patience, and by giving encouragement. An atmosphere of hopefulness should prevail at all times. Parents who have a realistic attitude of hope towards their child will be more willing to develop and adopt apparatus for him to use and toys for him to play with, and will realize how important is the stimulus to development which they can give the child.

Parents' associations have been formed in many countries where the abnormality is prevalent. These associations provide help, both social and economic, to their members, and most of them issue booklets or newsheets which explain the child's problems in nonmedical language, and contain helpful, practical hints (Lorber 1968b).

The child

Bowlby (1953) and others have shown that long periods of hospitalization result in deprivation of the infant and young child. This may be manifested by extreme apathy in the infant, and either apathy or aggression in the young child. As soon as his general condition allows, the infant should be picked up, nursed and talked to. Particular care should be taken when lifting him up to support his head and neck, because of his enlarged head and his lack of head control. He should not be left lying in his cot all day, with no stimulus of any kind. Colourful mobiles can be hung over his bed, close enough for him to see and reach. Even the young infant will respond to shapes made from tin foil as these move about and reflect the light. Where possible the infant's mother is admitted to hospital in order to help look after him.

Those who come in contact with the young child in hospital will take care to maintain as far as possible links with home and parents, by talking about them, by asking questions, and by finding out from his parents about his favourite toys and games.

When the child is discharged home it is suggested that he be brought for physiotherapy only as often as is necessary for his mother to be taught a home programme, which will change from month to month as he develops. As much of his treatment as possible is carried out at home. He will need intensive physiotherapy only when he is starting to stand and walk, after orthopaedic surgery, or if he has severe deformity.

The child's ability to learn about the world around him, and his ability to develop as an individual may be impaired by his difficulty in gaining head control, in developing balance in the sitting and standing positions, in moving from place to place, and in his lack of sensation. One has only to watch a normal child of 12 months scrambling over and under the furniture, reaching up into cupboards and pulling the contents down on top of himself, to realize how deprived of experience of the world the disabled child may be. Whether or not the child is mentally retarded, and a number of these children are, there is probably a degree of secondary mental retardation due to this inability to learn in a normal and uninhibited manner. Keeping up with other children, both mentally and physically, is one of his greatest problems. He needs great perseverence in order to do things which come naturally to other children. His learning may be further impaired by the failure of his parents to encourage in him a suitable independence.

Physically and mentally the child may be neglected by parents who have not the ability to cope with the situation, because it is after all a situation which demands a great deal from them. The child may develop pressure areas, or may be deprived, through his parents' lack of understanding of his needs, of contact with other children. These problems can sometimes be anticipated by the physiotherapist and talked over with the parents and with the social worker. Unfortunately in some cases the parents cannot cope with the strain of caring for their child and prefer him to be looked after in a special residential school.

As the child grows and develops he has to try to understand and to come to terms with his disabilities, according to his gradually broadening horizons, and there will be certain times when encouragement and support are more particularly needed. The doctor in charge of his treatment, or some other suitable person from the team looking after his management should set aside time for talking to the child at different stages as he grows up, particularly as he approaches adolescence. The child will know that there is someone of whom he can ask questions about his future, about his sexual function, the possibility of marriage and family life, and other questions about which he may need to talk.

These children often have what Durham Smith (1965) calls a brittle mental capacity, tending to be less adaptable to stresses and strains than other children. They often lack confidence, tend to be emotionally immature and to become very dependent. The handling of these children, particularly during their infancy and early childhood, is most important if they are to develop in a way which will allow them to live a happy and relatively independent life.

From his early infancy his parents are encouraged to handle him as far as possible as they would a normal child. By this is meant that he should be enabled to develop as many as possible of the normal milestones. It has been found in many cases much easier to teach a child to walk at 18 months than to wait until he is four or five years old and has lost the urge to walk which is so strong in the baby's second year. When these children are incapable of moving around by themselves their curiosity should be aroused as much as possible, and they need to be taught even such simple spatial concepts as being 'under' a table or 'in' a box. A padded board fitted with castors (figure 88) will allow a child to lie in prone and propel himself along the floor with his arms. The

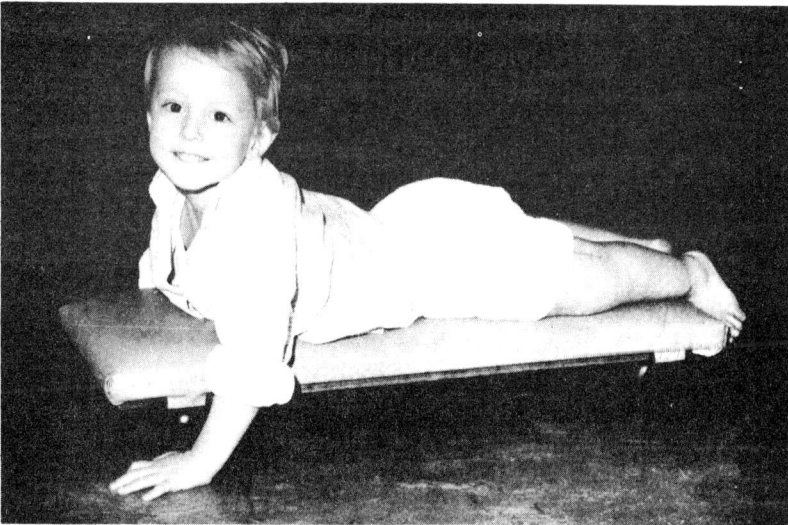

Fig. 88 Prone scooter. This encourages head and trunk extension and allows the non-ambulant child to be mobile.

Chailey Chariot (figure 89) or the Shasbah trolley which was adapted from it, were designed to enable these children to move about by themselves in the sitting position.

Although the chariot is a useful way of enabling the child to get about, it has one serious disadvantage. The child who spends a large part of his day in the sitting position, with his knees extended, quickly develops increased hip flexor contractures (particularly of iliopsoas and rectus femoris). Some degree of hip flexor contracture may well be impossible to prevent in many of these children. Nevertheless the child who uses a chariot should have his day carefully planned to include activities to counteract this tendency.

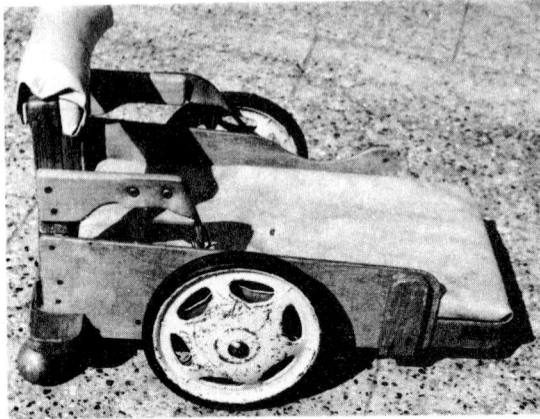

Fig. 89 The Chailey Chariot. Another means of gaining mobility for the non-ambulant child. (By permission of Chailey Heritage, Sussex, England.)

The child should be given the experience of moving through space and of falling, all with as little fear as possible. The child can be placed on top of a large ball, in sitting or in lying, with movement of the ball to stimulate his righting and equilibrium reactions and give him the pleasure of movement. A roller (figure 93) or a balance board is also a useful piece of equipment for improving confidence and balance in sitting and eventually in standing.

If fear is to be avoided great care must be taken during these and similar activities, because if he is seriously frightened, it will take much time and patience to restore his confidence, both in himself and in his physiotherapist.

Incontinence of bladder and bowel

The bladder is normally innervated from the sacral segments of the cord, therefore it is commonly paralysed in these children, particularly if the lesion is lumbosacral. These children suffer from overflow incontinence, which means that the bladder never completely empties, urine dribbling from it as it becomes full. The child does not have any sensation of fullness as he receives no sensory feedback from the denervated bladder.

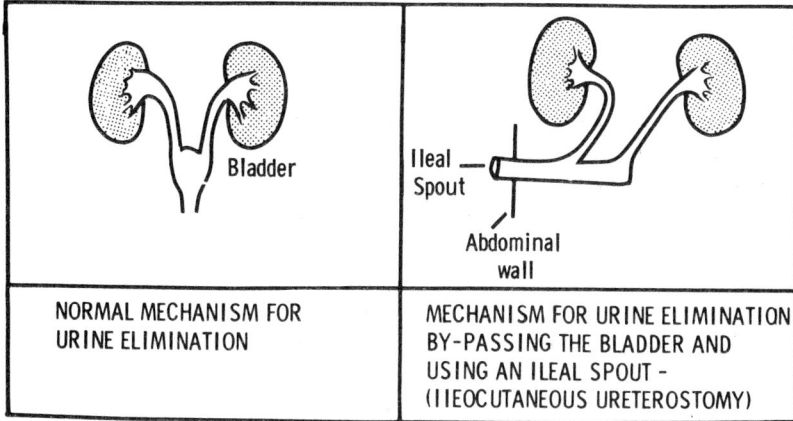

Fig. 90 Diagram of an ileocutaneous ureterostomy showing the means by which urine is diverted directly from the kidneys via an ileal conduit, thus by-passing the bladder.

Although boys may be fitted with collecting devices, many children now have an ileocutaneous ureterostomy or ileal loop diversion operation, afterwards wearing a bag in which urine is collected. This surgery (figure 90) involves the diversion of urine direct from the ureters, via a piece of ileum, to the skin, thereby bypassing the bladder. A primary cause of urinary tract infection is therefore avoided as urine can no longer be retained in the flaccid bladder leading to infection which may track back to the kidneys. Retention of urine in a paralysed bladder contributes to urinary tract infection and this is considered to be the greatest threat to the child's life after hydrocephalus has been controlled.

If one of the procedures above is not utilized, the child is condemned to an anti-social life in wet nappies, which is distressing both to him and to his parents, and which proves a great psychological handicap for the whole family.

In the period between infancy and the age when urological

surgery is performed regular manual expression of the bladder may be required. The child lies with his hips and knees flexed to take tension from his abdominal muscles and a dish is placed to collect the urine. Pressure is applied gently and firmly with the hand in a downwards and backwards direction. This is repeated until the bladder appears empty. Some consider that this procedure carries a risk of causing a back pressure on the kidneys and do not recommend it for these children.

If the child has a urinary diversion operation the collecting bag is held in place by a belt. Unfortunately this belt is sometimes a cause of pressure areas around the waist, especially in hot climates, but these may be prevented by lining the belt with lambswool. The child is taught to care for and empty his urinary apparatus himself when he is old enough. Once the apparatus is fitting correctly there is no reason why the child should not be allowed to go swimming, although he or his parents must make sure the bag is emptied before he goes into the pool.

Bowel-training presents few problems with most children. Despite the flaccid bowel, with perseverence on the part of his parents, the child will usually manage a regular bowel evacuation. His diet may need to be regulated to prevent either constipation or loose stools, and many children need to take an aperient regularly. A few children are difficult to train. A child may appear to have loose stools because he dribbles faeces throughout the day, but this may instead be caused by chronic constipation, and should therefore be corrected by an aperient rather than by an anti-dysenteric. Sometimes the failure in bowel-training can be due to the rush of the early morning, as the mother tries to get the family fed and off to work and school, as well as trying to find time to toilet-train her disabled child. In these cases it can be suggested that there is no reason why the child's bowel action should take place in the morning, and he should be trained in the evening instead, when there may be more time.

Deformity

Deformities in these children are common, difficult to treat and may be so severe as to hold back the child's developmental progress. Secondary deformities may not be as severe as congenital unless they are left untreated for a long period of time. Once a deformity has become established, it will progress, eventually becoming fixed as the child develops. One of the most severe deformities in a large number of infants is the kyphosis noticed from birth in the region of the spina bifida. It is progressive as the child grows, with a compensatory lordosis developing above the kyphosis. The erector spinae, because of their relatively anterior position, act as flexors and add a further deforming force.

A true congenital dislocation of the hip may be seen in these children as in otherwise normal children. An arthrogrypotic type of fixed talipes equinovarus deformity is also seen in some children with myelomeningocele and is very resistant to conservative treatment. Figure 91 shows a list of acquired deformities and their possible causative factors.

It seems that a number of the deformities mentioned could be prevented by intensive care from the child's birth onwards. He may be born with certain deformities due to muscle imbalance, such as talipes equinovarus, but there is no need for these to become worse, and indeed they should begin to improve from the day treatment starts. Deformities due to unopposed muscle action and posture which will develop as the child develops and moves about can very often be prevented by conservative means in infancy, followed by surgery to correct the imbalance when the child is old enough.

A muscle chart is done soon after the baby's birth (figure 92) from which can be established any potential deformities which may occur due to the baby's particular distribution of paralysis. From then on, prevention is a matter of foresight and care.

His mother is taught how to give the baby daily treatment, consisting of full range passive movements, stimulation of active corrective movements, where these exist, and the application and care of light plaster splints where these are necessary to prevent deformity due to unopposed muscle action. A small cradle or a pillow at the end of the bed will prevent the bedclothes pushing a flail or calcaneus foot into equinus. When the baby's mother is taught how to do passive movements, care must be taken to teach her the normal range of movement in order that she will not be too enthusiastic and damage the soft tissues around the joint. It is unwise to expect the mother to do these movements after only minimum instruction and the physiotherapist should spread her teaching over a reasonable period of time depending on the mother's skill.

```
┌─────────────────────────────────────────────────────────────┐
│ Feet.                                                         │
│                                                               │
│ Weakness or paralysis of                                      │
│ gastrocnemius and soleus    ────►   Calcaneo-valgus or        │
│ with active anterior                calcaneo-varus deformity. │
│ tibial muscles.                                               │
│                                                               │
│ Weakness or paralysis of                                      │
│ anterior tibial muscles     ────►   Equinovarus deformity.    │
│ and evertors.                                                 │
│                                                               │
│ Unopposed lumbrical action. ────►   Flexion deformity of      │
│                                     metatarso-phalangeal      │
│                                     joints                    │
│                                                               │
│ Total lower limb paralysis          Equinus deformity with    │
│ + pressure of bedclothes +  ────►   flexion at the metatarso- │
│ gravity.                            phalangeal joints and     │
│                                     tarso-metatarsal joints.  │
│                                                               │
│ Uncorrected calcaneus                                         │
│ deformity + pressure of     ────►   Flexion deformity of      │
│ bedclothes + gravity.               fore-foot.                │
├─────────────────────────────────────────────────────────────┤
│ Knees.                                                        │
│                                                               │
│ Unopposed sartorius action                                    │
│ leading to a lower limb     ────►   Flexion deformity.        │
│ posture of flexion, abduction                                 │
│ and external rotation.                                        │
│                                                               │
│ Unopposed hip flexion and   ────►   Flexion deformity.        │
│ adduction.                                                    │
│                                                               │
│ Unopposed quadriceps action.────►   Hyperextension deformity. │
├─────────────────────────────────────────────────────────────┤
│ Hips.                                                         │
│                                                               │
│ Total lower limb paralysis          Flexion, abduction,       │
│ + lower limb posture of     ────►   external rotation         │
│ flexion, abduction and              deformity.                │
│ external rotation.                                            │
│                                                               │
│ Unopposed flexion and               Dislocation of hip and    │
│ adduction.                  ────►   flexion/adduction         │
│                                     deformity                 │
├─────────────────────────────────────────────────────────────┤
│ Spine.                                                        │
│                                                               │
│ Hip flexor contracture.     ────►   Lordosis.                 │
│                                                               │
│ Imbalance of spinal muscul- ────►   Scoliosis                 │
│ ature.                                                        │
└─────────────────────────────────────────────────────────────┘
```

Fig. 91 The deformities which may occur and their possible causes.

ASSESSMENT CHART FOR SPINA BIFIDA CYSTICA

Date: ....

Name: .... Date of Birth:...............

Address: ....

Approximate level of lesion: ....

Muscle Power:

Left		Right
	Abdominals	
	Erector Spinae	
	Hip flexors	
	Hip extensors	
	Hip adductors	
	Hip abductors	
	Hamstrings	
	Quadriceps	
	Foot dorsiflexors	
	Foot plantarflexors	
	Foot invertors	
	Foot evertors	
	Toe extensors	
	Toe flexors	

Sensation:
(Tested by pinprick)

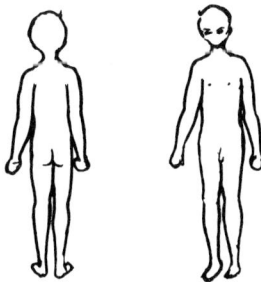

Contractures
and
Deformities:
....

Fig. 92 Assessment chart for spina bifida cystica.

271

Where there is already established deformity, treatment will be instituted as soon after birth as the baby's general condition will allow. In the case of talipes equinovarus and calcaneo-valgus, treatment will be as described in Chapters 1 and 2, although extra care will need to be exercised because of the poorly nourished skin and the lack of sensation. All plaster splints must be lined with orthopaedic felt or plastic foam, and particular attention is paid to skin under strapping should this be applied for an equinovarus deformity. Denis Browne splints probably should be avoided and strapping used in preference as this allows the foot to be mobilized.

Where there is unopposed toe flexor activity the toes will develop flexion deformities if they are not moved through a full range passively each day. All babies in the first few weeks after birth hold their hips in flexion, and it is not until they are several weeks old that their hips can be fully extended. Perhaps because of this, in the child with inactive hip extensors, it can escape notice that the hips are becoming more flexed. Particular attention is paid to the hip flexors and adductors in the early stages to prevent, as far as possible, contracture of these muscles, and to encourage as much hip mobility as possible. The prone position is useful for encouraging more extension in the hip, and the baby can be placed in this position for periods during the day.

Dislocation of the hip may be a congenital deformity or a secondary deformity due to unopposed hip flexor and adductor activity. Where the treatment regime is conservative, the child is subjected, often unsuccessfully, to long periods of recumbency and splinting, with possible effects of pressure ulceration, maternal deprivation, and slowed physical and mental development. Dislocated hips in these children may be reduced successfully, but maintenance of reduction is difficult and frequently impossible because of the continuing threat to hip stability posed by unopposed flexion and adduction, and by total paralysis of the lower limbs. The alternative is operative intervention, and an ilio-psoas transplant operation, such as the one devised by Sharrard (1969) may be performed. This surgery involves the transplanting of the ilio-psoas muscle through the ilium to the greater trochanter, this resulting in greater hip stability. The period of fixation in a plaster hip spica is followed by physiotherapy to mobilize the lower limbs, to encourage balance in standing and to develop the child's

ability to walk. If the hips are not reduced, and if they remain unstable, walking is difficult, the child will develop further flexion
contractures at the hips and a marked lumbar lordosis. Strain is
transmitted to his lumbar spine, and even if he does learn to walk,
he may eventually find that the effort is too much for him, and
will retire to a wheelchair instead.

Plaster splints

Light padded plaster splints are worn at night by a baby who may
be expected to develop contractures due either to unopposed
muscle action or to complete paralysis of muscles around a joint
combined with the effect of gravity. They are also worn by a baby
who has already acquired contractures, in order to stretch the soft
tissues. They may be applied antero-laterally to correct a
calcaneo-valgus foot, or posteriorly to hold a foot in a plantigrade
position. In this latter splint, the sole of the splint must be flat and
straight to prevent the foot developing a rocker shape, and the
medial border should also be straight to prevent the great toe from
abducting away from the midline of the foot. These splints must
be lined to avoid pressure areas on the sensitive skin. The feet and
legs are left free for a part of the day to allow as much movement
as possible to occur.

Sharrard (1971) suggests that night splinting is of little use in
correcting or preventing deformity where unopposed muscle
action is present. However, if splinting is worn also during part of
the day, and if it is combined with passive movements, it is this
author's experience that acquired deformities of the feet occur
with less severity than if the foot were left free. Similarly,
although splinting will not necessarily gain full correction of a
congenital foot deformity, nor will indefinitely maintain
correction where muscle imbalance exists, it will bring about
improvement in the position of the foot and maintain this improvement until surgery can be performed. Details of the surgery
performed for correction of deformity may be found in Menelaus
(1969) and Sharrard (1971).

Absence of sensation

Sensory loss does not always correspond with motor loss and is
difficult to assess accurately. Absence of sensation, both exteroceptive and proprioceptive, results in two major problems:

Risk of injury to soft tissues through the inability to feel pain, pressure and temperature.

Difficulty developing equilibrium reactions and a normal body image through lack of sensory feedback.

The skin of these children is prone to pressure areas and ulceration. The areas most affected are the bony points of the pelvis and the heels, and bony prominences of the feet and spine. Once the child starts to move about on the floor, the malleoli and the dorsum of the feet and toes become prone to friction burns and ulceration. Ill-fitting plaster splints, boots or calipers may cause pressure areas. Careless fitting of a boot may result in a great toe being flexed within the boot, and the child may walk around for some time without complaining of pain. Soft tissues of the lower limbs and the bones themselves may be injured or broken because the child is unaware of the position of his limbs. Warmth and swelling of a leg may be the only indication of a fracture.

Splints must be lined with orthopaedic felt or plastic foam material. When the child is ready to stand he is fitted with a pair of lambswool-lined boots which open and lace-up from the toes. Ordinary boots are too difficult to fit correctly on an anaesthetic foot.

The child's poor or absent proprioception makes learning to balance in sitting and standing difficult. He does not know where his lower limbs are in space unless he looks at them, and he will have to be taught to note the position of his feet when he is learning to stand and walk.

Normally an infant will investigate and discover the various parts of his body in a definite sequence. By five months he will have discovered his feet, and he will lie on his back and play with them. The myelomeningocele infant will have to be persuaded to play with his feet as he will have no sensory feedback to help him find them himself.

Problems of sensation are added to by the poor circulation found in paraplegic children. The normal pumping action of the muscles being poor or non-existent, circulation in the lower limbs may be very deficient. Should ulceration occur, the skin will heal very slowly and may need a graft to restore its integrity. In some cases infection occurs and may necessitate amputation (Sharrard

1971). In the cold weather these children suffer chilblains and trophic changes in the skin because of the sluggish circulation, and again ulceration may result.

Parents are warned of the difficulties involved in skin healing and advised to check the skin carefully as a routine each day. When the child is able, he will take over this task himself, which is probably not possible until he is at least seven years old, and this will depend on his intelligence and ability to accept responsibility. In the winter the child is dressed in warm clothes of wool or cotton, many synthetic materials being unsuitable as they may cause friction on the skin. Leggings, trousers, warm stockings may be worn, and when the weather becomes very cold, leggings may be made of quilted material. The child must be kept clear of hot water bottles, radiators and fires because of his lack of temperature sensation.

Disorder of movement

Lloyd-Roberts (1971) suggests the following system of grading of the paralysis in these children:

Grade 1: Flaccid paralysis of the lower limbs. The level of the lesion is from T12 to L1 downwards.
Grade 2: Hip flexion and adduction are present, and knee extension is present to some extent. All other muscles in the lower limbs are paralysed. The level of the lesion extends from L4 downwards.
Grade 3: Some muscles in the lower leg are paralysed. The level of the lesion extends from S1 downwards.

As has been noted, the child's development is hindered by the time he must spend in hospital undergoing surgery for his myelomeningocele mass, his hydrocephalus, his urinary tract incontinence, and for his dislocated hips. In his first few months he may spend several periods in hospital, and even with care on the part of the staff, there will be times when he will not be free to move about. All of these factors will result in a degree of motor retardation quite apart from the motor disability which results from lack of muscle contraction secondary to the neurological deficit. Soare and Raimondi (1977), following their study of 173 children with spina bifida, pointed out that all the children scored lower than their siblings on perceptuo-motor functions. They suggested that this may be due to the decreased stimulation associated with prolonged hospital stay, decreased opportunity for exploration or primary brain damage.

The myelomeningocele child will be slow to develop head control, particularly if he has hydrocephalus. However, head control will develop more quickly if he is picked up, carried about and nursed, than if he is left lying in his cot. It is interesting to note that normal African babies whose mothers carry them about all day on their backs seem to develop head control more quickly than European babies who are wheeled about in prams. The myelomeningocele baby, partly because of his long stay in hospital, partly because he is more awkward for his mother to handle, frequently lacks the stimulus of being picked up and carried.

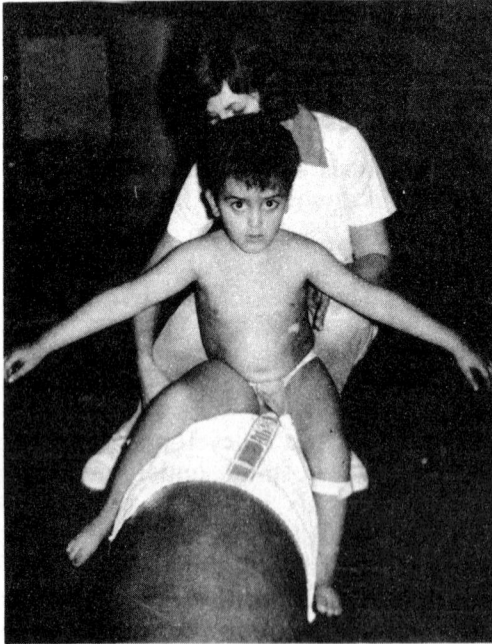

Fig. 93 Facilitation of equilibrium reactions using a roller.

He will not develop balance in sitting until he has developed head control, and even then he will be slow to gain balance because the paralysis of his lower limbs limits the effectiveness of his equilibrium reactions. He will have to learn to use his arms and trunk in order to balance (figure 93).

The normal child pulls himself to standing at nine months and begins to walk at approximately 13 months. At this stage of development the urge to stand and walk is very strong. Unfortunately many of these disabled children lack not only the physical ability to initiate these functions themselves but also lack the incentive or the drive to do so. It is essential that the child is helped to achieve standing and walking as near as possible to the time when he would normally be expected to achieve them. If standing and walking are left until he is older, the child has probably become accustomed to a life in which locomotion is accomplished with relative ease in a chariot or mobile chair and has developed fears and anxieties which make it extremely difficult for him to be encouraged to stand and walk. It is also important for standing to be instituted early in order to minimise muscle and bone atrophy (Curtis 1972).

In the infant, movement is encouraged in several ways, by localized stimulation such as gentle pinching, slapping or brushing of muscle groups, or by mechanical vibration, by stimulating such important basic movements as rolling over and righting the head, and by putting him in positions which encourage the required movements. The most important movements to stimulate in the infant in order that he may be prepared for functions such as standing and walking are head and trunk righting, trunk extension, and rotation within the body axis. In the absence of muscle power, extension at the hips and knees and a plantigrade foot position must be obtaincd and maintained by passive movement, surgery and splinting. In stimulating the development of balance, it is essential that appropriate movements are stimulated in the head and upper limbs, and in that part of the trunk which has muscle function.

Lying in prone over a foam wedge (figure 47) or over the therapist's knee (figure 45) will help the infant develop head control and trunk extension. He will learn to weightbear on his hands as he reaches out to play with his toys. These functions will all prepare him for walking with sticks or crutches, when he will need good trunk extension and the ability to weightbear through his hands.

Rolling over is stimulated from the trunk with a towel, or from the legs, the infant's attention being drawn to a colourful toy. Crawling or the maintenance of four point kneeling are encouraged by the use of a crawler or with a towel held under the baby's abdomen supporting him. His legs must be well protected by long pants and socks in order to avoid friction burns.

A great deal of emphasis is placed on strengthening his arms in preparation for walking with apparatus. He may be wheelbarrowed when he is old enough and strong enough to take his entire weight on his hands, but the physiotherapist must hold his thighs rather than his lower legs or feet in order not to put unnecessary strain on his osteoporotic bones. In sitting the child will learn to push down on his hands in order to lift himself from the floor, but he may need small wooden blocks under his hands if his arms are too short to afford him much movement.

The baby must not be kept in a lying position for any longer than necessary. In sitting he will be able to develop an interest in his surroundings which he will not do if he lies facing a ceiling or a blank wall. When he has sufficient head control he may be sat up against pillows in the corner of a sofa, in a car seat, or in a plastic blow-up chair. When he is old enough he can propel himself around sitting in a Chailey Chariot. These periods of sitting must be alternated with periods spent in prone over a wedge or on a prone scooter, as prolonged sitting will increase the tendency towards flexion contractures at the hips and knees.

When the child is ready to stand, and this should be some time before 12 months of age, apparatus may need to be provided which will give him support and confidence and allow him to play. A standing table will be useful at home, as he will stand and play, and by shifting his weight as he plays he will develop some balancing ability. Some form of splinting for the legs will probably be necessary for most of these children before they will be able to stand.

Deciding on the apparatus necessary for a particular child at this stage is very difficult and cannot be decided merely upon knowledge of his grade of paralysis. It is unfortunately to some extent a matter of trial and error, although Spiers (1972) suggests that it may be preferable to start with too much apparatus and gradually discard unnecessary parts as the child's disability becomes more evident. A child with some paralysis or weakness confined below the knee may manage to stand in short below-knee irons, or may be better able to manage in the beginning with long-leg calipers until he develops more balancing ability. A child with extensive paralysis may require extensive support in a Shrewsbury splint (figure 94) or in a parapodium (figure 95). This should soon be changed to a pelvic band jointed on to calipers (figure 96) or to calipers alone once the child has developed some hip stability.

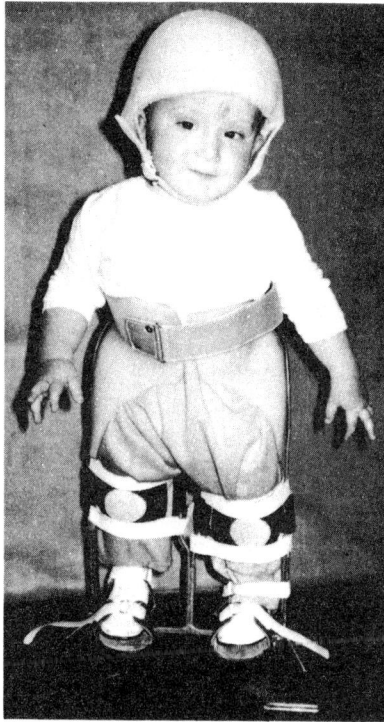

Fig. 94 The Shrewsbury splint.

In standing he will have to learn to balance by transferring weight with his trunk if he has extensive lower limb paralysis, and the stimulus to any adjustment of balance will have to come from sensory feedback from the muscles and joints of his trunk instead of from his lower limbs. There are many activities which the physiotherapist will use for training balance and gaining confidence in standing with these children. These may include: standing with hands on the wall, moving one hand, then both hands, on to differently coloured marks; standing with hands on physiotherapist's shoulders trying to push her over; standing with hands on a large ball while the physiotherapist moves the ball backwards and forwards and from side to side gently. These and other activities must emphasize the need for the paraplegic child to keep his weight forwards, and stress the fact that if he does fall he must fall forwards on to his hands.

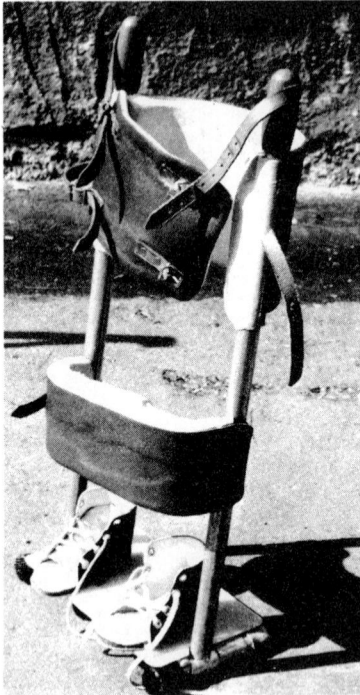

Fig. 95 A Canadian parapodium.
(By permission of Chailey Heritage, Sussex, England.)

Walking should be expected of every child, even if only for part of the day, no matter how high the lesion. Provided deformities are corrected, and the child has suitable intelligence, and provided attempts to encourage walking are made early enough, most of these children will be capable of walking quite effectively. For some, the effort may prove too great and they may eventually decide a wheel-chair offers the greatest possibility of mobility, but all of these children must be given the opportunity to walk if they want to, and all must be enabled to maintain the standing position, even if this requires extensive apparatus.

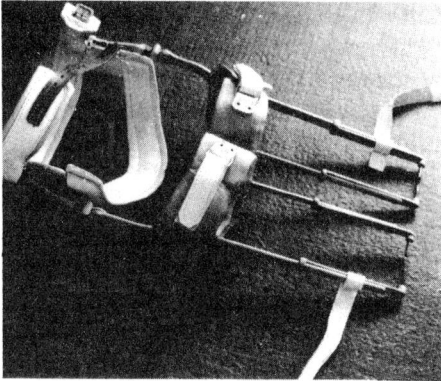

Fig. 96 Pelvic band and calipers.
(By permission of Chailey Heritage, Sussex, England.)

A child with severe disability may learn to walk pushing a weighted pram, a large wooden toy on wheels, or a specially made walker, or he may do better in the parallel bars. If the latter are used the child must be taught how to push down with his hands as he walks, otherwise he may try to pull up. He may learn better by walking in front of the therapist pushing down on her hands as he takes a step. Eventually he will walk with crutches or sticks (figure 97). There is no stick or crutch which is suitable for every child with this type of disability and while some children manage well with quadripod sticks, others will do better with crutches with a small ski tip placed instead of the usual ferrule.

Other children will learn to walk in a Shrewsbury splint, its great advantage being in the ability of a severely disabled and perhaps mentally retarded child to be ambulant while retaining full use of his hands. This splint is composed of a pair of leg irons with chest, pelvic, thigh and tibial bands, the leg irons being attached to bootees on footplates. The splint is rigid from the chest band to the bootee footplates in order that the child will not waste energy which should be transmitted directly to the footplates.

The only movement allowed is the pivot at the footplates. The child walks by transferring weight to one plate, rotating his trunk towards that side, then transferring weight to the opposite plate. The plates are returned to their starting position by springs. Most of these children need to wear crash helmets while in their Shrewsbury splints, although the splint is stable under normal circumstances. This apparatus should not be considered as any but a temporary means of getting a child standing and walking. As soon as possible the child should progress to apparatus which allows greater mobility and a more normal gait.

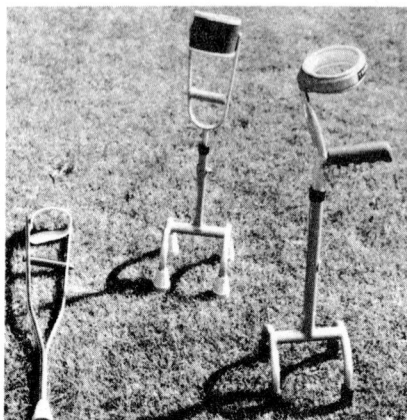

Fig. 97 A selection of crutches.
(By permission of Chailey Heritage, Sussex, England.)

A child wearing calipers must eventually be taught how to get up from the floor. Some of these children will learn to manage stairs on their feet, but many resort to sitting down and pushing on their hands.

Most children in calipers will learn to walk using a four-point and a swing-through gait, the latter being preferred by all children who have developed the confidence to use it because of the extra speed it allows. The child should not be hurried at this stage and care must be taken that he does not lose confidence. He cannot be made to walk before he has the desire to do so, but once he has reached this stage he will need all the help and patience his parents can give him.

Swimming is a good sport for these children once their incontinence has been overcome. They are taught to float, to swim, and to get in and out of the water, and as they develop proficiency can participate in races against each other. Archery and ball games provide other outlets for their sporting aspirations.

Children with high myelomeningocele lesions frequently lack normal respiratory movement due to spinal and thoracic deformity, weak abdominals and poor sitting posture, and may require daily breathing exercises at home in order to improve respiratory function. If the child is prone to respiratory tract infection his parents will give him postural drainage at home when it is necessary.

The physiotherapist must check the child's apparatus for length and fit at regular intervals, as ill-fitting apparatus will cause deformity and pressure ulceration. She will also check that whatever apparatus the child has is effective, and must remember that 'braces should be used to enlarge not limit a child's horizon' Ferguson 1968).

Assessment

The baby is assessed by the physiotherapist as soon after birth as practical, and he is reassessed at intervals throughout his childhood. The assessment may be done under the following headings: movement, sensation, deformity, development.

It is probably not necessary to do a complete and detailed muscle chart in the neonatal period, but rather an assessment of movement. The picture frequently changes following surgery to repair the myelomeningocele and assessment of muscle activity is made before and after surgery, as well as at intervals during the child's development. Movement is assessed by observation of the infant when he is awake and irritable before a feed. If necessary the various primitive reflexes such as crossed extension, and plantar grasp may be elicited as these will demonstrate the presence or absence of movement in certain areas. This assessment of movement is important as a guide to possible deforming influences. Sharrard (1971) suggests that percutaneous faradic stimulation may demonstrate the presence of an active muscle capable of producing a particular deformity where it is difficult to elicit an active contraction.

Deformities and contractures are noted as either present or potential, and present deformities are described and photographed.

Sensation is tested by the baby's response to pin-prick and is also recorded on the chart. However, this test has doubtful value as a guide to function. Testing sensation with a pin may elicit a response, but it is almost impossible to be accurate as to the level of sensory loss. Furthermore, as Sharrard (1972) points out, it is difficult to distinguish between a reflex movement and a movement which indicates that the sensation has reached the brain. Evoked cortical responses, which are the subject of study at the moment, may give better information.

Motor development is assessed within the first few weeks, then reassessed at intervals throughout childhood. The most important points to note are the development of head righting, of trunk extension, the ability to roll over and sit up, of eye-hand control and manipulation, of the parachute reaction of his arms and equilibrium reactions. As the child grows older, self-help and the use of his apparatus is assessed, as well as his ability to move about, to walk and to play. Where the child is either motor retarded, spastic or ataxic, perhaps as a result of damage to his brain caused by hydrocephalus, a more detailed developmental assessment, along the lines suggested in Section II, Chapter 1, will be necessary.

SUMMARY

The physiotherapist has two main objectives in the treatment of children with myelomeningocele.

Prevention of further deformity, of pressure ulceration, of secondary mental retardation, and correction of deformity already present at birth.

Development of basic motor skills, normal body image, effective balance reactions, head control, interest in his surroundings, strong arm and trunk muscles, and a method of weight-bearing ambulation as soon as possible. Physical treatment must therefore commence at birth and be a continuing process.

Whatever is involved in physiotherapy, whether for the baby or for the older child, it must be good fun. It must not degenerate into a set of meaningless exercises and passive movements. The physiotherapist must have sufficient understanding of children and must understand the importance of her own personality if she is to be able to make the child accomplish something while still enjoying himself.

The physiotherapist must work in close conjunction with the child's parents and later with his school-teacher, but teamwork involving several people is essential in the management of these children. In many cities there are special clinics to which the parents may bring their baby and where he can be seen by those of the team whose help he needs at that stage. This ensures that all aspects of the child's welfare are kept under observation. His parents benefit from this co-ordinated approach as conflicting advice is avoided. Periods of hospitalization are decreased as several investigations are carried out where possible at one admission. Such a clinic, together with the parents' associations which have been formed in several countries, can be a place where an atmosphere of hopefulness and encouragement prevails, and where both parents and child can draw comfort and guidance.

References

Bowlby, J. (1953) *Child Care and the Growth of Love.* London: Penguin.

Curtis, B. H. (1972) Principles of orthopaedic management in myelomeningocoele. In *Symposium on myelomeningocoele*, Am. Acad. Orthop. Surg. Assoc. St. Louis: Mosby.

Durham Smith, E. (1965) *Spina Bifida and the Total Care of Myelomeningocele.* Illinois: Thomas.

Ferguson, A. B. (1968) *Orthopaedic Surgery in Infancy and Childhood.* Baltimore: Williams and Wilkins.

Lloyd-Roberts, G. C. (1971) *Orthopaedics in Infancy and Childhood.* London: Butterworth.

Lorber, J. (1968a) The child with spina bifida. *Physiotherapy,* **54**, 11, 390.

Lorber, J. (1968b) *Your Child with Spina Bifida.* London: Association for Spina Bifida and Hydrocephalus.

Menelaus, M. B. (1969) *The Orthopaedic Management of Spina Bifida Cystica.* Edinburgh: Livingstone.

Patten, B. M. (1953) Embryological stages in the establishing of myeloschisis with spina bifida. *Amer. J. Anat.* **93**, 365.

Sherrard, W. J. W. (1969) Posterior ilio-psoas transplantation. in *Operative Surgery,* **8**. London: Butterworth.

Sharrard, W. J. W. (1971) *Paediatric Orthopaedics and Fractures.* London: Blackwell.

Sharrard, W. J. W. (1972) The kyphotic and lordotic spine in myelomeningocele. In *Symposium and Myelomeningocoele*, Am. Acad. Orth. Surg. Assoc. St. Louis: Mosby.

Sharrard, W. J. W., Zachary, R. B. and Lorber, J. (1967) Survival and paralysis in open myelomeningocele with special reference to the time of repair of the spinal lesion. *Develop. Med. Child Neurol. Suppl.* **13**, 35.

Soare, P. L. and Raimondi, A. J. (1977) Intellectual and perceptual-motor characteristics of treated myelomeningocele children. *Am. J. Dis. Child.* **131**, 199–204.

Spiers, B. W. (1972) Personal Communication.

Further Reading

Brocklehurst, G., Gleave, J. R. W. and Lewin, W. (1967) Early closure of myelomeningocele with special reference to leg movement. *Brit. Med. J.* **1**, 666.

Buvisson, J. S. and Hamblen, D. L. (1972) Electromyographic assessment of the transplanted ilio-psoas muscle in spina bifida cystica. *Develop. Med. Child Neurol.* **1**, **4**, Suppl. 27.

Edbrooke, H. (1970) The Royal Salop Infirmary 'Clicking Splint'. *Physiotherapy*, **56**, 4, 148.

Hamilton, E. L. (1972) Development in techniques for ambulation for spina bifida children. *J. Canad. Physio. Assoc.* **24**, 1, 17–19.

Hare, E. H., Lawrence, K. M., Payne, H. and Rawnsley, K. (1966) Spina bifida cystica and family stress. *Brit. Med. J.* **2**, 757.

James, C. C. M. (1970) Fractures of the lower limbs in spina bifida children. *Develop. Med. Child Neurol.* **12**, Suppl. 22.

Lloyd-Roberts, G. C. (1971) *Orthopaedics in Infancy and Childhood*. London: Butterworth.

Lorber, J. (1970) *Your Child with Hydrocephalus*. London: Association for Spina Bifida and Hydrocephalus.

MacKeith, R. C. (1971) A new look at spina bifida aperta. *Dev. Med. Child Neurol.* **13**, 277–278.

Martin, M. C. (1964) Physiotherapy in relation to myelomeningocele. *Physiotherapy*, **50**, 50.

Mustard, W. T. (1952) Ilio-psoas transfer for weakness of hip abductors, *J. Bone Jt. Surg.* **34A**, 647.

Sand, P. et al (1973) Performance of children with spina bifida manifesta on the Frostig developmental test of visual perception. *Percept. Mot. Skills* **37**, 539–546.

Sandifer, P. (1967) *Neurology in Orthopaedics*. London: Butterworth.

Scobie, W. G. Eckstein, H. B. and Long, W. J. (1970) Bowel function in myelomeningocele. *Develop. Med. Child Neurol.* **12**, Suppl. 22.

Chapter 6

Congenital Limb Deficiencies

There has been some difficulty in finding a classification for these children which will include all the varieties of limb deficiency or *dysmelia*. Frantz and O'Rahilly (1961), Henkel and Willert (1969) and others have attempted classifications depending upon morphology or clinical observation, but the results have been long lists of names, meaningless to those without a classical education, and still not embracing all the many varieties of deficiency which may be seen.

Two terms in common usage are phocomelia and amelia. Rubin (1967) describes *phocomelia* (figures 98 and 99) as an incomplete development of the limbs. *Amelia* (figure 100) infers complete absence of a limb. The varieties seen range from amelia of one limb to complete amelia of all four limbs.

The causes of this type of developmental failure are usually unknown, although it has been shown to be the result of certain drugs taken by the mother in the first weeks of pregnancy. The developmental breakdown probably occurs during the fourth to the eighth gestational week, at the time when the limb buds are forming.

The effects of the drug thalidomide are now well known. The affected children suffered a variety of congenital abnormalities including complete or partial absence of limbs, disorders of other systems, amongst them cardiac and intestinal abnormalities, and facial anomalies. The thalidomide tragedy focussed attention on all children with limb deficiencies and stimulated research into prosthetic design and management. The problems described below are particularly applicable to those families in which a severely limb-deficient child has been born, although they will be present to varying degree in all similarly affected families.

THE PROBLEMS

Acceptance

The parents of a child born with a limb deficiency suffer profound shock. They need to make considerable adjustment in order to cope with their grief and disappointment, and their feelings of guilt and shame. The parents' inability to come to terms with their

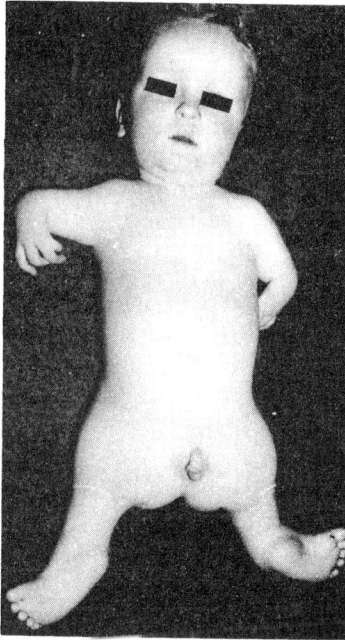

Fig. 98 Phocomelia (Thalidomide syndrome).

child's problems may lead them to reject him, either unconsciously or overtly, and consequently to over-protect him in an attempt to keep him dependent even when he is old enough to be assuming some independence. Unconscious rejection may lead the parents to seek help in the form of artificial aids for the child which they will never use, and practical suggestions which will never be put into practice. It is not enough just to teach a child to be independent, as those responsible for the management of these children have found out, but it will be the mother's attitude which will in the end determine how independent her child will be.

It is said to be fear and anxiety which lead to rejection, and these parents need expert counselling to help them see their problems in a realistic light, to gain some knowledge of the assistance they will receive, and to be reassured that they need feel no guilt about their child's deficiencies. Whether or not they will be able to lose their feelings of shame probably depends to a large extent on how the infant is accepted by relatives, friends and the community. Shame is connected with the disappointment all parents must feel if their newborn baby is not all they had hoped for, if they are not able to experience the pride of showing him off to their relatives and friends. A mother's efforts to cope with her feelings may suffer considerable setback if she boards a bus and finds herself surrounded by curious stares from strangers whose sympathy sets her apart in isolation.

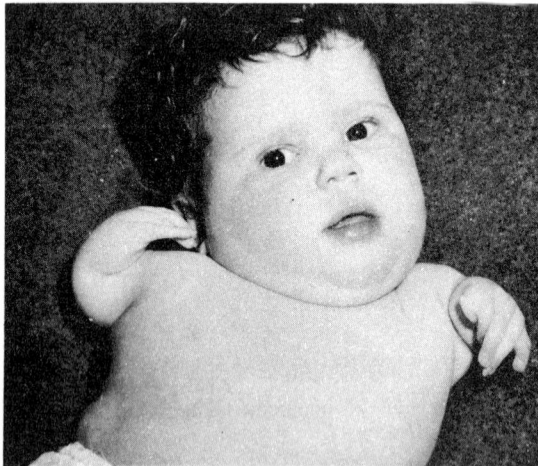

Fig. 99 Phocomelia of upper limbs only (Thalidomide syndrome).

The child, as he develops, will have to learn to see himself in a realistic light, and to accept himself as having certain limitations. As a small child he will probably have idealistic dreams of his future and it is necessary for the parents to be honest with him. One phocomelic boy was heard to say 'I'll be able to do it better when my arm grows.' As he develops he will have to learn to persevere towards more realistic goals. The child should be encouraged from as early an age as possible to have a positive attitude towards his life, as this will help him deal with the new problems which will arise as he grows older. From an early age he has to accept being stared at, and he will suffer to some extent from the failure of other people to accept his disabilities, although as a child he will find himself readily accepted by other children. He will also have to overcome his fear. Fear of falling is often considerable in these children whose balance is so difficult to achieve, whether this is due to lack of arms or to the child's inability to feel connected with the ground while wearing a lower limb prosthesis. Children with lower limb deficiencies plus hip instability suffer considerable balance problems. However, it is lack of mobility which appears to be the greatest handicap in these children, and the lower limb deficient children who suffer most in this respect.

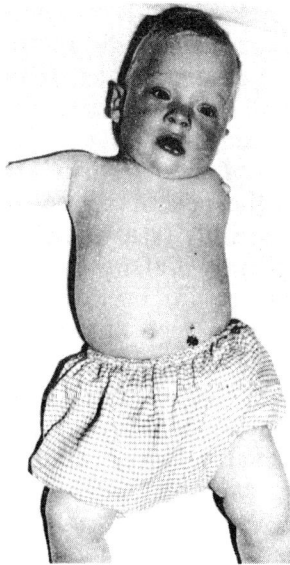

Fig. 100 Amelia of the left upper limb.

Development

All children with limb deficiency will suffer some delay in motor development. The delay may be localized, as in the child with absent fingers, whose development of prehension will be delayed, or more general in the case of a child with one or more limbs involved. The most handicapped will be the child with total amelia.

Normal motor development demands amongst other things intact skeletal and muscular systems, and in the presence of defects in these systems development will be both delayed and abnormal unless treatment is directed at overcoming the difficulties.

A child with no legs will not be able to sit or to develop skills in sitting unless he is provided with an external aid which will hold him erect. A child with no arms will be slow to develop trunk control and equilibrium reactions, and therefore balance, and he will get himself to standing much later than the normal child. His knowledge of the world around him will be incomplete as he has no hands with which to explore either himself or his surroundings. However, although the lack of hands may seem a severe deterrent to the sensitive exploration of the world around the child, the feet can develop remarkable dexterity and sensitivity if he is encouraged to use them. If he has neither hands nor feet, he is taught to use his lips and tongue as vehicles for sensory awareness and exploration. The use of the mouth or the feet as substitutes for hands is essential for the development of these children. There is apparently increased sensitivity at the tips of the phocomelic limbs and he will consequently prefer the use of these tiny limbs to any prosthesis which has so far been designed. No prosthesis, however sophisticated, can feed into the child's brain the knowledge that comes from sensation.

Problems arising from the delayed development of trunk control and equilibrium in phocomelic and amelic children cannot be overemphasized. Special balance training is required for the child with bilateral upper extremity amelia or phocomelia as arms are essential for balance especially when he first begins to stand and walk. A child with severe bilateral lower extremity deficiency will also develop balance slowly, partly because of a lack of sensory awareness. He will require special apparatus to enable him to develop balance in the upright position, and emphasis in treatment must be on stimulation of head and trunk movement in response to alterations in his centre of gravity.

An important factor in normal child development is the view the child has of his surroundings as he grows. When he first begins to sit he can see what is around him at this level. When he is on the floor he sees under the table, but he cannot see what is on the table until he can pull himself to standing. He sees things from a higher level when he is picked up by his mother, but there are times when he sees only those things which are situated at his own level. The author one day noticed a small child trying to find his mother amongst a group of women in swimming costumes. He was attempting to recognize her by looking around him at his own eye level, and at this level all he could see were knees. Even in his distress he did not look upwards at the women's faces which would have made recognition much easier. The child who is slow to stand will see the world either from floor level or from the level of his mother's shoulder. If his prostheses are not lengthened gradually to keep pace with his chronological progression he will not view the world from all the different levels as does the normal child.

The development of a normal child proceeds, if unimpeded, in an effortless manner, one step leading on to the next, the child driven on to achieve the next skill, repeating each new skill until it is effective, then going on to the next. Thus it is easier to teach a handicapped child how, for example, to walk when he is at an age, a stage of development, at which the urge to walk is strong, than to wait until he is older when the urge is less strong. With this in mind it is important to try, with the aid of prosthetic devices, to help the child achieve his milestones when the natural drive to do so is present.

Deformity

As in the case of any infant born with a congenital defect there is always the possibility of other defects, and many children born with limb deficiencies have deformities associated with the deficiency. These deformities may include talipes equinovarus, talipes calcaneus, dislocated hips or spina bifida. Many of the deformities defy description, so bizarre are the structural abnormalities. If an existing foreshortened limb is also grossly deformed further problems of management arise, especially when it is necessary to make decisions about the fitting of prostheses.

There is also a risk of contractures, particularly in those children with foreshortened limbs. A child with a phocomelic upper limb may develop contracture of the anterior shoulder muscles through the repeated action of taking the limb to his mouth. Acquired contractures must be prevented so the child will have maximum range of movement and be able to take full advantage of whatever limb remnants he has and of any prosthesis which may be designed for him in the future.

Loss of surface area

Some of these children have such an extensive loss of surface area that marked interference with the body cooling system occurs. These children sweat heavily, and in warm weather and during exercise care must be taken to dress them lightly to allow maximum circulation of air to take place.

Choice of prosthesis

Most authorities agree that a limb deficient child be fitted with a prosthesis to coincide with the appropriate stage of his development. In this way a lower limb deficient child will begin wearing a prosthesis when he is ready to stand, usually between 12 and 18 months, and an upper limb deficient child when he has sitting balance at 6 to 8 months. The early fitting of a prosthesis will, it is hoped, make more likely its incorporation into the child's body image, and there is some evidence that apparatus is more readily acceptable at an early age even if it is rejected by the child when he is older.

The complexity of the apparatus depends in part on the maturation of his central nervous system. As he matures so he will be able to use a prosthesis of increasing complexity. This applies particularly to upper limb prostheses, but it is difficult at the moment to realize this aim as there are many difficulties of design to be overcome. Unfortunately, at this stage of technological development, the more complex the equipment the heavier it is. However, there are many centres throughout the world where attempts are being made at refinement in their design.

Basically, prostheses can be divided into two categories, the cosmetic and the functional, and frequently the cosmetic apparatus is provided for the parent's sake as much as for the child's. The fitting of a cosmetic limb, especially an upper limb, is often necessary to give the child's mother the confidence to take him out into the community. As the child grows older he will usually prefer the functional prosthesis, but at the present stage of prosthetic design most children prefer to use their upper limb remnants and remaining limbs, as these give more speed of movement and more dexterity due to sensory feedback. Functional upper limb prostheses remain an ideal to be achieved in the future. While lower limb prostheses present fewer problems, many children find their activities too restricted, and remove the prosthesis in order to be more mobile (Robertson 1971). The child with bilateral hip instability may prefer to be mobile in a wheelchair, rather than struggle to maintain his balance in his prostheses (Robertson 1971).

It is important to keep in mind that whatever device the child uses for the upper limb, any limb remnants that he possesses, no matter how small, must be left free and should not be enclosed within the apparatus, as these remnants may be used to operate the apparatus (figure 101).

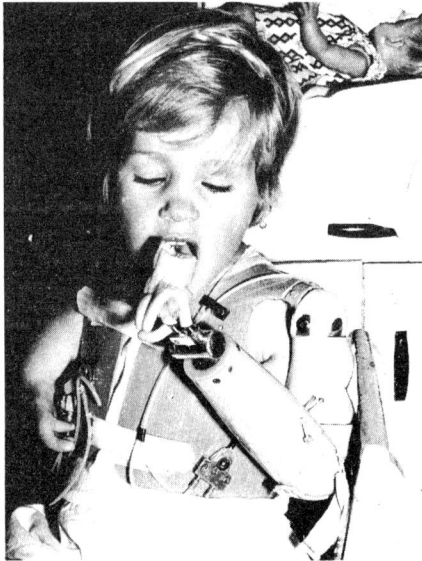

Fig. 101 Phocomelia. A functional prosthesis powered from a carbondioxide cylinder, and operated by the right phocomelic limb.

MANAGEMENT

A large team of people is involved in the care of these children: an orthopaedic surgeon, a limb-fitting specialist, a social worker, a physiotherapist and an occupational therapist. The child's parents and his school-teacher will also have important roles to play in his habilitation.

The infant's family will be seen by the social worker as soon as practicable after his birth, and her support will be continuous from then on, offering practical advice about financial assistance, schooling, and to some extent acting as co-ordinator between the various people responsible for the management of the child.

The physiotherapist will see the infant as soon as possible to assess what treatment is necessary to enable him to develop as normally as possible, and what must be done to prepare him for the prosthesis he will eventually require. She will begin to treat the infant by teaching his mother simple handling procedures to enable him to develop the appropriate motor control for his age, and her treatment will develop as the child develops.

Exploration

This is encouraged from infancy, with the child using his mouth, his feet or his hands in order to explore his own body and his surroundings. While he is an infant he will be put in positions from which he can see what is happening around him. A child with no arms, for example, may lie in prone, with a pillow under his chest allowing him to lift his head and trunk into extension. This allows him to look around and is effective for strengthing his trunk extensors.

Prehension

The hands are normally necessary for prehension, but the feet, lips or tongue may be effectively used in the absence of hands. The feet should be left free of shoes and socks except where these are really necessary. It may be difficult for the parents to accept this unconventional use of the feet for prehension and they may have to be persuaded to allow the child to use them in an unembarrassed manner. Toys will be selected or adapted to be held in the mouth, the upper limb remnant or the toes. The child will learn whatever movements seem most appropriate to his disability. He may, for example, learn to transfer a toy from one limb remnant to the other via his chin.

The attachments of an upper limb prosthesis are no substitute for upper limb remnants or toes, but the child may learn to use an artificial limb effectively for limited activities. The earliest apparatus, fitted when the child has good sitting balance, may allow bimanual grasp activated by shoulder girdle movement. An active terminal device such as a split hook on a conventional upper limb prosthesis cannot usually be operated by a child of less than two and a half years of age. Most of the prostheses in use at the present time, for amelic or phocomelic children, are powered by a carbondioxide cylinder, the valve being activated by on-off switches. These allow a variety of movements including elbow flexion and extension, forearm supination and pronation, and opening and closing of the split hook. The child may operate the switches with his limb remnants, his chin, or by shoulder movement. Some surveys, including a report by Robertson (1971) suggest that many of the children are unenthusiastic about upper limb prostheses if bilateral and powered by CO_2. The exceptions seem to be the children with severe bilateral upper and lower limb deficiencies who must depend on prostheses for any function at all.

The orthopaedic surgeon, together with a radiologist, will assess the extent of the infant's skeletal abnormality and his skeletal growth, and as the infant develops the surgeon will decide whatever splinting or reconstruction may be necessary in order to provide a suitable frame for a prosthetic device.

The occupational therapist will work with the physiotherapist in training the child to function at various stages of development, by using his unaffected limbs and his limb remnants. She will teach him how to hold a toy between his chin and shoulder if he is a complete amelia, in his feet if he has no arms (figure 102), or in the remnants of his upper limbs. He will learn to dress himself, feed himself and play, using his mouth and whatever limbs remain. The occupational therapist will help his mother make alterations to his clothing, will design equipment such as toothbrush and cutlery suitable to his needs. When he is fitted with a prosthesis for his upper limbs she will teach him how to use it, while the physiotherapist will be more concerned with the habilitation of the child wearing a lower limb prosthesis. Both therapists will work very closely with the child's parents, who will carry out much of the child's training at home.

PHYSICAL THERAPY

Assessment

The child's stage of development is assessed at regular intervals as this will be one of the major factors in his treatment. Specific assessment of the range and strength of his movements will be done at regular intervals and particularly before the prescription of a prosthesis is made. Once he has been fitted with a prosthesis, regular assessments of function, to determine how the child and his parents are managing, will be made in the child's home, where his capabilities will be more clearly seen than in the hospital (Robertson 1971).

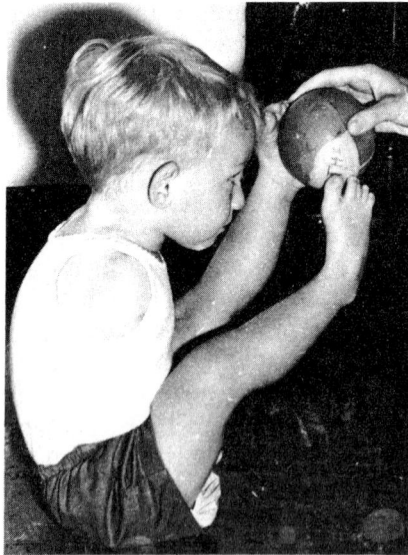

Fig. 102 Bilateral upper limb amelia. Training for balance and lower limb dexterity.

Mobility of limbs and trunk

The essential part of early treatment is concerned with preparing the child for maximum functional independence both with and without prostheses. Important for this maximum independence is a range of movement in several joints which exceeds the range normally found in a child or adult. This is achieved by encouraging activities that ensure the necessary length of the surrounding soft tissues. To this end treatment begins in infancy to maintain and where necessary increase the mobility of limbs and trunk. The upper limb amelic child will need to use his feet for dressing (figure 103), feeding (figures 104, 105 and 106), writing and toileting. The latter function, which requires that he reach his perineal area with his foot, requires a wide range of hip, knee and foot movement, much greater than is required in normal life. The child with phocomelic upper limbs will need a wide range of movement at the shoulder girdle in order to bring his small limb remnants as near to the midline and to his mouth as possible (figure 107).

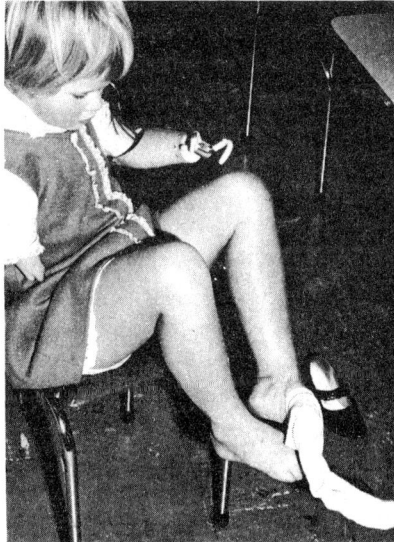

Fig. 103 Bilateral upper limb phocomelia. Dressing.

A general mobility is required as well as mobility of specific areas. It is difficult for a limbless child to move around, and this is partly a mechanical problem and partly the result of fear. General mobility is encouraged by teaching him to roll, rolling him in a towel when he is an infant, or down a sloping board when he is older. The upper limb amelic child will use this rolling to help

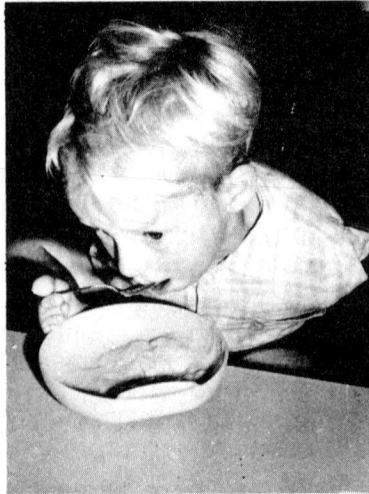

Fig. 104 Bilateral upper limb amelia. Eating.

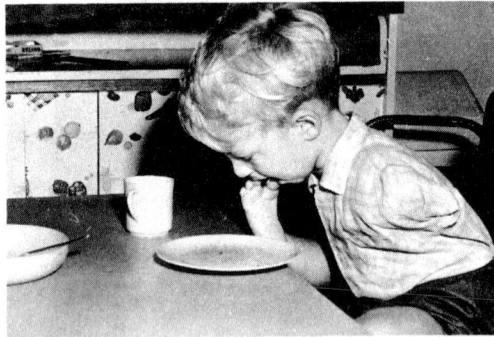

Fig. 105 Bilateral upper limb amelia. Eating.

him achieve the sitting position. In a small pool or in his bath, well supported by the physiotherapist or by floats, he can play using his remaining limbs, his trunk and head in order to move about. He will be able to move about the house on a prone scooter (figure 88) or a Chailey Chariot (figure 89). The upper limb deficient child will need to be taught such movements as standing up (figure 108) through half kneeling and squatting, making sure he can also do the movement in reverse, and walking on his knees.

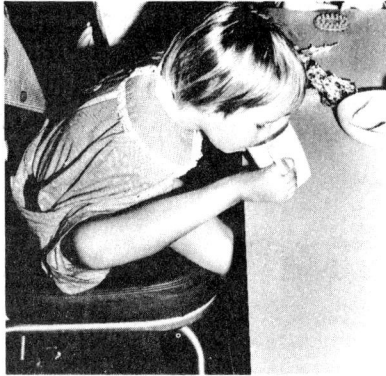

Fig. 106 Bilateral upper limb amelia. Drinking.

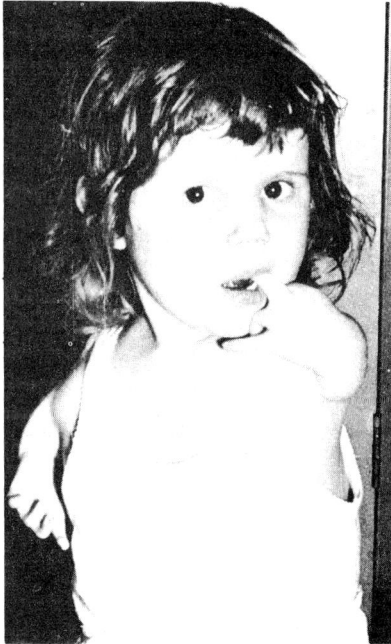

Fig. 107 Phocomelia. Hand to mouth.

As soon as the child with lower limb deficiency shows a desire to pull himself to standing he is given apparatus which will enable him eventually to learn a form of ambulation. This may be in the

301

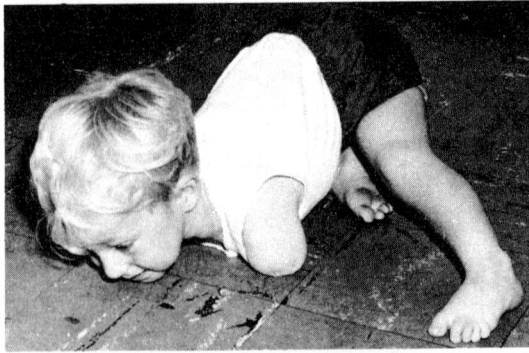

Fig. 108 Bilateral upper limb amelia. Part of the sequence of lying to sitting. Child is using his feet for leverage and is pushing backwards with his head and shoulders.

form of a simple lower limb prosthesis or pylon, or in the case of a bilaterally deficient child a pair of rigid legs on rockers which he will eventually be able to use for walking by using weight transference and trunk rotation (figures 109 and 110).

Muscle strength and endurance

If the child is to move and maintain postures against gravity despite his limb deficiencies he will need to develop muscle power and co-ordination in excess of that normally required by a child. Similarly, the better developed his strength and endurance the better use he will make of his prosthesis. His mother is taught some simple techniques for stimulating trunk and head movement against gravity, for developing weight-bearing on his hands as well as on his feet and for strengthening movements of the limbs and trunk.

Deformities

If maximum function is to be gained from dysmelic limbs it is sometimes necessary to correct existing deformities such as talipes equinovarus, where the lower limbs are involved, although each patient must be assessed individually. An equinovarus deformity will not be corrected, for example, if this position makes prehension with the limb easier. Correction of these deformities by splinting, however, is frequently disappointing and surgical correction may eventually be necessary. Deformities of the upper

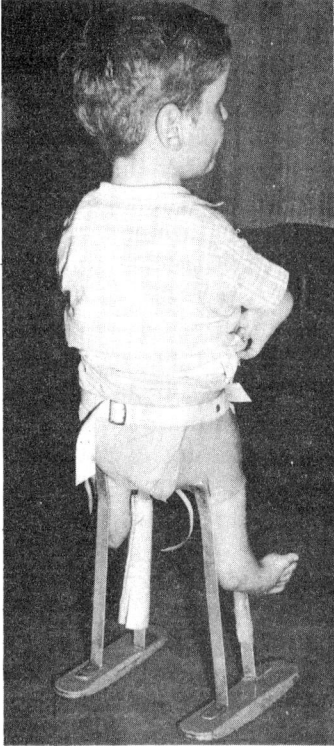

Fig. 109 Phocomelia. Early walking apparatus operated by weight transference and trunk rotation.

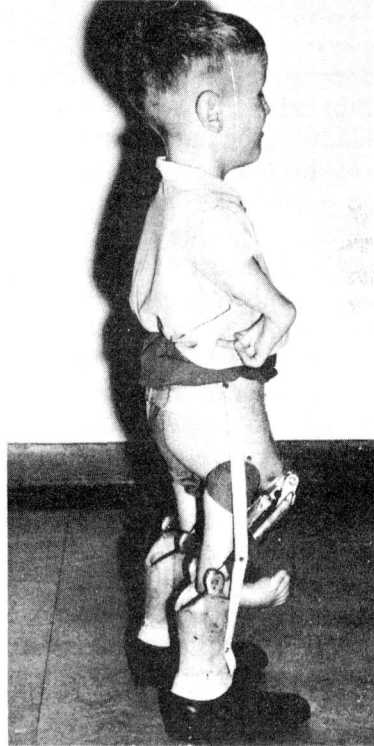

Fig. 110 More sophisticated walking apparatus allowing hip and knee movement.

limb are thought to be best left untouched until the child is older, when the usefulness of the limbs can be more accurately assessed, the child's own opinion being sought at this stage. The skeletal and muscular structure of phocomelic limbs is so relatively undifferentiated that accurate assessment of their potential is very difficult. Even a small limb remnant may be indispensable to the child's function.

Balance

These children, unless they have only minor deficiencies, will need help in order to develop balance. Equilibrium reactions may be stimulated in lying and sitting by using a beach ball or a balance board, with the child sitting astride a roller or held by the physiotherapist in such a way that a reaction from him becomes necessary. The lower limb amelic or phocomelic child who cannot otherwise sit, is placed in a 'flower pot' apparatus in which he learns to balance using his head, trunk and arms. Later he will require balance training in his prostheses. An upper limb amelic or phocomelic child must develop more effective trunk control in sitting and standing than his normal peers, as he must balance without the use of his arms. It is difficult for this child to stand up without the use of arms, and he will need very effective balance in kneeling and half kneeling, and in a squatting position. This child will be fearful of standing on his first few attempts. He has no protective extension of his arms when he falls, and he must make all his protective adjustments with his head, trunk and legs. This ability can be reinforced by standing and walking in the pool, some support being given by the water. He will be taught how to fall, beginning in upright kneeling, falling against the wall or against a large stabilized ball, falling sideways on to his shoulder thereby protecting his face. A crash helmet may be worn until he can walk without falling over.

The emphasis in balance stimulation must be on the stimulation of head and trunk movement as this is essential for the stability required for all functions.

SUMMARY

The limb deficient child has problems of emotional, intellectual and motor development stemming from the movement disorder produced by the absence or abnormality of his limbs. These problems will be principally in the areas of locomotion, balance and manipulation, but will extend much further into the development of the family unit and the child's ability to learn.

Physical treatment consists principally in stimulating the most effective development possible for the child, using prostheses where these are necessary for this development. Those responsible for the management of the child must be sufficiently adaptable and imaginative to be able to encourage unorthodox development of activities where this will enable the child to function more effectively.

References

Frantz, C. H. and O'Rahilly, R. (1961) Congenital skeletal limb deficiencies. *J. Bone Jt. Surg.* **43A**, 1202.

Henkel, L. and Willert, H. (1969) Dysmelia. *J. Bone Jt. Surg.* **51B**, 3, 399.

Robertson, E. S. (1971) *Follow-up Study into the Functional Abilities at Home and at School of Multiple Limb Deficient Children.* London: Queen Mary's Hospital.

Rubin, A. (1967) *Handbook of Congenital Malformations.* Philadelphia and London: Saunders.

Further Reading

Blakeslee, B. (1973) *The Limb Deficient Child.* Los Angeles: University of California Press.

Burtch, R. L. (1966) Nomenclature for congenital skeletal limb deformities, a revision of the Frantz and O'Rahilly classification. *Artificial Limbs*, **10**, 1, 24.

Kershaw, J. D. (1961) *Handicapped Children.* London: Heinemann.

Ladd, H. W. and Simard, T. G. (1972) Bilateral controlled neuromuscular activity in congenitally malformed children — an electromyographic study. *Inter-Clinic Information Bulletin*, **11**, 5, 9.

Lamb, D. W., Simpson, D. C., Schutt, W. H., Spiers, N. T., Sutherland, C. and Baker, G. (1965) The management of upper limb deficiencies in the thalidomide type syndrome. *J. Roy. Coll. Surg. Edin.* **10**, 102.

McCredie, J. (1974) Embryonic neuropathy. An hypothesis of neural crest injury as the pathogenesis of congenital malformation. *Med. J. Aust.* **1**, 6, 159.

MacDonnell, J. A. (1958) Age of fitting upper extremity prostheses. *J. Bone Jt. Surg.* **40A**, 655.

Marquardt, E. (1965) The Heidelberg pneumatic arm prosthesis. *J. Bone Jt. Surg.* **47B**, 425.

Pearson, F. A. and Spiers, B. W. (1966) Teamwork in the management of dysmelic children. *Physiotherapy* **52**, 6, 197.

Roskies, E. (1972) *Abnormality and Normality: The Mothering of Thalidomide Children.* Ithaca: Cornell University Press.

Sharrard, W. J. W. (1971). *Paediatric Orthopaedics and Fractures*. Oxford and Edinburgh: Blackwell.

Spiers, B. W. and Saunders, J. (1962) Aids for congenitally deformed babies. *Physiotherapy*, **48**, 346.

Swinyard, C. A. (1969) *Limb Development and Deformity: Problems of Evaluation and Rehabilitation*. Illinois: Thomas.

Whatley, E. (1962) The reactions of parents of handicapped babies. *Mental Health*, **21**, 93.

Wilson, A. B. K. (1965) Hendon pneumatic power units and controls for prostheses and splints. *J. Bone Jt. Surg.* **47B**, 435.

Section IV

Disorders of Bones, Joints, Muscles and Skin

INTRODUCTION

1. *DUCHENNE-TYPE MUSCULAR DYSTROPHY*

2. *MUSCULAR TORTICOLLIS*

3. *STRUCTURAL SCOLIOSIS*

4. *INFLAMMATORY DISORDERS OF SOFT TISSUES AND JOINTS*

5. *THE BURNT CHILD*

Introduction

The Chapters in this Section describe the disorders of bones, joints, muscles (excluding those of congenital origin) and skin suffered by children, and seen most commonly by the physiotherapist.

The role of the physiotherapist in the treatment of children with orthopaedic disorders has shifted emphasis considerably over the last few years. Much time used to be spent in treating children with knock knees, bow legs and flat feet, and children with Perthes' Disease and tuberculosis of the hip and spine, who spent a considerable part of their childhood immobilized on frames. Now *knock knees, bow legs* and *flat feet* are recognized as being usually only transient stages in the development of the normal postural mechanism. Diseases such as *tuberculosis* are disappearing, although not in underdeveloped countries. *Perthes' Disease* is now treated by allowing early ambulation in ambulatory braces or surgically rather than by long-term immobilization on a frame. *Poor posture*, commonly a combination of kyphosis, lordosis and round shoulders, is seen as a mostly transient stage in some adolescents, physical treatment drawing attention to a child already discomforted by constant nagging on the part of parents and teachers. For these children swimming, gymnasium and other activities are more acceptable than exercises which they will be poorly motivated to perform at home.

It is now realized that physical treatment is not necessary for most of these children, and that the physiotherapist's time may be more effectively spent in other areas of paediatrics. However, the author has included in this introduction some details relating to fractures, Perthes' Disease, knock knees, bow legs and flat feet — fractures because the physiotherapist may apply the fixation, Perthes' Disease because of the need to recognize the symptoms, postural disorders of the lower limbs because the physiotherapist will need to understand the degree of severity which may require orthopaedic consultation. For details about the clinical features and problems associated with tuberculosis of joints the reader is referred to Ferguson (1968) and Sharrard (1971).

FRACTURES

Children's bones respond to trauma with a pattern of injuries quite different from that of adult bones, except where osteroporosis is the predisposing factor. They are more pliable and therefore subject to greenstick fractures. However, if a fracture in a child *is* complete, the periosteum which is very strong frequently remains intact, thus aiding both reduction and repair. As a general rule, the younger the child is the more rapidly the fracture will heal. Children with muscle paralysis, such as those with myelomeningocele or poliomyelitis, and those who have had a prolonged period of immobilization, may suffer osteoporosis. In children with rheumatoid arthritis there may also be an associated osteoporosis. These children will all suffer an increased tendency to fracture even though the bones may only be subjected to minimal stress. Other children are born with multiple fractures and continue to suffer fractures on slight trauma, due to the familial disorder called osteogenesis imperfecta. Epiphyseal separation occurs only in childhood, and an injury which may cause a dislocation or a soft tissue tear in an adult may produce in the child the separation of an epiphysis, a few of which will result in growth arrest if uncorrected.

The physiotherapist may be required to apply the fixation for a child following a fracture — a fully enclosed plaster cast for a fracture involving a limb, traction for a femoral fracture, or a figure-of-eight bandage for a fracture of the clavicle. Except in the case of a child with multiple injuries, rehabilitation of full function upon removal of splinting proceeds in most cases quite naturally and requires no assistance. Most children progress their activities spontaneously, as their strength and mobility improve. The exception may be the child with a stiff elbow following a supracondular fracture of the humerus. Recovery of movement at this joint usually proceeds slowly, but the physiotherapist can devise ways of improving mobility which the child can practise at home. It is most important that all movement is within a pain-free range, and that no attempt is made to force the joint which will react by increased stiffness and permanent disability (Watson-Jones 1960, Sharrard 1971). Swimming and ball games using a large lightweight ball will encourage the child to regain movement himself, and are more suitable techniques for home treatment than exercises for the elbow itself, avoiding the irresistible tendency on the part of some parents, as well as physiotherapists, to force the elbow into a greater range.

PERTHES' DISEASE

Children with this disease in which there is a vascular necrosis of the head of the femur, present with a history of limp and pain. On examination the hip is found to lack full range of movement. Early treatment involves rest, sometimes in slings and springs, until the protective muscle spasm has disappeared. This is followed by early ambulation in ambulatory braces in which the legs are maintained in abduction and internal rotation. Some children require an innominate or femoral osteotomy to contain the femoral head within the acetabulum. Treatment is completed when the radiograph shows revascularization of the femoral head.

KNOCK KNEES, BOW LEGS, FLAT FEET

Knock knees, bow legs and flat feet are included below rather than in a separate chapter. Although they do not require physical treatment, they are common disorders in childhood and therefore seen frequently by the physiotherapist in patients attending for treatment of some other unrelated problem. In the course of her assessment of a patient she may note, for example, a severe degree of knock knee in a child in whom the deformity should have ceased to be apparent, and she will need to refer the child back to his doctor to whom she will report her findings.

Genu Valgum (Knock Knees)

Most children between the ages of 2 and 5 years have some degree of knock knee, many with associated flat feet, the latter due to the altered line of weightbearing. The deformity seems more common in children who are over-weight and in children who persist in sitting between their feet, a position which may stretch the medial knee ligaments. The severity of knock knee lessens as the child grows, although a small degree of valgus is normally present at the knee due to the relationship of the femur to the pelvis and the angle at which the femur joins with the tibia.

The degree of genu valgum is estimated by measuring the distance in centimetres between the medial malleoli with the child in supine and the medial sides of the knees in contact with each other. A measurement of more than 10 centimetres at the age of 3 years requires radiological investigation to exclude bony abnormality (Sharrard 1971).

Genu valgum may also occur secondary to paralysis of the lower limbs. It will occur where there is paralysis of the quadriceps and hamstrings due to the inability of these muscles to control the weightbearing alignment of the knee. Adequate splinting will prevent the knee being forced by the weight of the body into a valgus position.

Few orthopaedic surgeons prescribe splinting for children with knock knees, except where the condition is secondary to paralysis and likely to progress, in which case a long leg brace with a special knee pad will be necessary (figure 111). Some treat the associated flat feet, recommending a medial raise and elongation of the heel of the shoe, with the aim of transferring weightbearing more laterally. Others recommend no treatment, and advise parents that the stage is normal and transient, and that no treatment is required. In a small percentage of children the deformity does persist, probably due to an underlying growth disturbance (Ferguson 1968) and these children may require stapling of the tibial or femoral epiphysis or osteotomy as they approach skeletal maturity.

Genu Varum (Bow Legs)

In this deformity there may be lateral curvature of the tibia alone, or of both the femur and the tibia. Some degree of bow legs with flat feet is seen in small children when they first begin to walk, the whole leg being bowed outward, the bowing being more apparent than real. The deformity in this case is developmental and disappears within a short time, being replaced usually by a degree of genu valgum by the age of 3 years. However, genu varum may also be due to rickets, and is found in children with achondroplasia, osteogenesis imperfecta and Blount's Disease. There may also be an apparent rather than a true deformity in children with genu recurvatum (hyperextended knees) and those with medial rotation of the legs due to anteversion of the femoral neck.

The degree of bowing is measured with the child in supine and the medial malleoli in contact with each other. The distance between the medial femoral condyles is measured in centimetres.

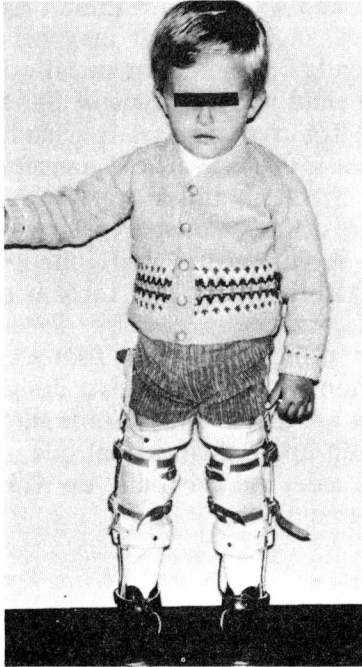

Fig. 111 Knock knee braces. Note the special knee pad which is extended medially to allow the straps to pull the knee towards the outside iron.
(By permission of W. Cumming.)

If the deformity is very severe it may need to be corrected surgically by osteotomy or by stapling of the lateral side of the femoral or tibial epiphysis. Otherwise no treatment is needed where the deformity is developmental, a fact which needs to be carefully explained to the child's parents.

Flat Feet

There are several types of flat feet seen in children. The difference between these types needs to be established as management will vary according to the causal mechanism.

Pes Planovalgus (developmental or inherited flat foot)

Some degree of flat-footedness is seen in all infants when they first begin to stand and walk, as a normal stage in the development of the postural mechanism. It may persist, and in these children it is frequently of familial or racial origin, and remains asymptomatic. If a child with this type of flat foot is referred to the physiotherapist for treatment, it is usually to reassure the parents, as treatment is of no avail and unnecessary as far as the child is concerned. Gradually this attitude towards the parents is disappearing as more orthopaedic surgeons realize the importance of explaining the developmental and inherited causes of the child's flat feet, reassuring them that there is no need for treatment.

The foot muscles in this type of flat foot are not weak, nor is the foot lacking in mobility, and exercises designed to strengthen or mobilize the foot are unnecessary. Some surgeons recommend that the shoes be built up on their medial side in order to prevent excess wear on that side, but this build-up will probably not influence the flat feet themselves.

Secondary Flat Feet

Flat feet may be secondary to genu valgum and varum, or to medial rotation of the legs due to anteversion of the femoral neck. In the latter case some recommend the child be taught hip external rotation exercises in standing, but although this will correct the pronated feet while the exercise is being done, it is impractical as a form of correction as the child will not remember to do it unless constantly reminded and it is unlikely that correction will be maintained between periods of practice.

Flat feet may also be secondary to contracture or spasticity of the calf muscles. Prolonged weightbearing on a foot in which the calcaneus is held in equinus by either spasticity of the calf muscles or contracture of the tendo Achilles, will cause the foot to 'break' at the mid-tarsal joints, the foot being made plantigrade by

314

dorsiflexion at these joints rather than at the ankle joint. This is relatively commonly seen in spastic children, and although this foot is unaesthetic in appearance it is surprisingly asymptomatic in childhood. If there is pain, it is usually due to the great toe being pushed into a valgus position by the medial weightbearing. This deformity may be prevented by surgical elongation of the tendo Achilles, or by the application of a skin-tight walking plaster with the toes in dorsiflexion. The toe dorsiflexion helps to inhibit the plantarflexion element of the abnormal extension pattern. The plaster is padded only at bony points in order to minimize movement within it. Any movement of the leg within the plaster will stimulate the hyperactive stretch reflexes and prevent inhibition of spasticity. The plaster is applied with the knee in a few degrees of flexion and the ankle in dorsiflexion. It is worn for 2 weeks, then reapplied for a further 2 weeks. It has been found to be very effective for some children (Hayes and Burns 1970) resulting in considerable inhibition of the spasticity throughout the entire body. The most important points in its application seem to be its length (i.e. including the knee as well as the foot) its skin-tightness, the dorsiflexion of the toes, its reapplication as spasticity is progressively more inhibited, and the ambulation and treatment of the child while weightbearing in the plaster.

Flat feet may also be secondary to muscle weakness such as may follow after poliomyelitis, when the tibialis anterior and posterior, both essential to maintenance of the medial longitudinal arch, may be weak or paralysed. The foot will be more stable and there will be less likelihood of strain to the medial ligament of the ankle if the child wears a short outside iron with an inside T-strap or a build-up on the medial side of the heel of the shoe.

Where there is insufficient tone to maintain the normal foot posture, the foot will collapse into a valgus position as soon as the child weightbears. This is seen in children during the hypotonic stage of cerebral palsy, and in those who have hypotonia due to other causes such as Werdnigg Hoffmann's Disease and benign hypotonia. Treatment is aimed at generally increasing tone (see Section II, Chapter 1) but an arch support inside the shoe will probably be necessary when the child begins to stand, in order to prevent structural damage to the growing foot.

Peroneal spasm causing flat feet

Peroneal spasm is thought (Lloyd-Roberts 1971) to be caused either by rheumatoid arthritis affecting the subtaloid joint and causing a localized painful spasm of the peroneal muscles, or to fusion of joints in the tarsus as occurs when there is a talo-calcaneal or a calcaneo-navicular bar, with associated shortness of the peroneal muscles.

Treatment in the latter case may not be necessary as the painful symptoms tend to disappear. If they persist, surgery in the form of a triple arthrodesis or excision of the bar, may be necessary when the child is old enough.

Painful flat feet

These are sometimes seen in adolescence, perhaps due to over-stretching of the plantar ligaments during the final growth and weight gain (Lloyd-Roberts 1971).

Wedging of the heels of the shoes is probably not acceptable cosmetically at this stage, but an arch support inside the shoe may help relieve symptoms, which will soon disappear anyway.

Congenital vertical talus

This uncommon disorder must be differentiated from talipes calcaneo-valgus which at first sight it resembles (figure 112). The foot is convex on the medial side, the head of the talus protrudes in the sole and there is rigidity of the sub-taloid joint.

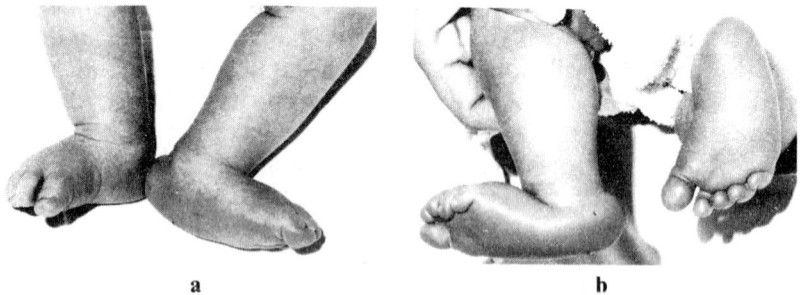

a   b

Fig. 112 The left foot has a vertical talus.
(By permission of the Royal Alexandra Hospital for Children.)

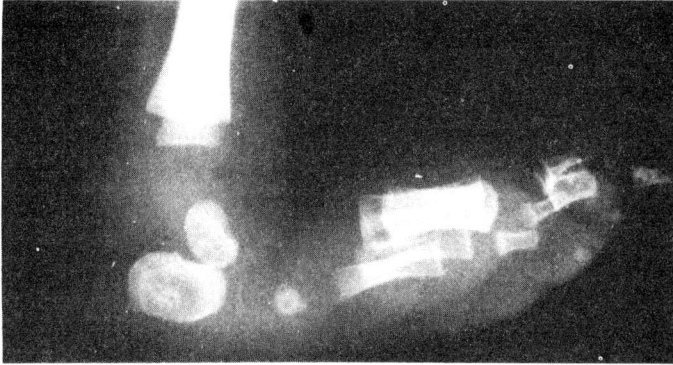

Fig. 113 A radiograph of the same foot showing abnormal bony relationships. (By permission of the Royal Alexandra Hospital for Children.)

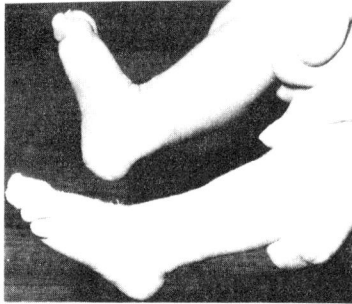

a

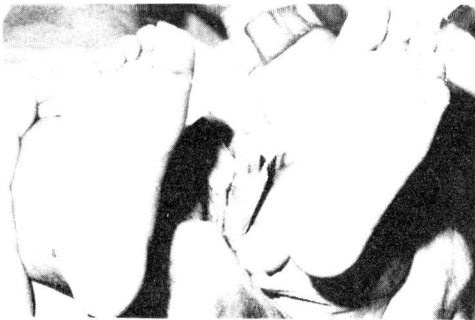

b

Fig. 114(a) and (b) These photographs show the altered position of the left foot after several applications of moulded plasters.
(By permission of the Royal Alexandra Hospital for Children.)

Radiographs show the calcaneus to be in equinus with the talus continuing in a vertical line from the tibia (figure 113). The talonavicular joint is dislocated.

This condition is treated conservatively by the application of a moulded plaster applied with the foot in plantarflexion and inversion (figure 114), or, if the child is not seen in early infancy, by surgery (Lloyd-Roberts 1971, Sharrard 1971).

References

Ferguson, A. B. (1968) *Orthopaedic Surgery in Infancy and Childhood.* Baltimore: Williams & Wilkins.

Hayes, N. K. and Burns, Y. R. (1970) Discussion on the use of weight-bearing plasters in the reduction of hypertonicity. *Aust. J. Physiother.*, **16**, 3, 108.

Lloyd-Roberts, G. C. (1971) *Orthopaedics in Infancy and Childhood.* London: Butterworth.

Sharrard, W. J. W. (1971) *Paediatric Orthopaedics and Fractures.* Oxford and Edinburgh: Blackwell.

Watson-Jones, R. (1960) *Fractures and Joint Injuries.* Edinburgh: Livingstone.

Further Reading

Asher, C. (1975) *Postural Variations in Childhood.* London: Butterworth.

Farrier, C. D. and Lloyd-Roberts, G. C. (1969) The natural history of knock knees. *Practitioner*, **203**, 789.

Helfet, A. J. (1956) Treatment of flat feet. *Lancet* **1**, 262.

Lloyd-Roberts, G. C. and Spence, A. J. (1958) Congenital vertical talus. *J. Bone Jt. Surg.* **40B**, 33.

Meyer, J. (1977) Legg-Calvé-Perthés' Disease. A study of the efficacy of three methods of treatment. *Acta Ortho. Scand. Suppl.* 167. Copenhagen: Munksgaard.

Roaf, R. and Hodgkinson, L. J. (1963) *The Oswestry Textbook for Orthopaedic Nurses.* London: Pitman.

Rose, G. K. (1958) Correction of pronated feet. *J. Bone Jt. Surg.* **40B**, 674.

Ibid. (1962) Correction of pronated feet. *J. Bone Jt. Surg.* **44B**, 642.

Chapter 1

Muscular Dystrophy

One of the most common conditions producing muscle weakness in children is *muscular dystrophy*. There are a number of inherited disorders called muscular dystrophy (figure 115), and all are characterized by progressive degeneration of muscle.

Spinal muscular atrophy (for example Werdnig-Hoffman and Kugelberg-Welander diseases) is another inherited condition seen in childhood in which there is muscle weakness. This condition must be distinguished, however, from muscular dystrophy, as the muscle weakness is secondary to anterior horn cell degeneration, whereas the primary defect in muscular dystrophy is unknown.

The Duchenne type dystrophy is described here as it is the most common dystrophy seen in paediatric physiotherapy departments, and because it provides an example of the problems seen in children with progressive muscular weakness. Treatment of children with other forms of dystrophy and with spinal muscular atrophy will be along similar lines to the treatment described below.

DESCRIPTION

This disease is characterized by progressive weakness and wasting of muscles. It is seen in males, and is transmitted as a sex-linked recessive characteristic with a high mutation rate. Clinical features are usually evident within the first three years of life, and the disease progresses until the patient is unable to walk, which may occur near the age of 12, or in early adolescence. The child dies from respiratory infection or cardiac failure some time in his second or third decade.

The muscle weakness is relatively symmetrical and begins proximally in the pelvic girdle, shoulder girdle and trunk. The hands usually maintain some useful function until the later stages of the disease, although the extreme weakness of the arms and the muscles around the shoulder girdle makes it very difficult for the child to make use of his hands without mechanical assistance. Pseudohypertrophy is seen to some extent in almost every patient, in the calf muscles, quadriceps, gluteal and deltoid muscles, and occasionally in other muscle groups (figure 116).

X-Linked Muscular Dystrophy

    Severe (Duchenne type)
    Benign (Becker type)

Autosomal Recessive Muscular Dystrophy

    Limb-Girdle types
    Childhood muscular dystrophy (except Duchenne)
    Congenital muscular dystrophies

Facioscapulohumeral Muscular Dystrophy

Distal Muscular Dystrophy

Ocular Muscular Dystrophy

Oculopharyngeal Muscular Dystrophy

Fig. 115 Types of muscular dystrophy. (From Walton, J. N. (1969) *Disorders of Voluntary Muscles.* Baltimore: Williams & Wilkins.)

Progressive muscle weakness combined with the effect of gravity results in soft tissue contracture, and eventual restriction to a wheelchair hastens the development of contractures and deformity. Contractures of the hip flexors, ilio-tibial tract and calf muscles occur relatively early and result in the typical posture and walk. Once confined to a wheelchair, hip and knee flexion contractures, and inverted, plantarflexed feet causing an equinovarus deformity, usually become very marked. Weakness around the trunk plus the effect of gravity in the sitting position cause the spine to telescope into a scoliotic deformity which may become extreme, further interfering with respiratory function. These deformities, although not preventable, probably do not need to occur to such a gross extent as is unfortunately sometimes seen.

In the past the intelligence of these children was thought to be unaffected, but several authors have described mental back-wardness and apathy in a significant number of their patients (Worden and Vignos 1962, Walton 1969). Some authors comment that in those children who are retarded, intellectual impairment may precede the onset of weakness, which suggests that in-tellectual impairment is not related to the physical handicap.

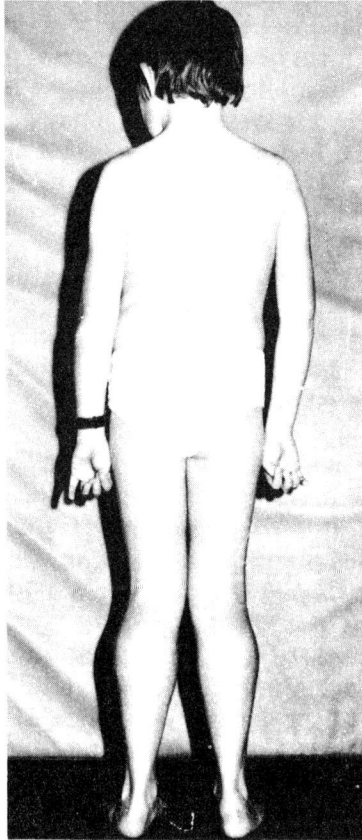

Fig. 116 Duchenne muscular dystrophy. Note the apparently hypertrophied calf muscles and the valgus feet due to contracture of the calf muscles.

321

PATHOLOGY

There is doubt in the minds of pathologists about the most significant pathological changes. There is a decrease in the number of muscle fibres, enlargement and atrophy of fibres, necrosis, signs of phagocytosis, infiltration by fat cells and increase in connective tissue. The muscles are eventually reduced to fat and connective tissue. In the later stages, some degree of osteoporosis of the long bones is found, probably due to disuse.

Whether or not muscular dystrophy is a primary disease of muscle is being questioned. Dubowitz (1968) suggests the possibility of some form of disordered innervation of the muscle, which would mean that myopathic changes may be under the influence of the nervous system. McComas *et al* (1970) in their studies demonstrated factors which suggest a neural basis for the disorder. Moosa (1974) comments that the presence of a factor in dystrophic serum may cause an increased release of creatine-phosphokinase (CPK) from dystrophic cells.

DIAGNOSIS

Diagnosis is made as a result of the clinical manifestations and knowledge of the family history, and is confirmed by the results of certain tests.

In an estimation of *serum enzymes*, serum creatine-phosphokinase (CPK) is found to be elevated, not only in the affected child but also in the asymptomatic carriers. *Muscle biopsy* demonstrates the typical changes seen in myopathy. *Electromyographic studies* demonstrate a characteristic pattern common to all forms of myopathy.

It is considered essential to offer genetic counselling to parents of a dystrophic boy. Gardner-Medwin (1977) points out the mother is a carrier of the gene in two-thirds of all cases and will have a one in four chance of producing an affected child in each subsequent pregnancy. The importance of such counselling taking place as soon as possible indicates the need for early recognition and diagnosis of the disease.

CLINICAL FEATURES

A delay in motor milestones in infancy is often evident. The child presents to his doctor, by the age of 3, with a history of frequent falls, of difficulty walking up stairs and running. When he gets up from the floor he does so in a characteristic way first described by Gower. He rolls to one side, pushes up to four foot kneeling,

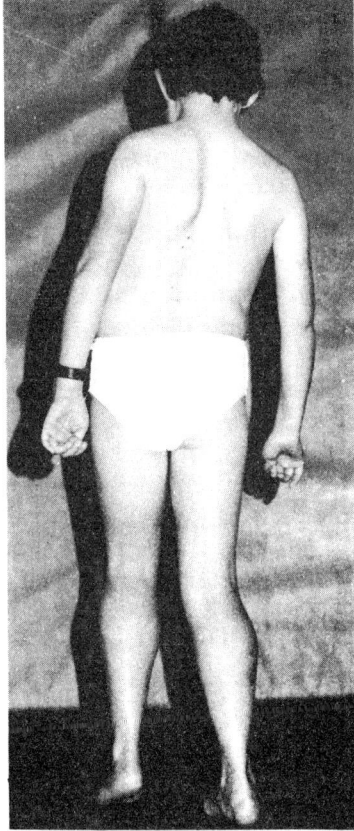

Fig. 117 Duchenne muscular dystrophy. Note the shoulders thrust backwards to maintain balance, the tilting down of the pelvis to the left side, the lack of ankle dorsiflexion.

extends his legs, finally pushing his body to the erect position by walking his hands up his legs. This manoeuvre is due to weakness of the extensor muscles, particularly the gluteals, and is also seen in other myopathic disorders, and in spinal muscular atrophy.

323

He walks with a waddling gait on a wide base, due to weakness of the gluteal and trunk muscles which causes loss of pelvic control and stability, and therefore poor balance. As the disease progresses, he walks with a marked lumbar lordosis, his shoulders and upper trunk thrust backwards (figure 117). His gait becomes high-stepping, due to weakness of the anterior tibial muscles, and his heels do not reach the ground because of the gradually increasing contracture of his calf muscles.

MANAGEMENT

The principal aims for all concerned with this child are to enable him to live a satisfactory and happy life, avoiding loneliness and boredom and to give him a means of education and an interesting active childhood. Few of these children reach a stage where they can earn a living, even in a sheltered workshop. Respiratory infections must be avoided, as also must fractures which may occur as a result of trauma to osteoporotic bones. Treatment should mean giving support to his parents as well as to the child, giving practical assistance and emotional support when they are needed.

Treatment therefore is partly *preventive* and partly *supportive*. It should be kept in mind that it is probably impossible to prevent either respiratory illness or deformity in the later and terminal stages of the disease. The word 'preventive' is used to indicate the importance of preventing such secondary complications from occurring in the younger child, causing him distress and making him immobile before he need be.

Assessment

It is necessary to assess the child regularly as a guide to possible apparatus and to treatment, but the assessment should not be done in such a way that might depress or upset the child. It should not appear to him as a confirmation of his increasing weakness and disability. A method of assessment has been suggested by Vignos, Spencer and Archibald (1963), which is done at three-monthly intervals. It may be used as a general guide to treatment as it indicates approximately the rate at which the child's disability is progressing.

Grade 1.   Walks and climbs stairs without assistance.

Grade 2.   Walks and climbs stairs with aid of railing.

Grade 3.   Walks and climbs stairs slowly with aid of railing (over 25 seconds for eight standard steps).

Grade 4.   Walks unassisted and rises from chair but cannot climb stairs.

Grade 5.   Walks unassisted but cannot rise from chair or climb stairs.

Grade 6.   Walks only with assistance or walks independently with long leg braces.

Grade 7.   Walks in long leg braces but requires assistance for balance.

Grade 8.   Stands in long leg braces but unable to walk even with assistance.

Grade 9.   Is in wheelchair. Elbow flexors more than antigravity.

Grade 10.   Is in wheelchair. Elbow flexors less than antigravity.

Muscle charting is too specific to be necessary as a guide to treatment. Weakness of its fixators and synergists makes it too difficult for a particular muscle to be tested accurately. A myometer is suggested (Edwards and Hyde 1977) as a possible means of obtaining quantitative data on muscle strength.

It is important to assess *function* as this gives a clear picture of disability and acts as a guide to treatment. Such functional assessment may be done by the physiotherapist once each school term, after she has visited the child's home, talked to his parents and to his school-teacher. She makes her own observations of such activities as walking, sitting to standing, standing to sitting, standing balance and effective use of hands, and keeps a record of these observations. Videotaped assessments combined with written or taped commentaries may provide a more accurate picture of functional states than written statements.

Of course, assessment is also carried out during each treatment session as an indicator of the effect of treatment and as an immediate guide to the details of treatment.

Respiratory function tests have an important place in the management of these children. A spirometer or peak flow meter may be used to assess the strength and fatiguability of respiratory muscles, as well as variations in vital capacity. Forced expired volume in 1 second (FEV_1) is tested using a vitalograph (see page 456).

Preventive Treatment

Prevention of respiratory illness

Rationale. Respiratory failure is a common cause of death in these children. Weakness and paralysis of the accessory muscles of respiration, particularly the abdominal muscles, latissimus dorsi and sternomastoid, make effective inspiration and expiration and therefore expulsion of mucus from the airways, difficult or impossible. Little can be done to avoid this in the terminal stage of the disease, when the child is confined to bed with little muscle power. At this stage, the only voluntary muscles capable of active contraction may be the diaphragm and facial muscles. Careful preventive measures in the early stages, however, will prevent the child from developing severe infections which would require bed rest with subsequent deterioration in his general condition. Because of the rapid deterioration which always follows periods of immobility, the dystrophic child will not be confined to bed during such childhood illnesses as chicken pox or measles, unless this is considered by his doctor to be essential.

Chronic alveolar hypoventilation has been reported in children with muscular dystrophy (Buchsbaum et al 1968). Hypoxaemia, retention of carbondioxide and respiratory acidosis lead to confusion, blurred vision and headache.

Methods. Daily breathing exercises for about 5 minutes attempting to obtain full expansion of the lungs may be done at home with the supervision of his mother. Emphasis should be on diaphragmatic breathing. In the early stages, adequate ventilatory function may be gained by swimming, and by games such as blowing a ping-pong ball around obstacles, in which case it is important that the therapist ensures that the child makes long controlled expirations. The child may be encouraged to play a wind instrument. Instruction in methods of postural drainage and assisted coughing is given to his parents, to be done when necessary. The criteria for necessity, the development of a cough or an upper respiratory tract infection, will be carefully explained to his parents. The length of time for postural drainage should be approximately five to ten minutes, although it is done for longer if necessary, and it should be done three or four times a day, depending also on necessity. The child is positioned in prone if he can tolerate it, and in side lying, in the manner described in

Section V, Chapter 4, for drainage of the lower lobes, unless specific segments need to be drained separately. Vibrations and breathing exercises with emphasis on full expiration will help to clear the secretions from the airways. In the later stages, the child may need routine daily postural drainage, a portable suction apparatus for the removal of secretions from the pharynx and a portable I.P.P.B. apparatus.

Prevention of soft tissue contracture and deformity

Rationale. One of the greatest problems facing the physiotherapist is the rapidity with which contractures progress once they have reached a certain point.

Muscle weakness occurring in one group of muscles leaves the opposing group free to pull the joint or limb into a deformed position. Since they are acting in a relatively unopposed manner these muscles eventually compensate and become contracted. Contractures once started progress very rapidly as the position of the limb becomes more mechanically favourable to the unopposed muscle group. Gravity favours the flexors in upright positions, and the weakness of the lower limb extensors which occurs early in the development of the disease increases the tendency toward flexion deformity. If the child is not encouraged to move about and to stand for periods of the day, time spent in sitting will also add to the tendency of the lower limb flexors to contract. So there is a trio of circumstances, unopposed muscle action, gravity and posture, which, acting together, rapidly produce deformity. It then becomes a fight against distortion of the skeletal system which the physiotherapist cannot hope to win.

Unfortunately some children in the early stages develop contractures which may become severe enough to limit activity even before muscle weakness is marked. Provided the child is kept mobile and upright it is possible to delay the early development of disabling deformity, although eventually as the disease progresses it becomes unpreventable.

However, it is difficult even in the early stages, to maintain soft tissue length in these children. A child at home for the school holidays, whose parents have not been thoroughly instructed by the physiotherapist may arrive back for the new term with contractures which are already too difficult to correct. Muscles

327

tighten so slowly and relentlessly that the therapist may not notice that she is gaining less range as the weeks pass. Periodic tests of joint range with a goniometer may be useful as a guide to the progress of deformity.

Whether or not it is of benefit to stretch contracted soft tissues manually once the contractures have become well established is controversial. It is doubtful that anything is achieved, and the procedures are time-consuming and painful. It the physiotherapist has the strength to affect the soft tissues, it is more likely that they will rupture before they will elongate. The soft tissue which is contracted is only partly muscle fibre. It is also composed to a greater or lesser extent of fibrous tissue, which has no elastic properties.

Methods. Activities which encourage the fullest range of movement possible plus the maintenance of an erect posture for as long as possible will delay the development of contractures and deformity. The therapist guides the child's activities and makes sure he moves his limbs to the limits of their range. Movements should involve active contraction of the muscles antagonistic to the potentially tight soft tissues, and movements involving extension are emphasized, with resistance or assistance from the therapist or from a pulley system, and by the general activities suggested below.

The therapist will need to use her ingenuity to work out ways of getting maximum involvement of the child in the activities she suggests. She must beware of boring him to either apathy or rebellion by giving stereotyped exercises which have no interest for him. There is enough variety in normal activities to give a basis from which to start and there is rarely need for treatment sessions devoted entirely to exercises.

The child is taught to maintain the length of his calf muscles himself, by standing with his pelvis forwards, his arms on his desk or on the wall, making sure his heels remain on the ground with his knees fully extended (figure 118). A period is spent either at home or at school lying in prone, which will help to maintain the length of the hip flexors (figure 119). For the older child, lying prone on a frame, such as the Rossfeld frame (figure 120) which can be leant against a school desk or a small tilt table, may be more acceptable, as the child is in a better position to see his teacher and the rest of his class. A frame has the advantage of holding the child in what is virtually the erect position, while still encouraging extension of the head and trunk.

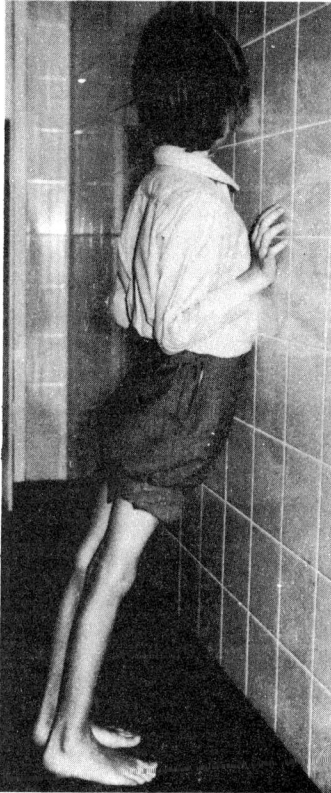

Fig. 118 A method of maintaining length in the calf muscles. The child should push his pelvis forwards as far as possible, with his heels on the ground.

Parents are taught how to maintain length of the calf muscles, ilio-tibial tract and hamstrings, and should spend a few minutes each day performing each stretch approximately 10 times. The parent's techniques must be reassessed frequently as it is important that these stretches are done correctly. The ilio-tibial band is stretched in prone, the hip being maintained in full extension while the leg is adducted (Vignos, Spencer and Archibald 1963) (figure 121). The hamstrings are stretched with the child in supine, his heel resting on the therapist's shoulder. The knee must be kept

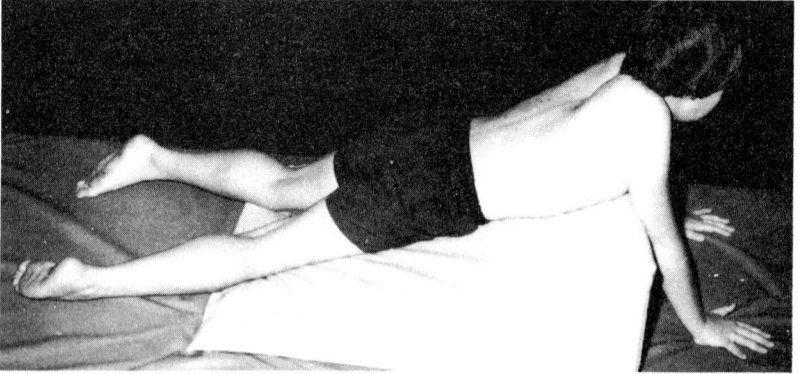

Fig. 119 Modified push-ups done over a wedge will encourage extension of the trunk and head as well as maintaining the length of the hip flexors.

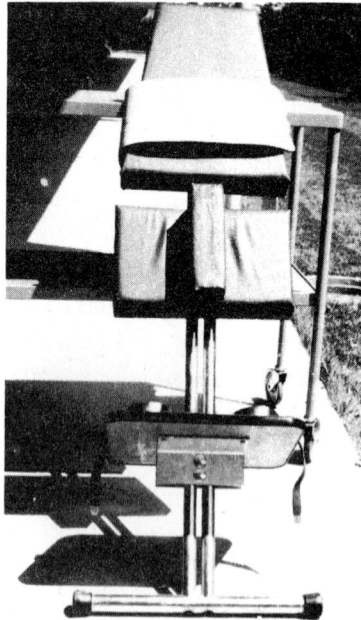

Fig. 120 The Rossfeld prone board. The child lies in prone and the board is leant against a school desk. The table should not have castors as shown here.

extended as the hip is flexed to approximately 60 degrees. The hold-relax technique (see Appendix 5) may be used if the child has sufficient muscle strength (figure 122).

Nevertheless, there is a point at which passive stretching will have little or no effect, and at this stage it is difficult to think of ways of preventing the gradual shortening of soft tissues.

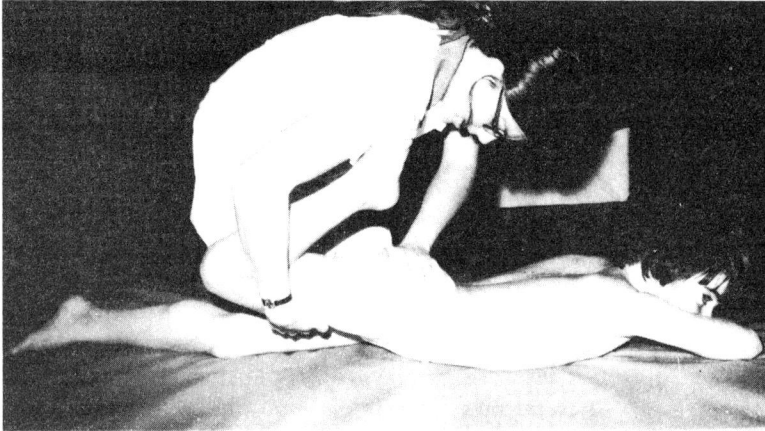

Fig. 121 A method of stretching the ilio-tibial tract by adducting the extended hip. Firm pressure should be given downwards on the pelvis to minimise movement at the lumbar spine.

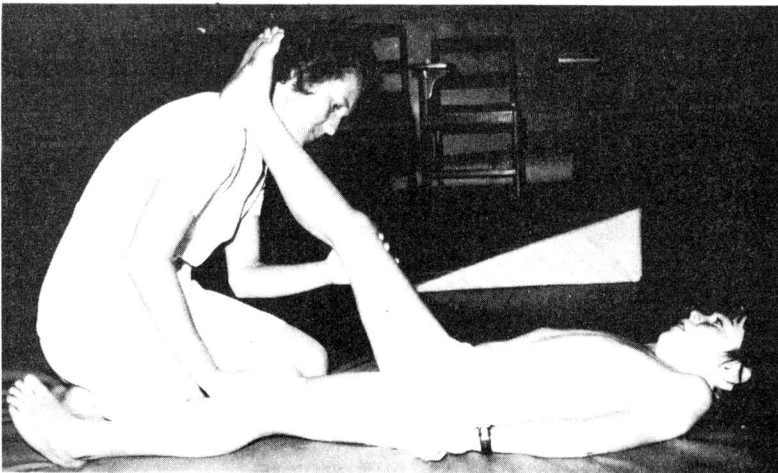

Fig. 122 Maximal contraction of the hamstrings followed by relaxation in an attempt to maintain their length.

Prevention of Immobility and Inactivity, both Mental and Physical

Rationale. It is probably possible to gain some increase in strength and activity when treatment first begins, as the child may have some disuse weakness if he is not referred to the physiotherapist until weakness is noticeable. The habit of exercising should be developed early in his life. The child is kept as active as possible without causing him fatigue. Games and activities need to be carefully thought out, so they will be a challenge to the child rather than a set of gymnastics to be carried out for the benefit of the physiotherapist. Inactivity is detrimental to these children, and a bored disillusioned child tends to be inactive, especially if it also an effort for him to move.

It is essential that the child develops in his life varied interests and an enthusiasm for hobbies which he will be able to continue once his activities are severely limited.

Methods. Swimming and games in the pool are activities which encourage mobility, endurance and respiratory control. The child's time in the pool is carefully planned to include the necessary activities without the element of fun being excluded. A group of children can play ball games with a ping-pong ball which is blown towards the goal. Flippers on the feet provide assistance to the knee extensors. Kicking practice with a board encourages spinal extension as well as active movement of the legs. Tunbridge and Diamond (1966) suggest sandhill climbing as a means of developing endurance. Activities with the assistance or resistance of a pulley system will exercise the abdominal muscles, the trunk extensors and lower limb extensors. Wrestling on mats on the floor can be enjoyed by even a moderately disabled child, and boxing a punching bag encourages balance in sitting, upright kneeling or standing. Tying knots with the guidance of a boy scout manual keeps the fingers dextrous, and modelling in clay or plasticine can be encouraged at school.

Part of each day, at least 30 minutes, should be set aside at home or at school for vigorous games and activities to encourage strength, mobility and respiratory function.

Splinting and Surgery

The use of splinting and surgery is controversial. There are basically two approaches to the management of the child at the stage when he is falling a lot and able to walk only along the flat. The first suggests that the child may be kept on his feet for an extra few years by surgery to divide contracted soft tissues such as tendo Achilles and tensor fascia lata. Surgery must be followed within twenty-four hours by weightbearing in plaster, and as soon as possible by the application of lightweight long leg calipers which give support under the ischial tuberosities (Spencer and Vignos 1962, Vignos 1975 and Siegel 1975a).

The second approach, discussed by Gardner-Medwin (1977) suggests that, provided the wheelchair *increases* the child's mobility, it may be preferable for the child by bringing to an end his struggle to stay on his feet. An electric powered wheelchair is essential for a child who lacks the upper arm strength needed to propel a chair. Vignos, Spencer and Archibald (1963) and Tunbridge and Diamond (1966) have found that the children in their care are able to stay on their feet for longer with the aid of calipers, and therefore the stage of dependency in a wheelchair is delayed.

A moulded leather or plastic jacket (Tunbridge and Diamond 1966, Sharrard 1971) or a corset (Vignos, Spencer and Archibald 1963) may prevent the development of severe scoliosis once the child is confined to a wheelchair. It is also important to ensure that the seat of the chair is very firm to prevent lateral tilting of the pelvis. Dubowitz (1977) suggests that the backrest should be angled backwards 5 or 10 degrees. This presumably prevents gravity exerting a directly vertical force upon the spine. Gibson and Wilkins (1975) suggest that a lumbar lordotic posture helps to prevent lateral curvature of the spine by locking the posterior intervertebral facets. They therefore recommend fitting moulded inserts to the wheelchair in order to induce this posture.

Supportive Treatment

For parents

The physiotherapist tries to establish a good relationship with the child's parents as soon as possible after treatment is started. It makes a considerable difference if the parents feel there is one person who is sufficiently outside their circle of family, friends and neighbours to be contacted about problems which may arise.

Many of the practical problems can be dealt with by the physiotherapist, or by an occupational therapist. However, there will be other problems, both social and economic, and these are referred by the therapist to the social worker. Emotional problems stemming from guilt at being a carrier affect many parents, and these feelings may need to be talked out with the social worker or with the physician.

Home visits will be made at intervals to determine what mechanical aids may be needed to solve practical problems. If it is possible these problems should be anticipated. Parents often have a tendency to endure what there is no need to endure. This occurs either because they are not aware of the facilities available, or because problems arise long before they are noticed to be problems. For example, the parents of a 12 year old boy had been lifting him in and out of the bath daily for some time and without complaint before anyone thought to ask how the child was being washed. Only when a hydraulic hoist was made available, did the parents, looking back over the preceding weeks, remember how difficult the situation had been.

Parents need guidance about the child's diet and this guidance should begin in infancy. Inactivity, overeating and an inappropriate diet are probably the principal causes of the obesity frequently encountered in these children. It is advisable that low carbohydrate high protein eating habits are developed early in life. Where an older child has already developed obesity, consultation with a dietician should be advised.

What the child does for pleasure at home will depend to some extent on the nature of recreation within the family. It is sometimes necessary to give some guidance in suitable activities for the child to pursue. Whatever activities he does engage in at home, he should not remain long in one position but should be as mobile as possible. For this reason long periods in front of the television may have to be curtailed. However, the physiotherapist must be careful not to interfere in the life of the family, remaining available to answer questions rather than giving advice where it may not be wanted. Families differ in their needs for help and the therapist must not be so insensitive as to ignore cries for help or to intrude unnecessarily upon the family's privacy.

For the child

The child himself requires encouragement. He may be negative and uncommunicative. He will become depressed if he sees he is achieving little, and if he works hard to accomplish so little, he will become even more downhearted. What he *does* achieve depends on how the physiotherapist organizes and carries out her treatment. She must grade assistance and resistance in such a way that the child feels he is doing his best and sees that he is accomplishing something at the same time. She should never ask him to do a movement which he cannot do. She should know his abilities well enough, through continuing reassessment, to be able to avoid a situation in which he has to struggle. He may, for example, be treated on a low bed rather than on a mat on the floor, as this will make it easier for him to stand up. The dystrophic child is faced with failure too often and the physiotherapist should try to demonstrate to him what he *can* do rather than what he cannot. She must try to maintain his confidence in himself, and can discuss this with his schoolmaster, who will be in a position to give the boy the necessary support and encouragement at school. He should not be over-protected either at home or at school, and should be helped to be as independent as possible.

SUMMARY

The child with Duchenne-type muscular dystrophy faces a childhood of gradually developing disability that will end in his death sometime during his second decade. It must be remembered that the muscle weakness in this disease is unpreventable and irreversible (Walton 1969). However, it seems possibile to minimize deformity and weakness in the early stages by keeping the child erect and active. In general, the best the physiotherapist can hope to do is to keep the child as happy and as active as possible, in the hopeful expectation that the disease will one day become curable.

References

Buchsbaum, H. D. et al (1968) Chronic alveolar hypoventilation due to muscular dystrophy. *Neurol.* **18**, 319–327.

Dubowitz, V. (1968) *Developing and Diseased Muscle.* London: Heinemann.

Dubowitz, V. (1977) Analysis of neuromuscular disease. *Physiotherapy* **63**, 2, 38–46.

Edwards, R. H. T. and Hyde, S. (1977) Methods of measuring muscle strength and fatigue. *Physiotherapy* **63**, 2, 52–55.

Gardner-Medwin, D. (1977) Management of muscular dystrophy. *Physiotherapy* **63**, 2, 46–56.

McComas, A. J., Sica, R. E. P. and Currie, S. (1970) Muscular dystrophy: evidence for a neural factor. *Nature* **226**, 1263.

Moosa, A. (1974) Muscular dystrophy in childhood. *Develop. Med. Child Neurol.* **16**, 97–111.

Sharrard, W. J. W. (1971) *Paediatric Orthopaedics and Fractures.* Oxford and Edinburgh: Blackwell.

Siegel, I. M. (1975) Surgery in the management of Duchenne muscular dystrophy. In *Recent Advances in Myology*, edited by W. G. Bradley, D. Gardner-Medwin and J. N. Walton. Amsterdam: Excerpta Medica.

Spencer, G. E. and Vignos, P. J. (1962) Bracing for ambulation in childhood muscular dystrophy. *J. Bone Jt. Surg.* **44A**, 234.

Tunbridge, P. B. and Diamond, S. (1966) Recent treatment of progressive muscular dystrophy. *Med. J. Aust.* **1**, 962.

Vignos, P. J. (1975) The comprehensive management of Duchenne muscular dystrophy. In *Recent Advances in Myology*, edited by W. G. Bradley, D. Gardner-Medwin and J. N. Walton. Amsterdam: Excerpta Medica.

Vignos, P. J., Spencer, G. E. and Archibald, K. C. (1963) Management of progressive muscular dystrophy of childhood. *J.A.M.A.* **184**, 2, 89.

Walton, J. (1969) *Disorders of Voluntary Muscles.* Baltimore: Williams and Wilkins.

Worden, D. K. and Vignos, P. J. (1962) Intellectual function in childhood progressive muscular dystrophy. *Paediatrics*, **29**, 968.

Further Reading

Anderson, R. S. (1971) Muscular dystrophy: Duchenne type. *Social Work Today*, **2**, 14.

Archibald, K. C. and Vignos, P. J. (1959) A study of contractures in muscular dystrophy. *Arch. Phys. Med.* **40**, 150.

Banker, B. Q., Victor, M. and Adams, K. D. (1957) Arthrogryposis Multiplex due to congenital muscular dystrophy. *Brain,* **80**, 319.

Bishop, A., Gallup, B., Skeate, Y. and Dubowitz, V. (1971) Morphological studies on normal and diseased human muscle in culture. *J. Neurol. Sc.* **13**, 333.

Bradley, W. G. (1971) Nerve, muscle and muscular dystrophy. *Develop. Med. Child Neurol.*, **13**, 528.

Diamond, C. (1968) Management of the dystrophic. *Rehabilitation in Australia,***6.**

Dubowitz, V. (1968) The myopathies. *Physiotherapy*, **54**, 11.

Dubowitz, V. (1971) Muscular dystrophy — where is the lesion? *Develop. Med. Child Neurol.* **13**, 528.

Dubowitz, V. (1976) Screening for Duchenne muscular dystrophy. *Arch. Dis. Childhd.* **51**, 249-251.

Hosking, G. P., Bhat, U. S., Dubowitz, V. and Edwards, R. H. T. (1976) Measurements of muscle strength and performance in children with normal and diseased muscles. *Arch. Dis. Childhd.* **51**, 957-963.

Inkley, S. R., Oldenburg, F. C. and Vignos, P. J. (1974) Pulmonary function in Duchenne muscular dystrophy related to stage of disease. *Am. J. Med.* **56**, 297.

Kottke, F. J., Pauley, D. L. and Ptak, R. A. (1966) The rationale for prolonged stretching for correction of shortening of connective tissue. *Arch. Phys. Med.* **47**, 45, 345.

Shaw, R. F. and Dreifuss, F. E. (1969) Mild and severe forms of X-linked muscular dystrophy. *Arch. Neurol.* **20**, 451.

Siegel, I. M. (1975) Pulmonary problems in Duchenne muscular dystrophy. *Phys. Ther.* **55**, 2, 160-162.

Vignos, P. J. and Watkins, M. P. (1966) The effect of exercise in muscular dystrophy. *J.A.M.A.* **197**, 11, 121.

Chapter 2

Muscular Torticollis

The term 'muscular torticollis' is used to indicate the torticollis associated with fibrosis of the sternomastoid muscle which is found in infants and young children, and to differentiate between this condition and torticollis associated with other factors, whether neurological (spasmodic torticollis) or structural (congenital hemivertebrae).

The infant with torticollis lies with his head side flexed to one side and rotated to the other (figure 123). He may be unable to rotate his head in the opposite direction beyond the midline. In many cases, but not in all, a sternomastoid tumour is evident. If it is present, it is noticed as an elongated swelling in the belly of the muscle, becoming obvious usually in the second or third week after birth, and usually disappearing before five or six months of age (figure 123). A degree of facial asymmetry will be present, and in some cases cranial asymmetry is severe enough to develop into plagiocephaly, although plagiocephaly is present at birth in a small percentage of these infants. This asymmetry may be very noticeable in the older baby or child, causing considerable anxiety to the parents.

AETIOLOGY

The cause of torticollis is unknown, but there have been several theories advanced. One commonly held hypothesis is that of intra-uterine malpositioning of the neck with resultant local ischaemia of the sternomastoid (Adams, Denny Brown and Pearson 1962). It has been noticed to follow after breech delivery, when the muscle may be subject to further trauma (Ferguson 1968). However, the fact that it has also been found in babies delivered by caesarian section (Coventry and Harris 1959) seems to refute the hypothesis of birth injury. Jones (1968) describes in detail the various theories of aetiology.

PATHOLOGY

There is also considerable confusion about the pathology of torticollis. Jones (1968) states that the most constant finding is fibrosis of the sternomastoid which may be present with or without a tumour. He also considers the tumour to be a localized phenomenon in an already fibrosed sternomastoid muscle.

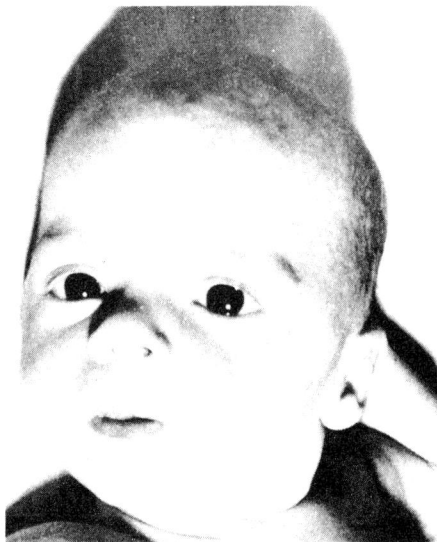

Fig. 123 Left torticollis with a tumour in the left sternomastoid muscle.

Sanerkin and Edwards (1966) describe an autopsy they performed on a two-day old premature infant with a sternomastoid tumour. In the sternomastoid they found haemorrhage, rupture and fragmentation of the muscle fibres with necrosis of some of the fibres, and disruption of the endomysial sheaths.

Adams, Denny Brown and Pearson (1962) commented that as the endomysial sheaths are destroyed there is fibrous tissue proliferation which prevents effective regeneration.

DIFFERENTIAL DIAGNOSIS

In all babies with torticollis, but particularly those without an evident sternomastoid tumour, the following diagnoses will be excluded by the baby's doctor.

Painful septic deep glands which will cause the baby to hold his head to one side.

Orthopaedic abnormalities, such as Klippel Feil syndrome and congenital hemivertebrae, which will result in a side flexed head posture. Visual defects such as diplopia due to strabismus, causing an ocular torticollis.

Plagiocephaly, in which the shape of the infant's head causes him to hold it in an asymmetrical posture without actual contracture of his sternomastoid.

Brain injury or developmental abnormality may be suggested in the young infant by persistent asymmetry of the head and neck, either as part of an asymmetrical tonic neck reflex or due to hypotonia.

PROGNOSIS

Although most of the cases of torticollis seen are infants, the onset of this deformity may develop or become accentuated at any age during early growth. Correction occurs in the majority of cases by six months of age. If the contracture persists, as it does in a small number of children, or if it appears in an older baby or child, the surgeon will perform a tenotomy of the sternomastoid and adjacent tight soft tissues. This procedure is usually not done before six months of age, and treatment is conservative until then. Surgery gives a successful result in most cases.

Once the head position has been corrected the facial asymmetry usually resolves. The baby's head moulds normally once it is free to rotate from side to side. Parents, often very anxious about this, may be reassured.

TREATMENT

Assessment

An initial assessment is made by the physiotherapist along the following lines.

The general appearance of the baby is noted, particularly the position of his head in relation to his trunk and limbs. The presence and extent of a sternomastoid tumour is palpated. The range of movement at the neck is tested by passively moving the baby's head in all directions and by attracting his attention to estimate the amount of active correction obtainable. The physiotherapist should note any apparent pain on movement or on palpation of the tumour. The degree of facial and cranial asymmetry is assessed by turning the baby's head to the mid-position with his face upwards.

His general development should be tested briefly, with note taken particularly of any persistent asymmetry of his limbs or trunk, any asymmetrical or abnormal reflex activity, such as presence of an asymmetrical tonic neck reflex, or asymmetry of a Moro, Galant or grasp reflex. If there is any doubt about development this should be reported to the baby's doctor, and a more thorough assessment made. This procedure is particularly necessary in those babies with no history of a sternomastoid tumour. The physiotherapist will occasionally find signs of possible brain damage in babies referred for treatment of what appears to be torticollis and it is important that she makes her findings known to the doctor so that treatment of what may prove to be cerebral palsy or some developmental disorder is begun early.

Rationale

There is some possibility that most cases of torticollis would resolve even in the absence of treatment (Coventry and Harris 1959). However, until controlled studies are done to establish the value of conservative treatment, it is in the best interests of the baby and his parents to institute a programme of passive and active correction.

It is difficult to devise a rational method of conservative treatment while the nature of the pathological process remains so uncertain. In the meantime it is assumed that in a young infant with a sternomastoid tumour but with little or no contracture of the sternomastoid, the purpose of treatment is to *prevent*, by stimulation of full range neck movement, the contracture of the muscle which may result from the fibrosis of the muscle fibres in the vicinity of the tumour. Where contracture is already established, the object is to gain full-range movement of the cervical spine by stretching the sternomastoid passively and by encouraging active correction by the baby himself. It is usually unnecessary to use splintage to hold the baby's head in a corrected position. However, a baby with plagiocephaly may require splinting by a cap and jacket (figure 130) for a short period in order to prevent his head rolling on to its flattened lateral surface.

Methods

Passive stretching

Technique. The baby is placed on a padded table in supine with the affected side away from the physiotherapist, who sits facing the table with the baby's legs and body under her arm. This hand holds his shoulder, thereby fixing the sternoclavicular attachment of the sternomastoid and allowing the side flexion of the head to perform the stretch. Her other hand holds his head, with care not to press on his ear, and pulls it towards her into as much side flexion as possible (figure 124). The stretch is repeated, this time with the addition of rotation (figure 125). Head rotation is encouraged by the mother, who should talk to the baby from one side.

It should be noted that the stretches may be done as one movement, rotation and side flexion together, but it is suggested that side flexion be done as a separate stretch, as it gives the baby a rest from rotation, which is often very uncomfortable, yet still allows the muscle to be stretched to some extent. It has been suggested that flexion should be added to the passive stretch (Hulbert 1950). However, the added discomfort caused to the baby, especially if there is a large sternomastoid tumour, makes the addition of the flexion element unjustified.

Precautions. It has been noted in some infants that the tumour appears painful within the first few weeks after birth, the baby crying when the swelling is palpated or the muscle stretched. The neck should therefore be handled gently, and the stretching done with minimal disturbance to the baby.

The physiotherapist need not give a maximum stretch to the muscle immediately, but should instead move the head until she feels the baby resist, then wait for him to relax, when she will be able to move it a little further. It is certainly not necessary for her to hold the muscle on the stretch with the baby screaming and struggling. If he is about to cry, she can relax the stretch a little, allowing him to move his head. When he has settled down, and his

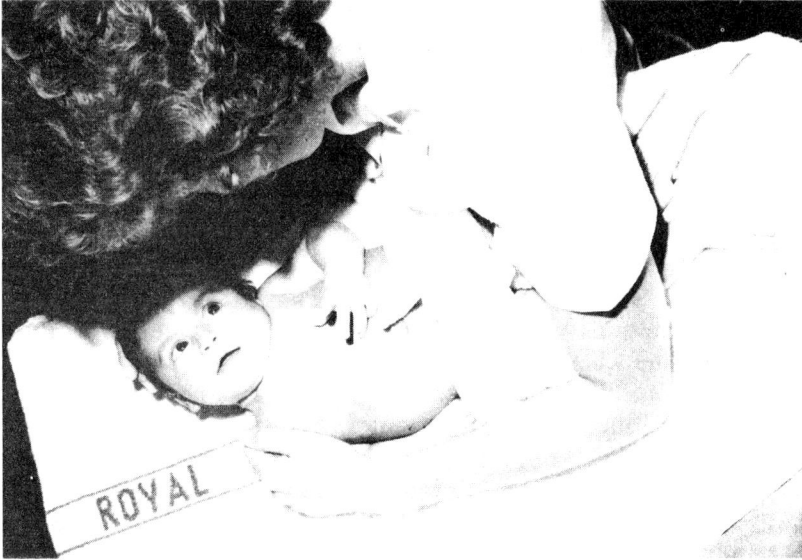

Fig. 124 Stretching the right sternomastoid muscle by side flexion of the head.

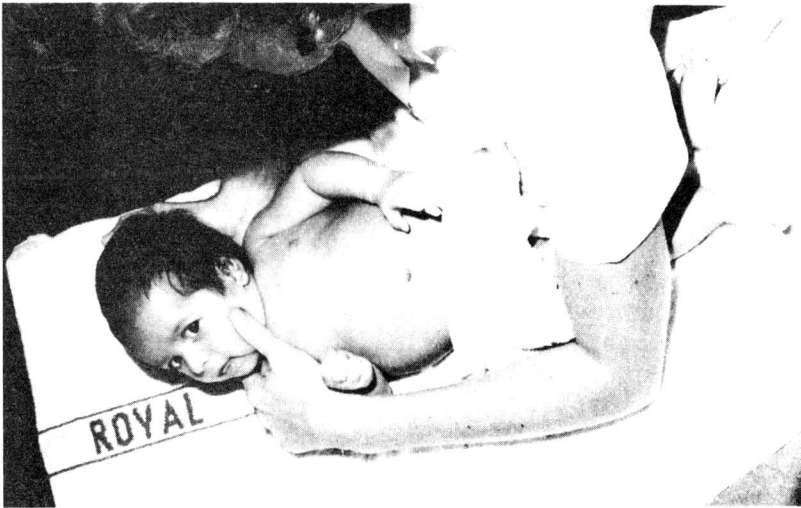

Fig. 125 Stretching the right sternomastoid muscle by side flexion and rotation of the head.

343

mother's help can be enlisted in calming and distracting him, the stretch can be reapplied. By doing this a five minute stretch may take much longer, but the delay is worthwhile as the baby will stay contented and unafraid.

The shoulder on the side of the contracture must be held gently on to the bed, and not forcibly depressed. A strong pull between the head and shoulder girdle may cause traction sufficient to injure the brachial plexus.

It must be emphasized that stretching must not proceed to the point where the infant is screaming and cyanosed. In some infants a large sternomastoid tumour probably presses against the blood vessels in the neck during rotation causing pain and cyanosis. With these infants the amount of rotation gained should only gradually be increased as the tumour becomes smaller.

Duration of passive stretch. Each stretch is done for approximately five minutes, but will probably take longer if the baby is allowed to move around and if the physiotherapist tries to keep him relaxed and happy. He should be seen by the physiotherapist several times in the first few weeks, until his mother is confident about her ability to continue treatment at home with weekly or fortnightly supervision by the physiotherapist.

Active Correction

Either before or after the stretching has been done, the physiotherapist spends some time in playing with the baby in order to encourage active correction and full-range movements of the head and neck (figure 126). In this way, his mother begins to learn how to play with him in order to achieve symmetrical behaviour and to stimulate his development.

As head control develops, lateral head righting is stimulated by holding the baby and moving him about to encourage rotation and side flexion (figure 126). Rotation may be stimulated on a ball, with the baby in prone or supine. As the ball is tilted to one side, the baby will rotate and side flex his head, especially if the stimulus of his mother's face on that side is added (figure 127). Once his head can be rotated to the midline, he may be placed in prone with brightly coloured toys hanging on one side to attract his attention, and his mother may talk to him and amuse him

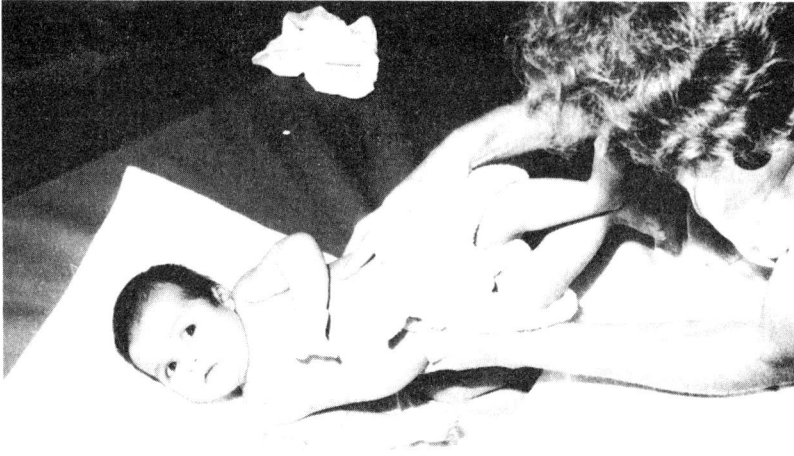

Fig. 126 A method of stretching the right sternomastoid which can be done by the parents while playing with the baby.

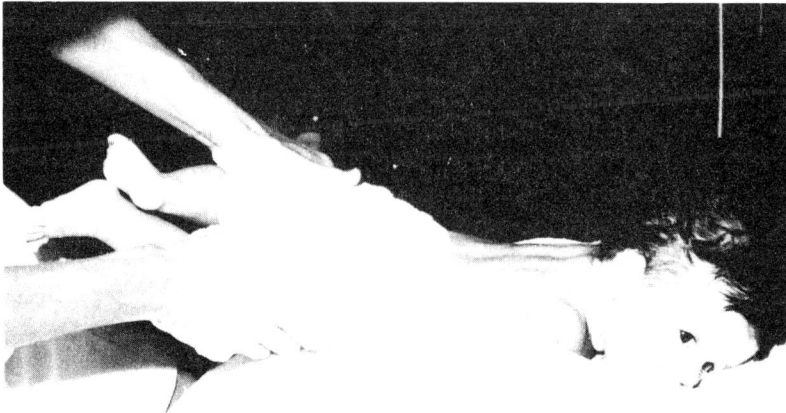

Fig. 127 Another method of stretching the right sternomastoid muscle with the baby in prone.

345

from this side. There are other ways of handling the infant in order to gain active correction and the physiotherapist should explore these herself.

In the author's opinion treatment may well consist only of these techniques of facilitating head movement, passive stretching of the sternomastoid being carried out as the baby is handled and moved about. However, the value of passive stretching as described above has not yet been measured against the value of active correction and handling and this should be a subject for further investigation.

It must be stressed that methods of encouraging active full range neck movement need to be practised by the parents with all infants who have a sternomastoid tumour, not only those with a recognisable torticollis.

Home Treatment

It is important for the physiotherapist to talk to the baby's parents on their first visit, and explain not only the purpose of treatment, but also some practical ways of making treatment at home as enjoyable as possible. Unfortunately, in a busy Paediatric Department, torticollis can be regarded as a relatively unimportant complaint, and the anxiety of the baby's family may be overlooked. Some mothers are nervous of handling their young infants, and may, when they leave the physiotherapist, be very anxious about the stretching of the sternomastoid and the stimulation which they are required to do at home.

The baby's mother is taught how to stretch the sternomastoid, and how to encourage the necessary movements but it is not enough for the physiotherapist to demonstrate these methods. She must persuade the mother to do them in front of her for a few minutes at every visit until it is certain that she is doing them correctly. She will require very careful teaching, and sympathetic understanding, for she may think she will hurt the baby when she does the passive stretch, and if he cries, her fears will be realized. If this part of the treatment becomes too upsetting for the mother it is probably better to discontinue the stretching and to put more emphasis on attempts at active correction.

On rare occasions mothers react by giving over-zealous stretches which do hurt the baby, and soon a cycle develops in which the baby begins to scream as soon as he is put down on the table. In this case it is better if the stretching is omitted from the home routine, and the baby taken more frequently to the physiotherapist, or again this part of the treatment may need to be discontinued altogether.

His mother is encouraged to treat the baby twice or three times daily for about ten minutes, and to make it a time to play and talk to him. A simple mobile made of pieces of aluminium foil suspended above his head, and other toys, will keep him amused at other times and encourage symmetrical behaviour. The importance of talking to him and of making noises to entertain him may need to be explained to some parents.

How treatment is fitted into the daily routine of the household may be left to the mother, but it is better not to time the stretching immediately before or after mealtimes. If it does cause pain or anxiety for the baby, there is no need to make his mealtimes miserable too, and he will soon learn to associate eating with the uncomfortable stretching.

If the baby reacts badly to the stretch, as it is described above, an alternative method can be used by his mother (Harrison 1968). The baby is held against his mother with the unaffected side uppermost, facing a mirror. His shoulder and head are held in the same way as in the original stretch, but it is the baby's body weight which applies the stretch. The advantage here is that he can be moved about gently and encouraged to relax, making it easier to put his sternomastoid on the stretch without too much discomfort. The mirror serves two purposes. The baby can recognize himself, and if he is too young to do this, the light on the mirror may attract his attention. The mirror also enables his mother to see clearly what she is doing (figure 128).

When he is in his cot, brightly coloured toys or foil shapes can be hung in front of him and to one side to encourage him to look around, and to get his hands and head to the midline. He would be slow to do this otherwise, and it is an important step in infant development. His cot should be placed in such a position that he can see what is happening in the room. He should be carried in a way which encourages him to turn his head in the direction opposite to his abnormal posture, and he may be nursed in a position similar to that suggested for stretching (figure 129). It is preferable for him to sleep on one side or the other, rather than in supine.

Cap and Jacket Splinting

Rationale

This method of splinting is no longer in use in most Paediatric Departments except occasionally for those babies with severely asymmetrical skulls, when it is useful to stimulate more normal head moulding. In most babies with torticollis the value of splinting is doubtful. It is said to hold the baby's head in a corrected position, and this it does to some extent, but it is doubtful that the amount of correction gained is worth the distress caused to the baby's mother, who resents such an overt demonstration of abnormality. Its advantage is that it does persuade the baby to look in a direction his muscle tightness would otherwise force him to ignore, but it is better that this should be gained if possible by more active means. The cap is sometimes prescribed by the surgeon following tenotomy of the

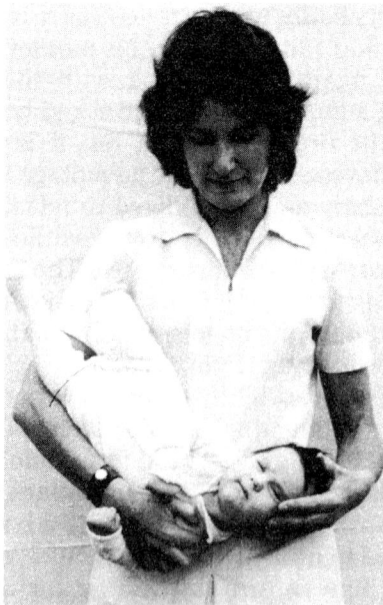

Fig. 128 Alternate method of stretching the left sternomastoid. (By permission of J. Harrison).

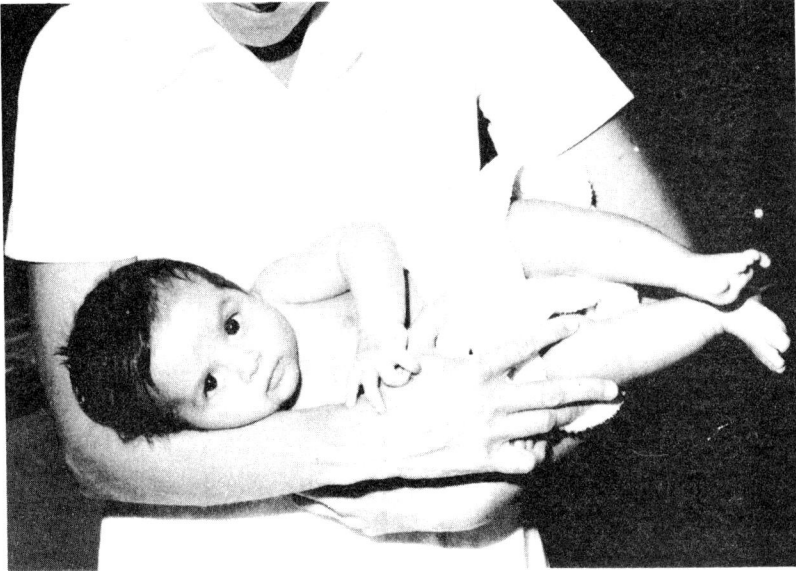

Fig. 129 A method of carrying a small baby with right torticollis.

sternomastoid, when it is worn for a short period until the child can hold his head in a symmetrical position (figure 130). Alternatively, a soft collar may be worn post-operatively for a few weeks to discourage the child from reverting to his habitual asymmetrical head posture.

Materials:
1 inch wide preshrunk webbing.
1 inch wide zinc oxide strapping.
Tincture Benzoin Compound.
2 jackets.
3 small buckles per jacket.
3 nappy pins.
Needle, cotton, pins.

The cap is made from webbing. The pieces are pinned together first, then sewn when it is certain the cap is a good fit. It must fit firmly or it will slip about on the head. Three webbing straps are attached. The anterior two control the position of the head and

349

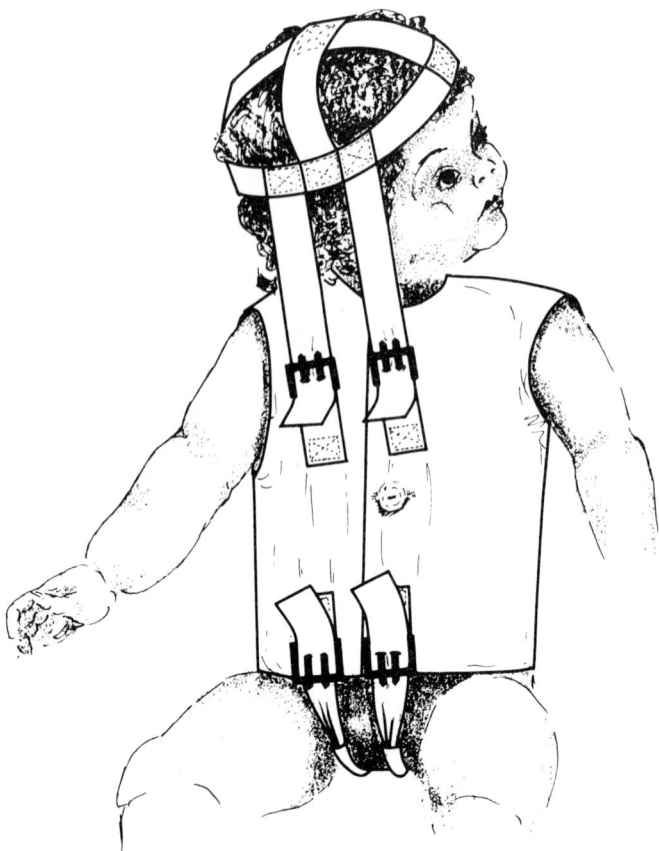

Fig. 130 Cap and jacket splinting. Alternatively the jacket may be pinned to the baby's nappy.

the posterior one prevents the cap being pulled down anteriorly. Two jackets are made which button down the front and must be long enough to attach to the nappy. When the jackets are made, buckles are attached, two on the front and one on the back. The front buckles are attached in such a way as to gain the most correction from the two straps which come, one in front of, the other behind the ear. The type of correction required can be altered by altering the position of the buckles and therefore of the straps. If the straps are taken down to the buckles placed on the same side of the jacket, more side flexion will be gained. If the straps are taken to the opposite side of the jacket, more rotation will be gained. If both side flexion and rotation are wanted, which is the case with most of these babies, the anterior strap is taken to the opposite side and the second strap to the same side of the jacket. The buckle for the posterior strap is placed anywhere in the midline at the back of the jacket, its function is merely to prevent the cap being pulled down anteriorly.

Application of cap:

Step 1. Strapping is applied to the cap, immediately in front of the ear on the side of the contracture. It is lined so it does not stick to the hair in front of the ear.

Step 2. Tinc Benz Co is applied in a narrow strip to the lateral side of the cheek and under the chin, where the strapping is to be attached.

Step 3. The cap is placed on the baby's head. When in place the strapping is attached to the cheek and under the chin. There should be no tension on the strapping. Its purpose is to prevent the cap being pulled down to the opposite side.

Step 4. The baby is dressed in the jacket, which is pulled down firmly, and attached to the nappy with safety pins. With an older child the jacket is anchored in place by groin straps in the absence of a nappy.

Step 5. The webbing straps are done up through the buckles, the anterior straps first, then the posterior. The baby's head should now be held in a side flexed and rotated position.

This cap will stay in place for one week, when it will be removed and reapplied. Generally the routine will continue until the infant can hold his head in the midline.

Advice to mother

The cap should not be removed completely. It may be slipped off sideways, leaving the strapping in place, so the baby's head can be washed. The webbing can be marked so the mother will know how firmly the straps should be done up. The cap can be removed twenty-four hours before the next appointment for re-application, when a clean one will be put on.

Surgical Treatment

If the contracture persists despite treatment, the surgeon may decide to do a tenotomy of the sternomastoid. It is usually performed just above the attachment of the muscle to the clavicle. Lloyd-Roberts (1971) and Sharrard (1971) describe the procedure.

Post-operative physiotherapy

Immediately following surgery, the child lies without a pillow, a sandbag preventing his head from returning to the asymmetrical position. The surgeon may prescribe cap and jacket splinting or a soft collar to be worn until the child can hold his head in the midline.

Stretches and active correction are started approximately thirty-six hours after surgery, with the aim of maintaining the length of muscle gained at operation. A child who is old enough to co-operate may assist by actively moving his head into side flexion and rotation as far as he can. It is often possible to gain almost full-range neck movement in this manner without having to use passive stretching. The child lies in supine and the physiotherapist holds his head and shoulder while he tries to move his head as far as he can against gentle resistance without causing himself pain. She helps him by holding his head in this position until he is ready to try to move it a little further. The two movements may be done separately. By attempting this active correction, which should result in relaxation of the tenotomized sternomastoid painful passive stretches against the resistance of an upset child are avoided. These movements must be done gently as the sutures will not be removed for several days, and a cosmetic well-healed scar is important.

After surgery, until he is allowed out of bed, the child should be positioned in the ward so he is encouraged to rotate his head in the direction required. If, for example, he has had a right sternomastoid tenotomy, it is necessary to place his bed in a position in which the other children and all the activity in the ward are on his right side.

As soon as he is allowed out of bed, the physiotherapist concentrates on developing normal righting reactions of his head, and on altering the abnormal body image caused by his abnormal head posture. There is no difficulty in overcoming the rotation element of the torticollis usually, unless the child has a visual defect, as he will bring his face forward as soon as he can. However, the side flexion element may persist for longer.

Head righting may be stimulated in sitting, standing and in other positions, by tipping him forwards and backwards, and from side to side. This may be done on a balance board, or by facilitating from the hands or legs. The child can be sat on a large ball, controlled movement of which will facilitate effective trunk and head righting. The feeling of being symmetrical may be reinforced for the older child, if, sitting on a stool in front of a mirror, he stretches up as tall as he can against the firm pressure of the physiotherapist's hand on the top of his head.

If he persists in holding his head to one side despite treatment, the physiotherapist should consider the possibility of acquired visual defect, which may only become evident when he has to hold his head in this altered position. In this case he should be referred back to his doctor for investigation.

SUMMARY

Torticollis is a disorder the aetiology and pathology of which are not understood. The effectiveness of physiotherapy in the treatment of infants with this deformity is therefore uncertain, but methods of treatment are suggested for use until satisfactory controlled trials are carried out. Emphasis is on careful explanation of techniques of passive stretching to the parents, plus discussion of the ways in which they may encourage active correction. Passive stretching should not leave the infant distraught and exhausted, or the mother guilty and anxious, but should be gently performed, with time allowed for the infant to become accustomed to this way of being handled. Physiotherapy following surgery is necessary and usually effective, and emphasis is particularly on the development of normal righting reactions, and of a more normal body image.

References

Adams, R. D., Denny Brown, D. and Pearson, C. M. (1962) *Diseases of Muscle. A Study in Pathology*. London: Kimpton.
Coventry, M. B. and Harris, L. E. (1959) Congenital muscular

torticollis in infants. *J. Bone Jt. Surg.* **41A**, 815.

Ferguson, A. B. (1968) *Orthopaedic Surgery in Infancy and Childhood.* Baltimore: Williams and Wilkins.

Harrison, J. (1968) Personal Communication.

Hulbert, K. F. (1950) Congenital torticollis. *J. Bone Jt. Surg.* **32B**, 1, 50.

Jolly, H. (1968) *Diseases of Children.* London: Blackwell.

Jones, P. G. (1968) *Torticollis in Infancy and Childhood.* Illinois: Thomas.

Lloyd-Roberts, G. C. (1971) *Orthopaedics in Infancy and Childhood.* London: Butterworth.

Sanerkin, N. G. and Edwards, P. (1966) Birth injury to the sternomastoid. *J. Bone Jt. Surg.* **48B**, 441.

Sharrard, W. J. W. (1971) *Paediatric Orthopaedics and Fractures.* Oxford and Edinburgh: Blackwell.

Further Reading

Chandler, F. A. (1948) Muscular torticollis. *J. Bone Jt. Surg.* **30A**, 556.

Chandler, F. A. and Altenburg, A. (1944) Congenital muscular torticollis. *J.A.M.A.* **125**, 476.

Ling, C. M. and Low, Y. S. (1972) Sternomastoid tumour and torticollis. *Clinical Orthopaedic and Related Research*, **86**, 144.

Macdonald, D. (1969) Sternomastoid tumour and torticollis. *J. Bone Jt. Surg.* **51B**, 3, 432.

Nelson, W. E. Vaughan, V. C. and McKay, R. J. (1969) *Textbook of Paediatrics.* Philadelphia, Toronto and London: Saunders.

Chapter 3

Structural Scoliosis

This Chapter is headed Structural Scoliosis in order that a clear distinction may be made between this serious, progressive and disabling condition, which is uncorrectable by any but surgical means, and sometimes not even by these, and the correctable, non-structural but postural lateral curvature of the spine. This latter may be found in some adolescents whose postural mechanism has suffered a temporary set-back due to a rapid growth spurt, and in children with one leg shorter than the other. In the latter children this asymmetry is corrected when the legs are made an equal length by the addition of a raise to the shoe, or by leg lengthening (Sharrard 1971) or leg shortening surgery.

Structural scoliosis does not just involve a lateral curvature of the spine, but also rotation within the spine itself. A simple test makes the difference between the two easily distinguishable. When the child with a postural lateral curvature bends forward to touch his toes in standing, the lateral curve disappears. In marked contrast, the child with a structural scoliosis continues to demonstrate a lateral curvature and the rotation element will be evident as a bony prominence on the side of the convexity (figure 131). This prominence is caused by the posterior displacement of the ribs on that side due to the rotation of the bodies of the vertebrae towards the side of the convexity. This causes the transverse processes on that side to be angled posteriorly. The ribs, because of their articulation with these processes, project backwards on the side of the convexity (figure 132). It is this rotational element that causes to a large extent the grotesque 'hunchbacked' picture which is unfortunately so typical. The rib cage deformity becomes increasingly more severe as the scoliosis progresses. The ribs on the concave side are prominent anteriorly and flattened posteriorly, while on the convex side they are flattened anteriorly and project in a hump posteriorly. The lateral curvature in which the rotation element is present is called the primary curve (figure 133). Above and below the primary curve are compensatory curves, which do not clinically contain a rotation element on forward flexion of the spine (Sharrard 1971).

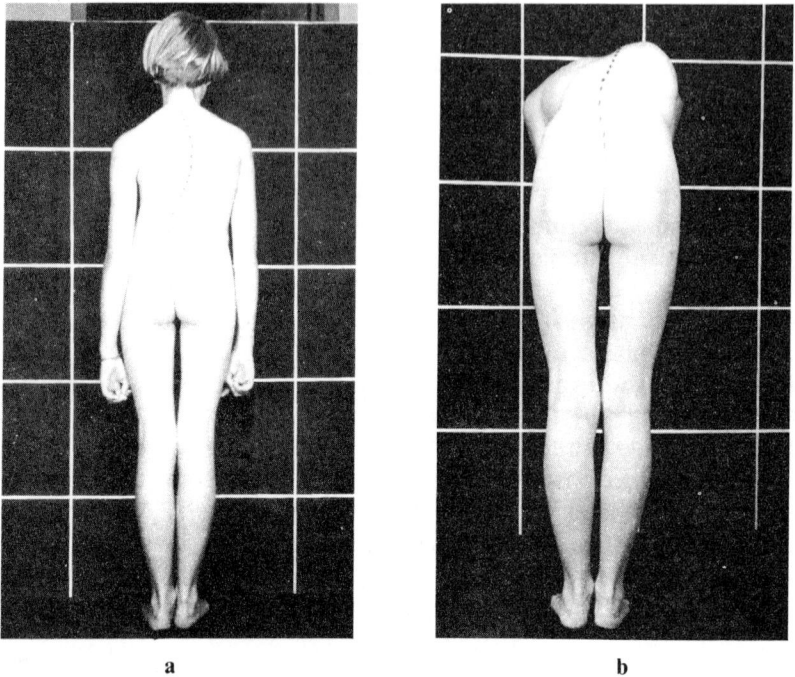

a   b

Fig. 131(a) Structural scoliosis with the primary curve convex to the right in the thoracic spine. (b) Bending forwards. Note the prominence of the ribs on the right side of the thorax.

Where deformity is severe the trunk muscles on the side of the convexity are at a mechanical disadvantage, and the degree of deformity is probably increased by the mechanical advantage of the spinal muscles on the concave side. Secondary complications eventually arise as the child grows if the scoliosis remains uncorrected. There may be considerable lung deformity, and some torsion of the pulmonary arteries and aorta may occur where the curve is severe, these factors causing cor pulmonale in later life (Sharrard 1971).

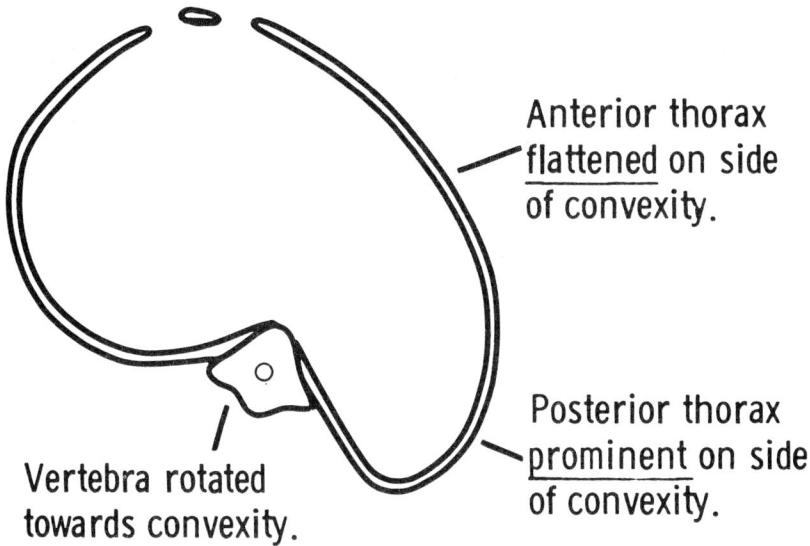

Fig. 132 Diagrammatic cross-section through the thorax of the child in figure 131, demonstrating the rib distortion.

AETIOLOGY

Scoliosis may be *idiopathic*, inferring the cause to be unknown. It may be *congenital* in a baby born with such congenital spinal defects as hemivertebrae. It is termed *paralytic* when it is due to spinal muscle imbalance such as may follow poliomyelitis, and this form of scoliosis is an almost constant finding in the later stages of progressive muscular dystrophy causing further respiratory complication. The spine in these dystrophic children collapses due to gradually increasing muscle weakness plus the effect of gravity, and eventually may become so misshapen that pressure areas are formed between the bony protuberances of the lower ribs and the pelvis. Athetoid cerebral palsied children with severe asymmetrical tonic spasms, spastic quadriplegic children with asymmetrical spasticity, spastic hemiplegic children, and children with neurofibromatosis may also demonstrate scoliosis.

TREATMENT

In the past there have been claims made that certain methods of physical treatment have an effect upon the scoliotic deformity, either halting or slowing its progression, or correcting the deformity. None of these has been proved effective, the curvature in most cases relentlessly progressing, although it sometimes becomes benign at adolescence. Some methods of surgery hold out hope for these children, and appear to correct the deformity in many cases. However, scoliosis remains a severely crippling and sometimes fatal disorder.

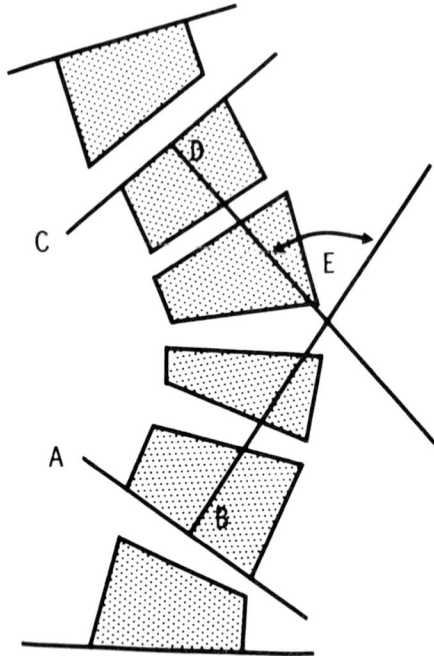

Fig. 133 Cobb's method of measuring the primary curve. A—Lowest vertebra whose inferior surface tilts to the side of the concavity. B—Perpendicular drawn from the inferior surface of the distal vertebra. C— highest vertebra whose superior surface tilts to the side of the concavity. D— Perpendicular drawn from the superior surface of the proximal vertebra. E— Intersecting angle measurement.

The physiotherapist has a part to play, however, in maintaining adequate respiratory function in these patients, particularly in those with progressing paralytic curves, and in giving advice to parents and child about activities such as swimming, which will maintain as much mobility as possible, not only in the spine, but in the whole skeletal system. It is probably true that activity helps maintain the child in the best possible general health, as well as helping him emotionally. That he should be kept as fit as possible, both physically and emotionally, is particularly important if he is to have surgery, as most methods involve considerable insult to the skeletal system, and are followed by long periods of hospitalization. Post-operatively the physiotherapist is responsible for the child's respiratory function, and for his eventual mobilization and rehabilitation.

Splinting

Probably the only forms of splinting which either control the scoliotic curve or correct it to some extent are variations of the Milwaukee brace (Blount, Schmidt and Bidwell 1958). The Risser jacket (Risser 1955) and Risser localizer plaster are effectively used to gain some correction pre-operatively and to maintain correction post-operatively (Risser 1964).

In the case of infants with congenital scoliosis the Denis Browne scoliosis splint (Brown 1956) is sometimes prescribed. Halo-pelvic traction has been devised for children with high curves, or where it is important to avoid pressure on the thorax (Garrett, Perry and Nickel 1961). No other splint, leather jacket or corset seems to have any effect on the curve or its progression.

Seat moulds and other methods of splinting chairbound scoliotic children are briefly mentioned in Chapter 1 of this Section.

Milwaukee brace

This brace provides the traction element which is most important in correcting the deformity, and this, combined with pressure over the point of maximum convexity, corrects the curvature to some extent and prevents secondary contracture of the spinal muscles on the side of the concavity (figure 134). Traction is exerted between the skull and the pelvis. The brace must be applied so that when pressure is on the occiput the mandible is free, therefore allowing the child to move his head, although in a limited way, and to eat comfortably. The degree of traction can be increased by increasing the length of the anterior and posterior rods, and adjustment for growth is made in the same manner.

In order that the brace will be a perfect fit, a plaster mould of the pelvic piece is made. This mould, upon which the leather pelvic piece will be fitted, is made with the child suspended by a halter from the head in order that as much correction as possible is gained.

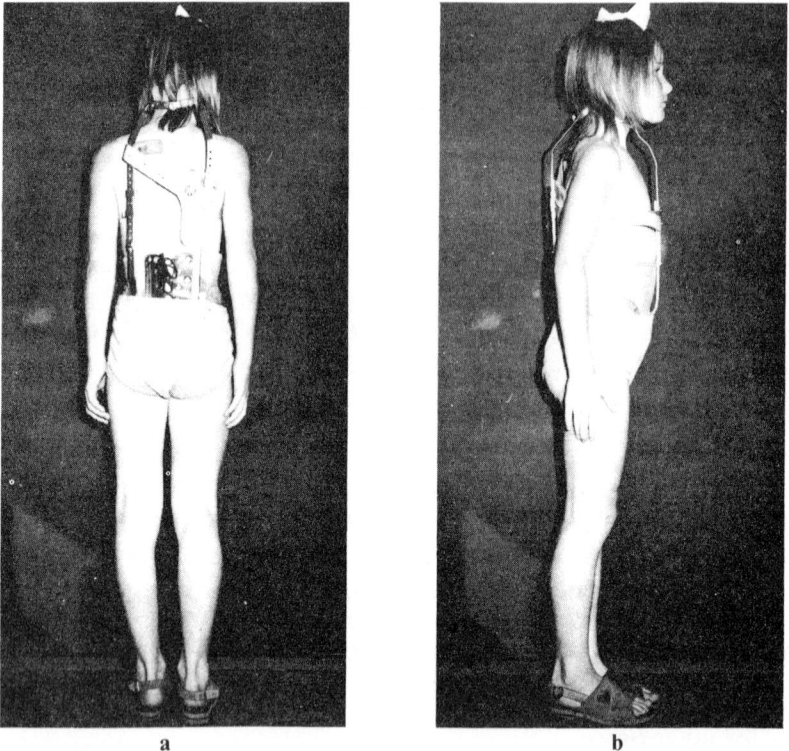

a   b

Fig. 134 Milwaukee brace. (a) Note the pad over the convexity of the primary curve. (b) Traction is applied between the occiput and the pelvis.

The brace may be worn during the day, or day and night, although the child is usually allowed out of it for bathing. It may also be prescribed following operative fusion of the spine in order to maintain immobilization (Sharrard 1971).

Denis Browne splint

Scoliosis developing in the first year of an infant's life tends to resolve in the majority of cases (Lloyd-Roberts and Pilcher 1965). Browne (1956) designed a splint in which the infant could lie with his spine curved in the direction opposite the deformity. While the infant is in this splint, his mother will make sure he has a mobile and toys hanging above him so he will have something upon which to focus his attention.

Risser jacket

This plaster jacket is applied with the child in supine on a special frame which allows traction to be given between the head and the pelvis. Padding is placed over bony prominences, and the jacket is made in two sections, cervical and pelvic, the latter incorporating the traction bands. The plaster should be particularly well moulded over the iliac crests. Traction is then applied through the head halter and the pelvic traction bands, a localizer pad made of several thicknesses of plaster over felt is placed over the rib prominence, and a jack gives pressure over this prominence postero-laterally. The plaster is completed by joining the cervical and the pelvic pieces together including the localizer pad. The child may be ambulant in this jacket.

Risser turnbuckle jacket

Traction is applied as above. The plaster extends from chin to pelvis, including the lower limb to the knee on the side of the convexity and possibly the arm as well on that side. When the plaster is dry it is divided, hinges are placed on the convex side and a turnbuckle on the concave side. Over approximately three weeks the jacket is hinged open and some correction of the curve is gained. Unfortunately, the child cannot be ambulant in this jacket.

Halo-pelvic traction

The use of this type of apparatus in a humid, hot climate where plaster jackets are poorly tolerated is described by Morton and Malins (1971). The apparatus consists of a metal halo which is attached by four pins which penetrate the outer table of the skull, a metal pelvic hoop which is secured by two long pins transfixing the innominate bone posterior to the anterior superior iliac spine along the crest to the posterior superior iliac spine, and four vertical extension bars. The operation is done in two stages, the extension bars being added a few days later. A small amount of distraction is achieved daily by turning the screws on the extension bars situated near the pelvic hoop. When satisfactory correction has been gained, the spine may be fused with or without the addition of an internal jacking device. The child is checked carefully as distraction progresses for neurological signs indicating cord or nerve traction — anaesthesia, paraesthesia, pain, or hyperactive stretch reflexes.

Surgery

Surgical procedures are described by James (1967) and Sharrard (1971). They include spinal fusion, if the child is over ten years of age, and soft tissue release. Various methods of internal fixation have been designed in order to gain correction (Harrington 1961, Dwyer 1969), and these are combined with spinal fusion.

Physical Treatment

The aim of the physiotherapist is the prevention, as far as possible, of those secondary problems which may arise as a result of the skeletal deformity — poor respiratory function and lack of general mobility.

Respiratory function

Poor respiratory function is common in these children and is due to the deformity of the thoracic cage and consequent poor rib mobility and lung expansion. The object of breathing exercises, which can be done daily by the child at home, is to develop respiratory function as effectively as possible despite the deformity of the thorax. That is, to mobilize the thorax and to obtain the most efficient ventilation possible. The child is taught diaphragmatic breathing, and basal and apical breathing. He will need to be supervised by his mother until he is old enough to be responsible for his own treatment, and she is taught how to give him postural drainage should he develop a respiratory tract infection. Swimming or similar activities will also improve respiratory function and may be sufficient treatment for many of these children. This routine is in a sense pre-operative as many of these children will eventually be candidates for surgery to correct and fuse their spines. Respiratory function is assessed at intervals (Section V, Chapter 4).

General mobility and strength

This is frequently poor, particularly in those children whose scoliosis is due to muscle weakness or paralysis. However, children with severe idiopathic scoliosis are seldom energetic, and suffer a secondary lack of mobility and strength due to their deformity. It must be emphasized that no amount of enthusiasm on the part of the physiotherapist will mobilize the spine of a child with structural scoliosis where the loss of mobility is due to the skeletal deformity, but a programme of activity designed to maintain mobility in a general sense is of benefit to most of these children. Swimming is recommended as one of the best ways of combining mobility and improved respiratory function with sport and pleasure, and these children can be taught how to swim different strokes, and how to swim under water. The therapist teaches the child exercises which will strengthen his trunk muscles, particularly his abdominals. A child in a Milwaukee brace is encouraged to be as active as possible, and at periods during the day to stretch up in his brace to make himself as tall as possible.

Pre- and post-operative treatment

Pre-operatively the physiotherapist measures the child's respiratory function and gives intensive breathing exercises with postural drainage if necessary for the few days before surgery. This is in order to maintain a clear airway and to ensure the child will be able to resume effective ventilation and an effective cough after surgery. The post-operative treatment depends upon the surgery performed. In general, an intensive period of breathing exercises is given for the first few days with care to encourage lung expansion in all areas. If necessary a respirator may be used to aid ventilation. As soon as possible the child is mobilized within the limits of whatever splinting he is in. It is not until all splinting is finally removed that the child can be fully rehabilitated, and this may be achieved by a period of exercise aimed at increasing mobility, strength, co-ordination and endurance, most of which can be accomplished by swimming practice and other activities which the child finds enjoyable.

SUMMARY

Scoliosis is a severely disabling progressive deformity, with distortion of the thoracic cage caused by rotation within the laterally curved spine. Treatment consists of splinting which corrects the deformity by applying traction to the spine, followed by surgery, which gains further correction by internal devices, and maintains this correction by spinal fusion. Physical treatment has no effect on the scoliotic deformity, but is an important adjunct in improving respiratory function and general mobility in these children.

References

Blount, W. P., Schmidt, A. C. and Bidwell, R. G. (1958) Making the Milwaukee brace. *J. Bone Jt. Surg.* **40A**, 526.

Browne, D. (1956) Congenital postural scoliosis. *Proc. Roy. Soc. Med.* **49**, 395.

Dwyer, A. F. (1969) An anterior approach to scoliosis. *J. Western Pacific Orthop. Assoc.* **6**, 1.

Garrett, A. L., Perry, J. and Nickel, V. L. (1961) Stabilization of the collapsing spine. *J. Bone Jt. Surg.* **43A**, 474.

Harrington, P. R. (1961) Treatment of scoliosis. Correction and internal fixation by spine instrumentation. *J. Bone Jt. Surg.* **44A**, 4.

James J. I. P. (1967) *Scoliosis.* Edinburgh: Livingstone.

Lloyd-Roberts, G. C. and Pilcher, M. F. (1965) Structural idiopathic scoliosis in infancy. *J. Bone Jt. Surg.* **47B**, 520.

Morton, J. and Malins, P. (1971) The correction of spinal deformities by halo-pelvic traction. *Physiotherapy*, **57**, 12.

Risser, J. C. (1955) Application of body casts. *Instruction Course Lectures American Academy Orthopaedic Surgery*, **12**, 255.

Risser, J. C. (1964) Scoliosis: past and present. *J. Bone Jt. Surg.* **46A**, 1.

Sharrard, W. J. W. (1971) *Paediatric Orthopaedics and Fractures.* Oxford and Edinburgh: Blackwell.

Further Reading

Cobb, J. R. (1948) Outline for Study of Scoliosis. *Instruction Course Lectures American Academy Orthopaedic Surgery*, **5**, 261.

Ferguson, A. B. (1968) *Orthopaedic Surgery in Infancy and Childhood.* Baltimore: Williams and Wilkins.

James, J. (1956) Paralytic scoliosis. *J. Bone Jt. Surg.* **38B**, 660.

Moe, J. H. (1961) Changing concepts of the scoliosis problem. *J. Bone Jt. Surg.* **43A**, 471.

Chapter 4

Inflammatory Disorders of Soft Tissues and Joints

Children affected with any of the disorders in this group suffer loss of function due to the inflammatory process involving the soft tissues, and in the case of rheumatoid arthritis, the bones and articular cartileges as well.

The loss of function is due to loss of range of movement, and this occurs as the result of pain, protective muscle spasm, contracture of soft tissues surrounding the joint, and in some cases of rheumatoid arthritis and haemophilia, to ankylosis of the joint. Loss of function is also due to muscle weakness and loss of co-ordinated movement of the limbs and trunk, and may also be due to disuse, or to emotional disturbances in an anxious child who feels himself to be an invalid.

It is in order to minimize or prevent loss of function that these children are referred to the physiotherapist for treatment.

JUVENILE RHEUMATOID ARTHRITIS (STILL'S DISEASE)

Terminology and classification of the chronic arthropathies of childhood are more difficult than they are in adult rheumatoid arthritis and they vary throughout the world. The condition called juvenile rheumatoid arthritis includes a diverse collection of chronic arthropathies (see figure 135) manifesting themselves in many different ways.

Juvenile rheumatoid arthritis differs from rheumatoid arthritis in several respects, including the occurrence of secondary growth disturbance, and its usual onset in the large joints.

Ankylosing spondylitis may begin with peripheral arthritis in childhood, making it difficult to distinguish from juvenile rheumatoid arthritis. It occurs mainly in boys from the age of 10 onward.

Juvenile rheumatoid arthritis manifests itself in children as

366

either a generalized systematic disease involving many joints, or as a disease apparently localized to a few joints with few systemic symptoms. Those children with a generalized disease may present with more obviously systemic symptoms than arthritic, with pyrexia, rash, general malaise, anaemia, and occasionally pericarditis, as well as the peripheral symptoms of warm swollen joints, tenderness, muscle spasm, pain, tenosynovitis, muscle weakness and wasting.

TYPES OF CHRONIC ARTHRITIS OF CHILDHOOD

JUVENILE RHEUMATOID ARTHRITIS

   Systemic onset

   Polyarticular
      Seronegative
      Seropositive

   Pauciarticular
      Early onset (predominantly girls)
      Early onset (predominantly boys)

ANKYLOSING SPONDYLITIS

ARTHRITIS SECONDARY TO OTHER INFLAMMATORY DISEASES

   Rheumatic diseases (eg. rheumatic fever, systemic lupus erythematosus,
      vasculitis, dermatomyositis, scleroderma)
   Other diseases (eg. Reiter's disease, psoriasis, inflammatory bowel
      disease)

ARTHRITIS RELATED TO OTHER PROCESSES

   Infectious diseases (eg. septic joint disease, osteomyelitis)
   Malignant disease (eg. Leukaemia, neuroblastoma)
   Non-inflammatory conditions of bones and joints (eg. trauma,
      avascular necrosis)

---

from Schaller, J. (1977) Juvenile rheumatoid arthritis. Post graduate Medicine 61, 1, 177-184

Fig. 135 Table showing types of chronic arthritis in childhood.

Rheumatoid arthritis is rarely seen in children of less than one year of age. Its aetiology is unknown, although there is some question whether it may be based on psychodynamic factors (Rimón, Belmaker and Ebstein 1977). Onset may be a gradual development of symptoms, or a sudden acute flare-up. Symptoms may exacerbate and remit throughout the course of the disease. In a large percentage of affected children stress, trauma, infection or inoculation can reactivate the disease, even in adult life (Stoeber 1977).

Prognosis in uncontrolled cases may be poor, with the child progressing to a stage where ill-health, blindness, deafness and eventually death overcome him. In less severe cases the disease may burn itself out, leaving the child with little disability.

No single laboratory test confirms the diagnosis of juvenile rheumatoid arthritis. In the acute systemic form, anaemia, elevated erythrocyte sedimentation rate and leukocytosis are prominent findings. There is a lower incidence of the rheumatoid factor than in adult rheumatoid arthritis.

Pathology

Nelson, Vaughan and McKay (1969) describe the pathology as being a chronic non-suppurative inflammation of the synovium. The earliest changes are periarticular oedema with little synovial reaction or joint effusion. However, synovial inflammation soon becomes apparent. The thickened synovium protrudes into the joint space, and may result in erosion and eventual destruction of the articular cartilage. If the disease progresses, synovial tissue will fill the joint space causing narrowing and fibrous ankylosis, and bony fusion may eventually destroy the joint.

Thus the swelling, a constant finding in affected children, is due to periarticular oedema, joint effusion, and synovial thickening. The loss of movement found on examination of the child may be due in the early stages to protective muscle spasm, but eventually to actual joint destruction and ankylosis. The inflammatory process extends to the tendons and tendon sheaths, and to the muscles. Osteoporosis may occur in the vicinity of the involved joints. Growth may be interfered with, being either slowed or hastened, and this is due to involvement of the epiphyseal centres. Any joint may be involved, but the most commonly affected in children are the wrist, metacarpo-phalangeal, ankle, subtaloid, knee, hip and temporo-mandibular joints, and the joints of the cervical spine.

Iridocyclitis, a potentially scarring eye disease, is an insidious complication, usually associated with involvement of only a few joints. Early recognition and treatment are essential to the preservation of vision.

Joint destruction once it occurs has generally been considered to be irreversible, partly because early studies (Bywaters 1937) showed cartilege to exhibit very limited powers of repair. There is some evidence that this may not be so. Bernstein et al (1977) describe 6 children with long standing rheumatoid arthritis and radiological evidence of severe hip joint damage, who were found to have radiological evidence of widening of joint space and remodelling of articular surfaces. The authors consider that control of the inflammatory disease was a necessary pre-requisite for the apparent hip joint restoration. A common factor was vigorous physiotherapy with emphasis on increasing muscle strength and ambulation and on avoiding wheelchair use. There is evidence from animal experiments (Thompson and Bassett 1970) that joint immobility results in degeneration and necrosis of cartilege in areas of articular compression and in the contact-free area.

Bernstein *et al* (1977) suggest that there may be an equilibrium between reparative processes and destructive processes, and that the growth potential of children may be the principal factor in shifting the balance toward repair if vigorous medical and physical measures are used.

DERMATOMYOSITIS

This disease is also characterized by a non-suppurative inflammatory process, involving widespread vascular changes in the connective tissue of skin, muscle, fat and small nerves. It is rarely seen before the age of two years. Its aetiology is unknown. The disease may develop slowly, with the usual presenting symptoms being muscle weakness which develops insidiously in the proximal muscles of the extremities, trunk and neck muscles, pain and tenderness. Weakness may also involve palatal, pharyngeal and oesophageal musculature. The clinical picture may be very varied, and include a rash, usually on the face, extensor surface of knees and elbows and dorsal surface of hands, and subcutaneous calcifications. All muscles may eventually be affected. Involvement of respiratory and swallowing muscles may lead to death.

Pathology

Nelson, Vaughan and McKay (1969) describe the most prominent lesion in children as a vasculitis involving capillaries, arterioles and venules in the connective tissue of the skin, subcutaneous tissue, muscles and gastro-intestinal tract. In the affected muscles, vasculitis is accompanied by infarction, atrophy of muscle fibres,

369

interstitial oedema with proliferation of connective tissue, while in the affected skin there is a thinning of the epidermis, oedema and vasculitis in the dermis.

The skin over the affected parts appears tight and shiny. Eventually it may atrophy and become bound down to sub-cutaneous tissues. The progress of the disease eventually slows, but although it may become inactive, the child may be left with marked residual disability due to contractures and deformity. It is to prevent or minimize this disability that he is referred for physiotherapy.

There is evidence of improved prognosis following cor-ticosteroid therapy (Sullivan et al 1972). The improvement which follows the initially high dosage allows the child to participate more actively in physiotherapy.

SCLERODERMA

This uncommon condition is a chronic inflammatory disorder of unknown aetiology affecting the connective tissue. It may affect the skin alone or involve internal organs as well. It is charac-terized by typical skin lesions called morphea. These lesions are at first either erythematous or atrophic, but later become indurated and may enlarge to involve an extensive area of the body. Fibrosis may occur and the skin may be bound down to subcutaneous tissues, with resultant contractures of the affected part. Fibrosis may also involve the heart, lungs, kidneys, gastrointestinal tract and synovium. The active disease may spontaneously arrest or continue as a chronic state for a long time. In some children it may be rapidly fatal. Physiotherapy is important in the early stages of the skin lesions to minimize contractures and loss of function.

Treatment of Inflammatory Disorders

The aim of treatment in a child afflicted with one of these disorders is the prevention or the minimizing of deformity with its resultant interference with function. All treatment is directed to this end, and it is hoped that the child will be referred to the physiotherapist in time for an attempt at prevention to be made. In severe manifestations of these disorders it may unfortunately be difficult to prevent some degree of disability occurring, because of the rapidity with which the inflammatory process may progress. Nevertheless, the various members of the health care team must strive for a positive attitude towards treatment, aiming for normal function and not setting limitations, either consciously or unconsciously, for the child.

Anti-inflammatory drugs, such as the salicylates, are prescribed for these children. Steroids are only given in certain circumstances, their side effects making them a contraindication for all but the most severe and uncontrollable cases. Pain as a warning signal may not be felt by the child following drug therapy and the therapist must bear this in mind during treatment. Pain is not a prominent feature in juvenile rheumatoid arthritis, and severity of pain is therefore not a good indicator of the severity of this disease or the activity of the disease process (Scott, Ansell and Huskisson 1977).

Physical treatment, for convenience of description, is discussed under three headings:

Relief of pain.
Stimulation of mobility, strength and function.
Teaching of a home programme.

Rest is important, particularly during exacerbations in children with rheumatoid arthritis, but rest does not mean immobilization. Periods of inactivity are not advisable for these children. They are instead encouraged to lead gently active lives with appropriate periods of rest, with the intention of preventing loss of mobility. Children with rheumatoid arthritis complain of 'stiffness' and a feeling of 'seizing up' when they get up in the morning, and after any period of prolonged immobility. Most physicians are in agreement that the child spend as little time in bed, especially in hospital, as possible. Similarly, if splinting is used, it is to rest a painful limb, not to immobilize it, and must be designed so it can easily be removed.

These are depressing disorders, and a concerted effort must be made to prevent the affected child from lapsing into a state of emotional invalidism out of proportion to his physical disability. Pain and the fear of it, plus muscle weakness, combine to make him anxious. Well-planned treatment, practical advice to his parents, and an encouraging approach from the physiotherapist will help him to be active and to develop emotionally and physically. Where pain and protective spasm are inhibiting movement they must be relieved. Where a child is too anxious to move freely, an astute physiotherapist will find ways of encouraging him. As much treatment as possible should be done at home, the parents being supervised by the physiotherapist at regular intervals.

Assessment and frequent reassessments are important in establishing the child's particular problems. Joint range is measured with a goniometer. Muscle strength is tested by charting of individual muscles where there is evidence of weakness. Muscle bulk is determined by measuring the girth of the limb with a tape measure. Function is assessed by observation of the child's movements. Objective functional testing is more difficult to devise, but tests are gradually being developed which will be useful for children with musculo-skeletal disabilities (MacBain and Hill 1973). Presence of pain is noted throughout treatment, whether at rest, or in a particular part of a range of movement.

Relief of Pain

Pain is not a constant finding in these conditions, but it does occur at one time or another, and in varying degrees of severity in most cases.

Pain results in protective spasm of the muscles surrounding the painful area, and because it is usually the flexors rather than the extensors which protectively spasm, the part involved is held in a position of flexion. Due to the inability of these muscles to relax and lengthen in reciprocation, movement is inhibited, the child being unable to move the part even if he wants to. Pain, or fear of pain, results therefore in protective spasm and loss of movement. It follows that all physical treatment must be painfree if the aim of treatment is to encourage the fullest most functional movement possible.

Pain during or immediately after treatment may indicate overstretching and damage to soft tissues, and this also will cause a limitation rather than the hoped for gain in range of movement. Moreover, painful treatment will certainly alienate the child who can hardly be blamed for rejecting further attempts of the physiotherapist to treat him.

Methods for the relief of pain and protective muscle spasm, apart from drug therapy, include rest, heat in the form of warm packs and wax, and cold in the form of ice packs.

Rest. It has been suggested above that rest does not mean immobilization. Where there is pain the child may need periods of bed rest, and a limb or part of a limb may be rested effectively in a light splint, which will help maintain the optimum position of the limb, rather than be nursed free in bed. Splints may be of plaster, aluminium or thermoplastic material. They should be padded and well-fitting, light and as simple as possible. When making splints, it should be remembered that the tendency is to flex a painful joint, and that some joints tend to assume positions which require the least effort against gravity. The ankle joint, for example, tends to fall into plantarflexion, and will therefore be splinted in a plantigrade position. The knee is splinted in extension, although not hyperextension. A knee flexion deformity is easily acquired in rheumatoid arthritis and causes great handicap. The foot must not be allowed to flex at the midtarsal joints or metatarso-phalangeal joints. When the hips are involved, the child will spend part of his rest period in prone. It is important that his feet are over the end of the bed to ensure a good position for his knees and ankles. The wrist is rested in an extended position and is not allowed to fall into ulnar deviation; the thumb in abduction with some opposition; the fingers in slight flexion. No joint is allowed to remain splinted day and night. It cannot be stressed enough that splinting is a means of resting a painful part of a limb. A splint is made so it fulfils this requirement yet does not allow the joint to become stiff or to assume an unnatural position. Once pain is no longer a problem the splint can be removed.

Heat. Care must be taken during any application of heat not to burn the delicate and sometimes atrophic skin of these children. It is a good precaution to test temperature sensation before the application of either heat or cold. *Warm packs* are probably the most practical and most effective form of applying heat. They can be applied at home to relieve pain and protective spasm and should precede the active part of treatment. Towels may be heated in the oven or in hot water, in which case they must be thoroughly wrung out, and they are wrapped around the part of the limb involved. They are changed every few moments as the heat soon dissipates, and the total period of application need not exceed seven to ten minutes, although this depends on the effect.

Heated wax is a useful means of applying heat to the hands, particularly in children with dermatomyositis, and the wax has the added effect of being a lubricant for the skin. This also can be easily done at home. The wax remains on the hands for approximately ten minutes, and is followed by active movement.

Cold. Sometimes cold is more effective for relieving pain and protective spasm in rheumatoid arthritis than heat, although care should be taken that the application of cold is not intolerable and that it does not cause the child to feel stiff. In a child with residual deformity due to soft tissue contracture, cold may be a useful means, if combined with mobilizing techniques (Appendix 5), of gaining more range of movement.

Cold is applied by terry towels which have been soaked in flaked ice and water and wrung out to remove as much moisture as possible. The towels are re-applied every minute for approximately five to ten minutes, in such a way that the part is kept constantly cold. If they are left on for too long they absorb heat from the body and the required effect is lost. The towels are wrapped around the part to be treated. In the case of hamstrings, for example, care is taken to apply the cold to the entire length of the muscle, and not just to the part nearest the joint. For the use of cold to be effective, mobilizing techniques, or techniques to increase muscle length and therefore joint range (Appendix 5), must be done either during the application of the towels, or immediately afterwards, before the effect of the cold has been dissipated. If cold is not employed in this manner, that is, in conjunction with these techniques, it cannot be expected to be effective.

Stimulation of Mobility, Strength and Function

It must be stressed that for both their physical and emotional development these children need to participate as fully as possible in normal daily activities. This means that parents must be made fully aware of what their child can do.

No matter how local and peripheral the inflammatory process may be in the child receiving treatment, the physiotherapist must remember to treat him as one complete unit whose entire function as a child is disturbed because of this one part which cannot perform normally.

Pain and protective spasm must be relieved, joint range increased, and muscles strengthened, and all by specific techniques directed locally at the affected part. All these techniques are a way of preparing the child for more normal movement, normal movement being essential for effective function. Treatment ends prematurely if it consists only of warm packs and techniques directed at the affected limb. It is useless to prepare the child in such a way without going on to encourage him to use his improved mobility and strength. The effect of such mobilizing and strengthening techniques becomes consolidated if the child is encouraged to use the affected limb in conjunction with the rest of his body in some normal functional movement.

Take, for example, a child with rheumatoid arthritis affecting a knee. He may need warm packs or ice to relieve protective spasm in his hamstrings, plus techniques to gain full-range flexion and extension of the knee and to strengthen his flexors and extensors. These modalities are very specific and are in preparation for the next part of his treatment in which he will be encouraged to use his knee in as normal a manner as possible in the movements necessary for normal function. Such activities as described below may be devised by the physiotherapist.

Sitting on a stool, moving around the stool as quickly as possible to face the other direction. Feet must be on the floor during weight transference. (To encourage weight transference and the ability to co-ordinate movement of limbs and trunk).
Sitting on a stool to standing, by pushing against a stick held by the therapist. (To encourage weight transference. The therapist can facilitate transfer in any direction by appropriate pressure on the stick.)
Standing on a large balance board while it is moved about by the physiotherapist. (For weight transference and co-ordinated automatic reactions.)
Walking in footsteps drawn on the floor. (For a gait with even steps and to encourage equal weightbearing on each foot.)
Walking in the rungs of a ladder laid on the floor. (For controlled knee movement.)

These activities are merely suggestions to illustrate how a child may be persuaded to use his knee in movements which involve his whole body. They give him something to think about, so he will not tend to favour the affected leg. They can be made simpler or more complex depending on the age of the child, the number of joints affected, and the severity of the involvement. Activities should make him transfer weight and move symmetrically and smoothly and they should be fun. The child may need to be shown what he is capable of doing, that is, he may need to be surprised by what he can do. However, whatever activity is given it must not produce pain.

For the child with pain, or for the very anxious child, provided he is not afraid of the water, *hydrotherapy* makes a useful adjunct to treatment. Water temperature should not exceed 34°C or it will be too enervating, and the child should not stay in the water longer than fifteen to twenty minutes. Activities again will need to be adjusted according to the child's disability, age and temperament. Movements and games in a pool can be great fun and are better if treated more as a swimming lesson than as treatment. The child is taught simple swimming techniques, kicking with a board and dog paddle, and these can be progressed to breaststroke swimming and the crawl, and to backstroke. By this stage he should be attending the heated pool nearest his home for professional instruction, or just to practise by himself. Swimming with the face in the water, ducking under the water to retrieve a toy, blowing a ping-pong ball along the surface all improve breathing control in children with some thoracic involvement. Children who experience pain in weightbearing joints on walking and who are otherwise confined to bed, may be able to stand and walk with the help of the buoyancy of the water. Games with other children can be devised to encourage certain movements which need to be practised. The Halliwick method of swimming (Reid 1976) provides an enjoyable combination of water activities and group involvement.

Splinting may sometimes be necessary to increase range and may be in the form of progressive serial plaster splints or wedged plaster cylinders.

Hand function. Where part of the hand is involved, particular care must be taken to preserve or regain full wrist extension, thumb abduction, pincer, palmar and ulnar grasp, and release. Full wrist extension is essential for such protective responses as the parachute reaction (Appendix 1), for sitting sideways on the floor, and for pushing up from a chair. Extension is also

376

necessary for normal grasp, particularly for a strong grasp. Such activities as described below may be used.

Playing with plasticine. (Emphasis on various types of grasp and on making different objects.)
Squeezing a plastic ball with retractible knobs. (For pincer grasp.)
Hammering wooden pegs. (For palmar grasp and radial extension.)
Screwing and unscrewing wooden nuts and bolts. (For palmar and pincer grasp combined with forearm movement.)
Dressing and undressing dolls. (For dexterity.)

Manipulative activities are given according to the child's age and preference, as well as his disability. They should not be aimless, and the child should see a definite result for his efforts. Peripheral mobilizing techniques, such as those described by Kaltenborn (1976) and Maitland (1977), may be useful in preventing loss of function. Where the physiotherapist and the occupational therapist work together, as they should with the management of a child with this type of disability, the development or restoration of hand function may be their joint responsibility.

His *postural development* should be carefully assessed as he grows, and deviations corrected by muscle lengthening or strengthening techniques, relaxation techniques and by methods of improving postural awareness.

Respiratory function. This will need to be assessed in those children whose thorax, whether joints or muscles, is involved. It has been pointed out above that disorders of growth may occur in children with severe rheumatoid arthritis, and these children, as well as those suffering from dermatomyositis and scleroderma will benefit from exercises and activities designed to increase the mobility and expansion of the thorax as well as increasing respiratory efficiency. Some children, especially those with generalized disease, require regular testing of their ventilatory efficiency, and this may be done as described in Section V, Chapter 4.) For these children, and for those who tend to be inactive, breathing exercises directed at expanding the lower ribs and the ribs laterally and apically, are done at home each day. Should infection of the lower respiratory tract occur, parents will have been taught techniques of postural drainage and so will be able to commence them as soon as necessary.

Teaching a home programme

It has been said above that the child should spend as little time as possible in hospital and this applies also to his visits to the physiotherapist. Treatment is planned so it can be carried out at home with a minimum of effort for the parents and with maximum amount of effect and pleasure for the child. The physiotherapist assesses the child at regular intervals, plans his treatment, teaches the parents how to carry out treatment at home, and regularly supervises this. It is sometimes necessary for the child to be treated by the physiotherapist more frequently when he is in hospital or if he is developing contractures or any other specific difficulty, but outpatient visits should be kept to a minimum. It has to be remembered that none of these disorders occurs briefly, and that it is unrealistic to expect parent and child to attend for treatment frequently over a prolonged period. Similarly, this is kept in mind when planning home treatment, which should be short and to the point, with the possibility of some varition in techniques to prevent the child becoming bored.

The child should sleep on a firm mattress with a small pillow, especially if he has cervical rheumatoid arthritis. His desk and chair should be of correct height so he may sit with flat feet on the floor and thighs and back supported. The desk should be high enough for him to be able to rest his forearms comfortably. He should be encouraged to be as active as possible, but to take periods of rest when necessary.

Parents are shown how to apply any necessary splinting, how to give wax to the hands, warm or cold packs, breathing exercises and postural drainage if necessary. They are encouraged to take him swimming in the local heated pool. Riding a tricycle or bicycle will also help the child keep mobile. He must be allowed to dress himself including buttons and shoelaces, even if it does take a little longer than necessary.

One of the major problems for the child particularly as he approaches adolescence, is his difficulty relating his desire to lead a 'normal' life with the need to exercise caution in everything he does. His appearance of normalcy makes his task even more difficult. In adolescence, his capacity to control his own body is threatened. He has difficulty developing the independence for which he yearns.

HAEMOPHILIA

This is a chronic, hereditary and incurable disease resulting from a congenital deficiency in blood coagulation factors. It is a sex-linked recessive disorder affecting males. The first signs of haemophilia do not appear until the third trimester of infancy, and sometimes not until the second or third year.

Haemorrhage occurs recurrently within any part of the body, but it is haemorrhages into the joints and soft tissues of the limbs which cause the most disability, and it is the weightbearing joints, particularly the knee, that are most commonly the sites of repeated haemarthroses.

Mechanism of Haemarthrosis. When trauma occurs in or around a joint, haemorrhage may be severe causing local swelling, pain, heat and tension, and pressure on nerves and soft tissues. As a result of repeated episodes the synovial membrane thickens and there will eventually be a lack of nutrition to the articular cartilage, the surface of which becomes irregular and pitted. There is a risk of ultimate subluxation and deformity. Muscles become fibrosed and with other soft tissues may contract. The most commonly involved nerve is the femoral, which is associated with haemorrhage into the sheath of the iliacus muscle (Goodfellow, Fearn and Matthew 1967), and which takes several months to recover function.

Treatment

It seems that joint destruction and deformity can be prevented or minimized in many cases by correct treatment, which involves the child's parents, as well as the physician and physiotherapist. The parents will have to be aware of the dangers to their child even in earliest infancy, and will have to exercise care in the selection of toys, and supervise his activities more than normal. Emphasis is on strengthening muscles surrounding the at-risk weightbearing joints in the hope of minimizing the likelihood of trauma to the area and of protecting the joints. Cryoprecipitate is frequently given as a prophylactic, enabling greater continuity of rehabilitation.

The child will usually be hospitalized after severe intra-articular haemorrhage. During this acute period of anti-inflammatory measures, administration of plasma, cold packs and, in the case of weight-bearing joints, bed rest is instituted, and continued until pain, effusion and protective spasm have subsided. The joint is rested in a functional position, the knee, for example, in extension. If a weightbearing joint is involved, the child will not be allowed to bear weight for at least one week, and then probably only with the protection of a caliper or splint. Once pain and effusion have subsided, gentle mobilizing active movements are commenced. Isometric contractions are effective for regaining some control over a muscle group prior to active movement. Mobilizing techniques are used carefully in a pain-free range. Treatment in a pool is a useful adjunct for mobilizing and ambulation. Strong active resisted movements are given to the uninvolved lower limb while the child is hospitalized in order to maintain muscle strength and therefore minimize the risk of repeating the trauma to the affected joint once the child is allowed out of bed.

Between episodes the child must carry out a short home programme of exercises designed to improve strength and to increase the effectiveness of the equilibrium reactions, and if possible, should continue with regular swimming practice.

SUMMARY

Inflammatory diseases affecting soft tissues and joints interfere with movement by causing pain and protective muscle spasm, soft tissue contracture and ankylosis. Physical treatment is aimed at enabling the child to grow and develop with a minimum of musculo-skeletal deviation and deformity. It consists principally of methods of relieving pain and protective spasm, and of encouraging movement.

References

Bernstein, B. et al (1977) Hip joint restoration in juvenile rheumatoid arthritis. *Arth. & Rheum.* **20**, 5, 1099–1104.

Bywaters, E. G. L. (1937) The metabolism of joint tissues. *J. Pathol. Bacteriol.* **44**, 247–268.

Goodfellow, J., Fearn, C. B. and Matthews, J. M. (1967) Iliacus haematoma. A common complication of haemophilia. *J. Bone Jt. Surg.* **49B**, 748.

Kaltenborn, F. M. (1976) *Manual Therapy for the Extremity Joints.* 2nd Edition. Oslo: Olaf Norlis Bokhandel.

Laaksonen, A. (1966) A prognostic study of juvenile rheumatoid arthritis. *Acta Paediatr. Scand. (Suppl.)* **166**, 98.

MacBain, K. P. and Hill, R. H. (1973) A functional assessment for juvenile rheumatoid arthritis. *Am. J. O. T.* **26**, 6, 326–330.

Maitland, G. D. (1977) *Peripheral Manipulation.* 2nd Edition. London: Butterworth.

Nelson, W. E., Vaughan, V. C. and McKay, R. J. (1969) *Textbook of Paediatrics.* Philadelphia, London and Toronto: Saunders.

Reid, M. (1976) *Handling the Disabled Child in Water.* Assoc. Paed. Chartered Physiotherapists, Birmingham.

Rimón, R., Belmaker, R. H. and Ebstein, R. (1977) Psychosomatic aspects of juvenile rheumatoid arthritis. *Scand. J. Rheumatology* **6**, 1–20.

Stoeber, E. (1977) Juvenile chronic polyarthritis and Still's syndrome. *Documenta Geigy*, Basle.

Scott, P. J., Ansell, B. M. and Huskisson, E. C. (1977) Measurement of pain in juvenile chronic polyarthritis. *Ann. Rheum. Dis.* **36**, 186–187.

Sullivan, D. B., Cassidy, J. T., Petty, R. E. and Burt, A. (1972) Prognosis in childhood dermatomyositis. *J. Pediatr.* **80**, 555.

Thompson, R. C. and Bassett, C. A. L. (1970) Histological observations on experimentally induced degeneration of articular cartilege. *J. Bone Jt. Surg.* **52A**, 435–443.

Further Reading

Adams, R. D., Denny Brown, D. and Pearson, C. M. (1962) *Diseases of Muscle.* New York: Harper.

American Academy of Orthopaedic Surgeons (1965) *Joint Motion. Method of Measuring and Recording.* Edinburgh and London: Livingstone.

Ansell, B. M. (1965) Rheumatoid disorders in childhood. In *Physical Medicine in Paediatrics.* London: Butterworth.

Baldwin, J. (1972) Daily living for the patient with juvenile rheumatoid arthritis. *J. Canad. Physio. Assoc.* **24**, 1, 12–16.

Banker, B. Q. and Victor, M. (1966) Dermatomyositis of childhood. *Medicine*, **45**, 261.

Blom, G. E. and Nicholls, G. (1954) Emotional factors in children with rheumatoid arthritis. *Amer. J. Orthopsychiat.* **24**, 588.

Boone, D. C. (1966) Physical therapy aspects related to orthopaedic and neurological residuals of bleeding. *Phys. Ther.*, **47**, 12.

Curwen, M. (1974) A guide to functional assessment of children with rheumatoid arthritis. *Physiother. Canada* **26**, 2, 78–79.

Chaplin, D., Pulkki, T. and Saarimaa, A. et al (1969) Wrist and finger deformities in juvenile rheumatoid arthritis. *Acta Rheum. Scand.* **15**, 206.

Cole, S. and Jones, P. (1976) Physiotherapy in haemophilia. *Physiotherapy* **62**, 7, 217.

France, W. G. and Wolf, P. (1965) Treatment and prevention of chronic haemorrhagic arthropathy and contractures in haemophilia. *J. Bone Jt. Surg.* **47B**, 247.

Greenberg, R. S. (1972) The effects of hot packs and exercise on local blood flow. *Phys. Ther.*, **52**, 273.

Gregg, S. (1972) Physiotherapy and the haemophiliac. *Proc. XIIth World Congress of Rehabilitation International.*

Kass, H., Hanson, V. and Patrick J. (1966) Scleroderma in childhood. *J. Pediat.* **68**, 243.

Kerr, C. B. (1963) *The Management of Haemophilia.* Sydney: Australian Medical Publishing Company.

Knott, M. (1967) Introduction to and philosophy of neuromuscular facilitation. *Physiotherapy*, **53**, 1.

Kornreich, H. K. and Hanson, V. (1974) The rheumatic disease of childhood. In *Current Problems in Pediatrics*, **4**, 6. Chicago: Year Book Medical Publishers.

Moore, D. M. (1964) Experiences with the use of ice for treatment of patients with arthritis. *J. Canad. Arth. Rheum. Soc.* **7**, 1.

Nordemar, R., Berg, U., Ekblom, B. and Edström, L. (1976) Changes in muscle fibre size and physical performance in patients with rheumatoid arthritis after 7 months of physical training. *Scand. J. Rheumatology*, **5**, 233–238.

Robbins, R. H. C. and Piggot, J. (1960) McMurray osteotomy. Regeneration of articular cartilege. *J. Bone Jt. Surg.*, **42B**, 480–488.

Schaller, J. and Wedgewood, R. J. (1972) J.R.A.: a review. *Pediatr.*, **50**, 6, 940–953.

Showman, J. and Wedlich, L. T. (1964) The use of cold instead of heat for the relief of muscle spasm. *Aust. J. Physiother.*, **10**, 85.

Chapter 5

The Burnt Child

'Few accidents can match a major burn in the speed with which the unlimited possibilities of youth are shrivelled and handicap replaces promise' (Cosman 1974). Cosman goes on to say 'burn is one of the most severe traumas that the body can survive and one of the most painful it can endure'. The extent of the disability may be wide-ranging, affecting a great deal more than the dermal covering of the body, and resulting in functional, cosmetic and psychiatric disability. The importance of skin should be carefully considered. Not only does it give protection and appearance, its integrity and elasticity are essential for all physical activity.

Children form a large part of the burn population, burns being a common form of injury during childhood. The causes include domestic accidents (electrical burns, hot water scalds, flame burns due to burnt clothing), the so-called 'battered baby' syndrome, and attempted suicide.

Electrical burns and hot water scalds are most common in infancy. *Electrical burns* may occur when a toddler is left alone in a room with a radiator. He may chew the cord or touch the bright element. *Hot water scalds* are sometimes referred to as the 'hot teapot syndrome' and usually occur when a toddler pulls a pot of boiling water down from the stove. The sites of injury in these cases are usually typical, and include the upper arm, forearm, neck and chest, and may result eventually in contractures of the anterior axillary fold, elbow and anterior surface of the neck. *Flame burns* due to ignited clothing principally affect legs and lower trunk but may be more extensive. *Abused children* may demonstrate hot water scalds or localised cigarette burns combined with evidence of other forms of assault. The majority of burns are said to involve 'the interaction of a poorly supervised child with a poorly supervised environment' (Cosman 1974).

Depth of burn wound

A burn may extend through the entire thickness of skin or damage or destroy only part of the skin. Burns are traditionally described according to degree. A third degree burn is a full thickness injury. First and second degree burns are partial thickness injuries.

A *first degree burn* is characterized by erythema and involves only the surface epithelium. It will heal within a few days. A *second degree burn* may be superficial or deep. The *superficial* burns are characterized by erythema, oedema, blistering and pain, and will also heal within two weeks, although with minor scarring. *Deep* second degree burns may result in destruction of the epidermis and upper levels of corium. These may heal without grafting in a few weeks provided no infection occurs. However, scarring may be considerable. Pain is experienced in both first and second degree burns, although there will be little pain with deep second degree burns where there is destruction of superficial nerve endings. *Third degree burns* involve the destruction of the skin with its appendages (hair follicles, sweat glands and sebaceous glands). Peripheral nerve endings are also destroyed. These burns will not heal spontaneously and will therefore require grafting.

Estimation of burn size

Burns in children encompassing more than 10% of the body area are said to be severe, and survival beyond 60% is uncertain. Estimation of the percent of total body surface involved is usually based on the 'rule of nines', in which the body surface is divided into anatomic areas, each constituting 9% or a multiple of 9% of the total body surface. This requires some modification for small children who need a greater percentage allowance for the head compared to the trunk and extremities.

Burn physiology

A large burn loses a considerable amount of fluid (in the form of water, electrolytes and serum proteins) both externally and internally through the walls of damaged capillaries. Oedema occurs initially at the site of injury and becomes generalized within a few hours. Loss of fluid into the interstitial and intracellular spaces results in elevated haematocrit and haemoglobin (called haemoconcentration).

Fluid loss leads to shock with vasodilation, increased capillary

385

permeability, increased fluid loss and diminished urine output. Eventually renal shutdown may occur. Hypotension and tachycardia may result finally in cardio-pulmonary arrest. The severity of burn shock is related to the size of the burn area rather than its depth. However, overall prognosis depends on depth.

A burn imposes an increased caloric loss upon the child. One of the causes for this is destruction of the protective epithelium with increased fluid loss. It is said that between 2000 and 3350 calories may be lost in evaporation from a burn of one square metre. Wound healing also places a greater demand on calories than normally required for growth and development. Added to this is the sick child's reluctance to eat.

While the wound lacks skin cover there is a great risk of sepsis. The necrotic mass of burned tissue, called the eschar, is bound by collagen fibres to the viable tissue below. Eventually, these two layers will separate, but until they do the space between them allows bacteria to proliferate.

If a burn is circumferential around a limb, the eschar may act as a tourniquet as oedema develops. Decreased arterial blood supply will result in pallor, numbness and inability to move the fingers or toes. Interrupted venous return results in swelling, cyanosis and pain as well as difficulty in moving.

Healing will eventually take place by scar tissue formation which has a tendency to contract. It is generally considered that early skin coverage combined with the early resumption of normal activity and continuous pressure is the best means of controlling excessive scar tissue formation and contraction.

Respiratory complications

Inhalation of hot air may burn the mouth, nose, pharynx and larynx as far as the upper trachea. However, heat is effectively removed from the air by the nose and larynx in most cases, so damage is rarely seen beyond the upper respiratory tract.

Nevertheless, smoke and fumes, especially in confined spaces, may injure the lower airways. The mucosal lining may be inflamed or destroyed in which case it will eventually slough off. The patient may cough up the plugs of necrotic tissue or they may block small airways.

Respiratory complications may include bronchospasm caused by inhaled smoke debris, dyspnoea, consolidation or collapse. In certain types of burns respiratory damage may lead to severe and rapidly progressive bronchopneumonia. Infection may occur due to blood or air-borne bacteria. An increased metabolic rate may add to the already present ventilatory inadequacy. If the chest is burnt, a tight eschar around the circumference of the chest may restrict breathing.

CARE OF THE CHILD IN THE POST-BURN PERIOD

The post-burn period can be divided into three stages according to Cosman (1974):

1. Initial shock and resuscitation (first 2 to 4 days).
2. Wound débridement and coverage (3 to 6 weeks).
3. Skin restoration and reconstruction (several years).

Growth and development of the child impose ever-changing requirements for both function and appearance. Hence the third stage will continue for a lengthy period.

In all stages, the prevention of complications is essential. Hence, nutritional support, antibacterial measures and physical treatment to ensure effective ventilatory function and effective movement of the limbs, trunk and head must be carried out throughout the entire period.

Aggressive resuscitation, replacement plasma therapy, nutritional supplement, topical antibiotics, surgical débridement and early skin grafting are resulting in the survival of many burned children, including those with a large percent of body area burned. A comprehensive burn management programme, to be effective in ensuring survival of the child and some quality in that survival, requires a team effort from parents, nurse, physiotherapist, occupational therapist, social worker and medical practitioner working together with a mutual understanding of the child's needs.

Immediately post-burn

Treatment consists of prevention of shock or resuscitation if shock is present, fluid replacement therapy, antibiotics and nutritional supplement. Maintenance of a good airway will be a major consideration, particularly in burns of face, neck and chest and where there is actual airway damage. Intubation may be necessary and in some cases tracheostomy may be performed, although this is a controversial point.

Bladder catheterization may be required to allow monitoring of urine concentration and output. Blood pressure and pulse are monitored frequently. Escharotomy may be required to relieve constriction of a limb or of the thorax.

Physical treatment will consist of treatment of already existing problems and prevention of suspected future problems. Techniques of treatment for specific ventilatory problems will be as described in Section V. However, there are some points specific to the care of the burnt child which should be mentioned.

Where *nasopharyngeal suction* is necessary to remove secretions, particular care must be taken to maintain a sterile procedure and to pass the tube gently because of the damaged mucosal lining. Where suction is performed via a tracheostomy, care must be taken not to dislodge any slough into the airway.

The intensive treatment which may be necessary in the so-called 'inhalation burns' must be adjusted according to the extent and site of all burnt areas. If secretions must be cleared from the chest, *vibrations* are necessary and if the chest skin is burnt, the therapist must wear sterile gloves. The pain caused by vibrations may actually inhibit respirations, so they should be avoided where possible.

Postural drainage may be necessary to mobilize secretions. Unless there is a specific lung area involved, elevation of the foot of the bed, with breathing exercises and instructions to cough may be sufficient. If the child must be positioned for a particular lobe, sufficient people should be present to enable the child's position to be shifted with a minimum of trauma. Posturing with the legs higher than the head may have to be avoided if neck and facial oedema is gross.

Where possible, *burnt limbs are elevated* to help disperse oedema. The arm is elevated on pillows and the end of the bed is elevated if the legs are involved. Unfortunately, the position of comfort will usually be a position conducive to contracture, so the child must be positioned to minimize the risk of contracture. If the neck is burnt, for example, the head is extended over a foam block. If the axilla is involved, the arm may be positioned above the head. Splinting may be necessary for particular segments of the limbs.

Active movement with assistance from the therapist is begun as soon as the child is admitted. These movements are also performed in his daily bath. On the whole the child will move little unless encouraged to do so. The combination of lying still and sepsis may cause significant bone decalcification (Koepke and Feller 1967). Lack of movement will also result in wound contracture and joint stiffness, disuse muscle weakness and depressed respiratory function. It is therefore essential that the therapist is able to encourage the child to move. He may need to be reassured that he will not damage his skin by moving. He may be allowed out of bed and walking if his general condition allows. If his hands are burnt, he may be allowed to remain independent in activities such as feeding if his hands are encased in sterile plastic bags.

Preparation for skin grafting

The main *objectives* at this stage are to prevent infection and encourage wound healing, in other words, to promote the best possible functional cosmetic skin covering. Infection will prevent successful skin grafting, and it must also be remembered that infection can threaten the child's life until the time when his wound is completely healed.

Débridement, which involves separation and removal of remnants of dead tissue, is carried out if necessary as soon as the child's general condition is stabilized. It may be done nontraumatically in a bath as well as surgically.

Daily or twice daily *active movements* in water and whirlpool baths help to separate remnants of dead tissue non-traumatically, reduce bacterial infection and stimulate capillary ingrowth, as well as facilitating dressing changes. An antibacterial agent, such as chlorhexadine, is added to the water, and the temperature should be approximately 35°C. The child spends 15 to 30 minutes in the bath. Room temperature should be warm, and after his bath the child may be dried under heat lamps. It is generally considered impractical to maintain sterility of the bath but some suggest the use of disposable plastic liners, and certainly the bath should be cleaned after use.

The child may resist hydrotherapy. This anxiety may be relieved if he is encouraged to become involved in the various procedures, such as filling the bath, and if he is allowed to play with his own bath toys. A television set in the room may also divert his attention.

Following the bath, the burn eschar may be probed with forceps and trimmed. An antibacterial cream such as silver sulphurdiazine, or embryonic membrane, is applied directly to the wound, sealing it from the air.

Early *surgical débridement*, followed by skin grafting, is said by its advocates to minimize sepsis, provide early skin cover, allow early resumption of normal activity and decrease time spent in hospital.

If the burn does not involve the full thickness of skin, granulation tissue will form on the surface of the wound as the burn eschar separates. If epithelium has survived, it will grow to the surface and across the granulation tissue and this results in wound healing.

Skin grafting

Skin grafting will be necessary in the case of a full thickness burn. Autogenous split thickness skin is taken from an unburned part of the child's body, called the donor site. The graft tissue is placed over the wound, either completely covering it in the case of a relatively small area, or in strips a few millimetres apart in the case of a larger area. 'Meshed' grafts with multiple perforations are also used, and are said to allow the skin to stretch. Further skin grafting will be necessary as the child grows because scar tissue and skin grafts do not grow at the same rate as the child. Elastic pressure supports are applied as soon as healing and grafttake permit. They are worn at first in conjunction with splinting.

Physical treatment following skin grafting

Deep breathing and *coughing* must be stimulated following surgery. If the chest skin is involved, the therapist must wear sterile gloves. Posturing and turning a child with extensive burns may require 3 or 4 people in order that sufficient care can be taken of the newly grafted areas and the donor sites. Pain will inhibit respirations so vibrations are only given if really essential for clearing the chest. *Nasopharyngeal suction* will stimulate the cough reflex and eliminate secretions if the child is reluctant to cough or expectorate, but it should not be done unless really necessary as it adds to the child's discomfort and fear. Elevation of the foot of the bed must be avoided if neck and facial oedema are present.

No movement of the newly grafted area is allowed for several days (5 to 10 days). Immobilization is gained by thermoplastic splinting or skeletal traction. When the donor sites have healed (in approximately 7 to 10 days) *hydrotherapy* may recommence. Movements should not be too vigorous. It is suggested (Koepke and Feller 1967) that movement may, in some cases, stimulate contracture band formation on flexor surfaces, resulting in a band of scar tissue. The extremities should not be dependent too soon after grafting or microhaemorrhage will occur beneath the graft. Standing can be gradually assumed with elastic supports if the legs are involved, and the child should have his legs elevated when he rests.

Burns to the hand

Burns to the thin elastic skin on the dorsum of the hand present a particular problem as the extensor mechanism and joint capsules are very vulnerable. The common deformity following a burn to this area results from hyperextension of the metacarpophalangeal joints and flexion of the interphalangeal joints. As soon as possible after admission, the hand is splinted to a functional position. The thumb should be in an opposed position with a large web space, the wrist extended 30°, metacarpophalangeal joints flexed 70°, proximal and distal interphalangeal joints extended. The arm is elevated to relieve oedema, and active movement is encouraged several times a day. Following skin grafting the hand is immobilized for 7 to 10 days before movement can be recommenced and then splinting will need to be continued at night and when he is resting during the day. Activities with relevance for the child are better than exercises. He should be encouraged to feed and dress himself and to play using his hands. Excess stretch to the extensors should be avoided as it may cause the tendons to rupture.

Wound healing, hypertrophic scarring and contracture

Two of the most frustrating sequelae of burns are contractures and hypertrophic scars. A child may demonstrate a satisfactory appearance upon discharge, following either spontaneous healing or skin grafting, yet only a few weeks later scar hypertrophy may already be leading to severe deformity.

Joint contracture and *scar contracture* both pose a serious problem during the healing stage which commences immediately after injury and continues throughout the entire post-recovery period for a minimum of six months. Both are facilitated by a number of factors including the child's preference for certain 'comfortable' positions and his reluctance to move. Scars anterior to the flexor surface will, if uncontrolled, lead to severe contracture.

Scar hypertrophy occurs anywhere except those areas of the body in which the skin is splinted by its attachment to underlying structures. It tends to form a bridge across the crease lines of the body.

Hypertrophy occurs following both spontaneous healing and skin grafting. Skin grafting actually decreases hypertrophic scar formation but scarring will still develop between the normal skin and the graft, or between adjacent grafts. The graft limits the excessive proliferation of connective tissue and by its natural pressure prevents to some extent the formation of the whorl-like or nodular arrangement of collagen fibres characteristic of a hypertrophic scar (Larson 1973) and unlike the normal parallel arrangement of collagen fibres.

The risk of scar contracture and hypertrophy will be present throughout the phase of scar maturation, during which the scar is actively growing.

Both hypertrophic scarring and joint contracture are frequently accepted as the natural course of events following burns. However, it is becoming apparent that these sequelae can be significantly altered and controlled with special techniques involving continuous controlled pressure with custom-made splints and anti-burnscar elastic supports. These give non-surgical control of scar contracture and hypertrophic scar formation.

Custom-made splints. Splints (usually of thermoplastic material) are applied soon after admission to maintain the appropriate body position for function. The position of uninvolved as well as involved joints must be considered in order to prevent soft tissue shortening. Unfortunately, the child's preferred position will be one of flexion, and splinting must be used to maintain the extension necessary to prevent contracture and to allow function to be eventually regained. Such splinting is particularly important where burns involve the hands, axilla and neck. Once wound coverage has been attained, appropriate positioning is maintained by splinting and pressure garments (elastic supports).

Anti-burnscar elastic pressure supports (Jobst*). These are worn for twenty-four hours a day until the scars are mature (approximately 6 to 12 months). They promote flatness and smoothness of the healing tissue (figures 136–138). They are usually applied a few weeks after skin grafting before scars begin to form.

Emotional and behavioural complications

Pain and increasing perception of the extent of the injury usually becomes most evident after the fourth day and is then present constantly. In this early stage, the child's relative isolation and the continuous interruptions of treatment procedures add to his confusion. How the child copes with the mental and physical agony following the burn depends partly on his pre-burn personality, and partly on how those caring for him can cope with their own feelings and give encouragement and motivation to him. He may develop stress ulceration of the stomach or duodenum or bizarre signs such as amnesia or opisthotonos. His behaviour may regress.

The staff caring for him also suffer emotional distress and this, combined with anger at having to cause pain, may cause them to withdraw from the close contact with the child which he so desperately needs. The nurse and therapist must be able to gain the child's co-operation in painful treatment and cope constructively with the child's response to pain. Changing a dressing or giving active movements to a hysterically screaming child, knowing that one is increasing his pain, requires that the nurse and therapist understand fully the reasons for the treatment being given. If they also realize that fear and anxiety increase pain, they can divert their own thoughts to ways of easing these.

The therapist should be firmly reassuring to the child and make sure she explains each step of treatment so he will know what is happening. The establishment of a daily routine of therapy often gives the child emotional support and helps to allay anxiety.

*Jobst® Anti/Burnscar. Available from Jobst Institute, Inc., P.O. Box 653, Toledo, Ohio 43694, U.S.A.

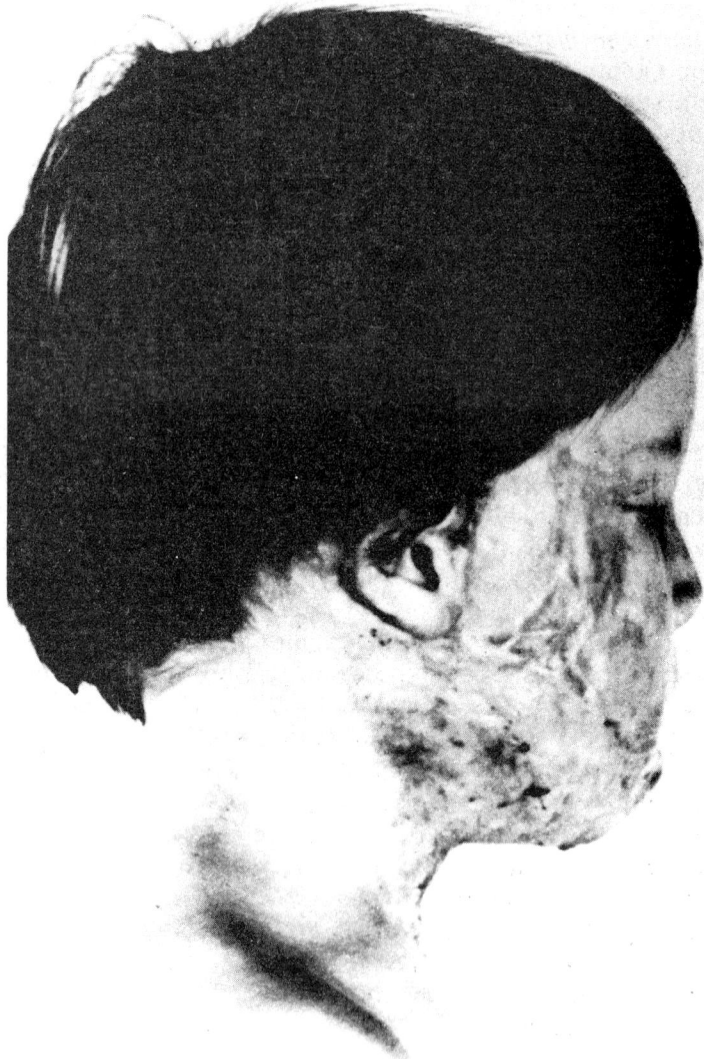

Fig. 136(a) A burned child prior to wearing the Jobst®anti-burnscar **support.** (Reprinted with permission of the Jobst Institute, Inc.)

394

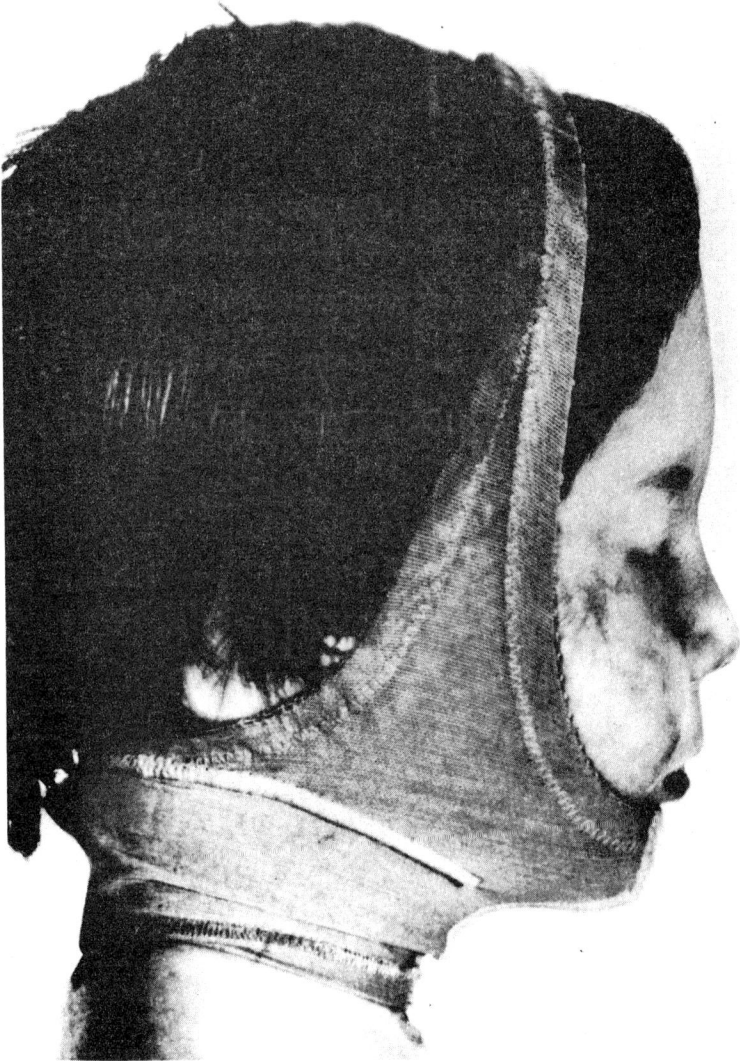

Fig. 136 (b) The child wearing a half mask.
(Reprinted with permission of the Jobst Institute, Inc.)

Excessive staff changes must be avoided as the child may react
badly to this, thinking he has driven his therapist away from him.
Savedra (1977) studied the coping strategies of 5 children aged

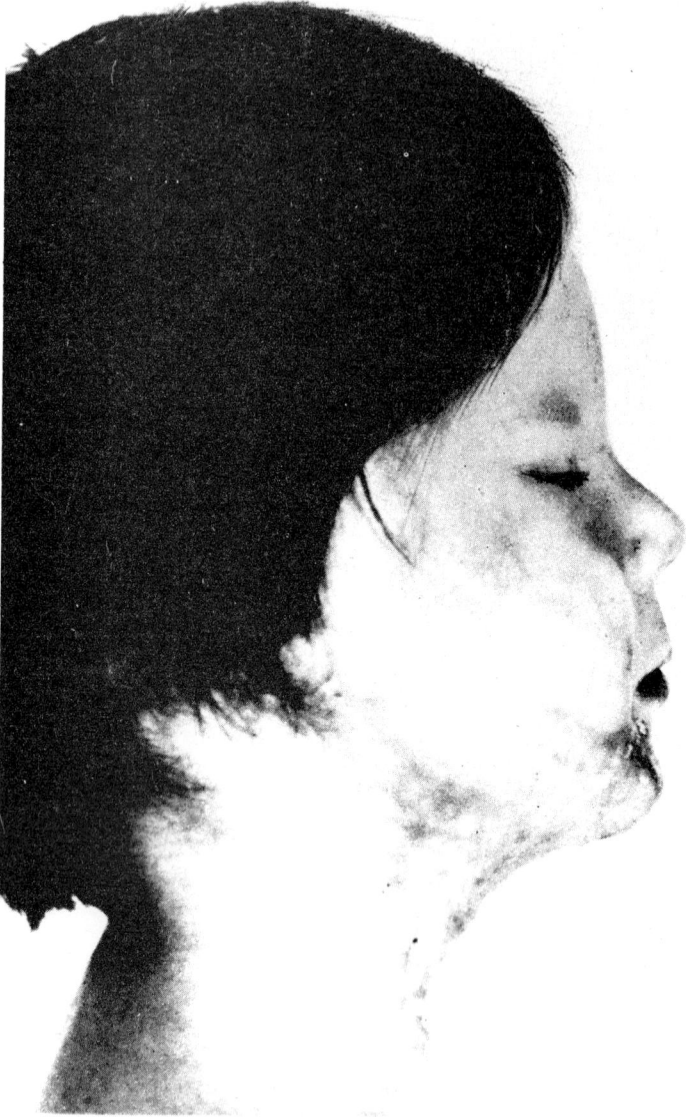

Fig. 136 (c) After wearing the half mask for one year.
(Reprinted with permission of the Jobst Institute, Inc.)

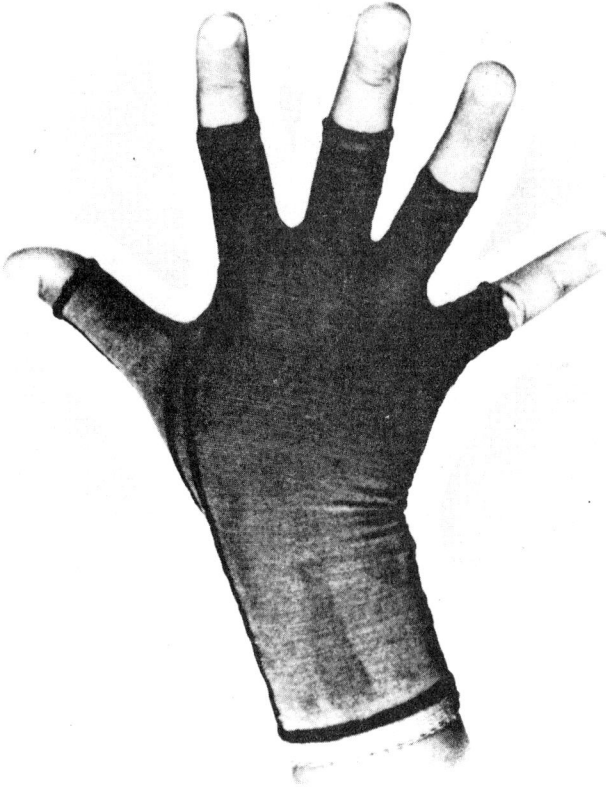

Fig. 137 A custom-fitted Jobst®glove.
(Reprinted with permission of the Jobst Institute, Inc.)

6–9 years, hospitalized with severe burns. They included the following:

Reduction of threat with efforts made to lessen the expected pain ('Don't hurt me').
Postponement (asking that another child could have his bath first).
By-passing the procedure (asking nurse to 'pretend' to do the dressing).
Creating a distance between himself and the threat (kicking legs to keep the nurse or therapist away).
Dividing attention (having hand held, story reading, talking).
Sleep

397

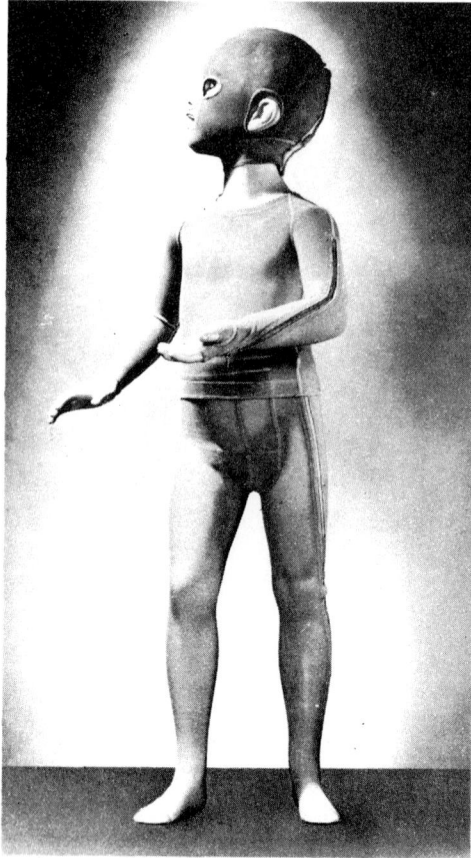

Fig. 138 Custom-made Jobst® anti-burnscar supports.
(Reprinted with permission of the Jobst Institute, Inc.)

Responses to crying of others (intolerance of other children crying).

Leaving hospital is a major hurdle for the burnt child and his family, more so if the child is disfigured, and efforts must be made by the parents, with help from social worker, child guidance counsellor and therapist, to re-establish family routine as soon as possible.

The child's skin must be protected from the sun as it will burn and blister easily. The skin should be patted dry after a bath rather than rubbed. The importance of pressure garments must be impressed upon the parents before the child leaves hospital. Parents and child are taught how to care for these garments and avoid staining and other damage. Parents may need to encourage the child to be active, by playing active games or doing exercises. The child's progress will depend a great deal on the motivation, help and encouragement given by the family.

SUMMARY

Burns constitute a severe and common trauma in childhood. The sequelae may be long-lasting and may affect the child's motor function, personality and general development. Emphasis in physical treatment is on the prevention of permanent disability by the encouragement of active functional movement, by splinting and pressure supports, and by careful advice to parents and child.

References

Cosman, B. (1974) The Burned Child. In *The Child with Disabling Illness. Principles of Rehabilitation*. Philadelphia: W. B. Saunders.

Koepke, G. H. and Feller, I. (1967) Physical measures for the prevention and treatment of deformities following burns. *J.A.M.A.* **199**, 127.

Larson, D. L. (1973) *Prevention and Correction of Burn Scar Contractures and Hypertrophy*. Shriners Burn Institute, University of Texas Medical Branch, Galveston, Texas.

Savedra, M. (1977) Coping with pain. Strategies of severely burned children. *Canad. Nurs.* Aug., 28–29.

Further Reading

Achauer, B. M., Bartlett, R. H., Furnas, D. W. et al (1974) Internal fixation in the management of the burned hand. *Arch. Surg.*, **108**, 814–820.

Alhopuro, S., Sundell, B. and Ritsila, V. (1976) Late complications of scalding in children. Treatment and prevention. *Annales Chirurgiae et Gynaecologiae*, **65**, 151–153.

Brown, J. M. (1977) Respiratory complications in burnt patients. *Physiotherapy*, **63**, 5, 151–153.

Burke, J. F. (1971) Isolation techniques and their effectiveness. In *Contemporary Burn Management*, edited by H. C. Polk and H. H. Stone. Boston: Little Brown.

Eckhauser, F. E., Billote, J., Burke, J. F. and Quinby, W. C. (1974) Tracheostomy complications in massive burn injury. *Am. J. Surg.* **127**, 418–423.

Evans, E. B., Larsen, D. L., Yates, S. (1968) Preservation and restoration of joint function in patients with severe burns. *J.A.M.A.*, **204**, 91.

Gilder, N. (1977) Treatment of burns in a general hospital. *Fisioterapie*, Sept., 5–7.

Hales, M. (1977) Physical treatment and rehabilitation for burns. *Physiotherapy*, **63**, 5, 157–158.

Malick, M. H. (1975) Management of the severely burned patient. *Br. J. O. T.*, **38**, 4, 76–80.

Newton, W. and Bubenickova, M. (1977) Rehabilitation of the autografted hand in children with burns. *Phys. Ther.*, **57**, 12, 1383–1387.

Quinby, S. and Bernstein, N. B. (1971) Identity problems and adaptation of nurses to severely burned children. *Amer. J. Psych.*, **128**, 1, 90–95.

Van der Spuy, J. W. (1977) The changing face of burns. *Fisioterapie*, Sept, 3–4.

Willis, B. A. (1973) *Burn Scar Hypertrophy*. Toledo, Ohio: Jobst Institute.

Section V

Disorders involving the Respiratory Tract

INTRODUCTION

1. *THE DEVELOPMENT AND MECHANICS OF RESPIRATION*

2. *RESPIRATORY DISORDERS IN THE NEONATAL PERIOD AND IN INFANCY*

3. *RESPIRATORY DISORDERS IN CHILDHOOD*

4. *SPECIFIC TECHNIQUES OF PHYSICAL TREATMENT*

Introduction

Infants and children with respiratory disorders are referred to the physiotherapist in order to improve their respiratory efficiency, and the treatment of most of these children involves three basic aims — to clear airways obstructed by accumulated secretions or aspirated material, to re-expand a collapsed segment of lung, and to improve the mechanism and control of breathing. These aims are directed at fulfilling the major objective of ensuring adequate transmission of gases to and from vital organs such as the brain. There are certain specific techniques used by the physiotherapist in the treatment of these problems of increased secretions and inefficient ventilation, and these are described in Chapter 4. The treatment of children with cystic fibrosis and asthma are described separately and in detail as the problems to be handled by the physiotherapist are complex.

In treating both infants and children, the anatomy of the bronchial tree must be carefully considered, plus the effect of the child's habitual posture upon the siting of accumulated secretions. For example, an infant or a bed-ridden child with pneumonia will be more likely to develop pooling of the secretions in the right upper lobe, although this may also occur elsewhere, whereas the child who spends his time in the upright position is more likely to accumulate secretions in the right lower lobe, the right main bronchus being straighter than the left. The development of the respiratory tract must also be considered. The infant with his relatively undeveloped and inefficient bronchial tree may suffer far more serious consequences of infection or aspiration than the older child or adult.

There is an important element of prevention involved in the physical treatment of these infants and children (figure 139). Diseases such as bronchiolitis, aspiration, bacterial and viral pneumonia may be complicated by atelectasis and the stagnation of infected secretions if the obstruction caused by the secretions becomes complete. These complications may also occur following attacks of asthma in which mucous plugs may effectively obstruct airways. Bronchiectasis may develop as the result of the effect of infected mucous secretions on the walls of the bronchioles if these secretions are allowed to remain. The child with cystic fibrosis may develop atelectasis, pneumonia or bronchiectasis as a result of a failure on the part of the normal clearing mechanism to remove tenacious secretions. Emphysema may develop in children, as in adults, as a result of chronic respiratory disability. Figure 140 lists the various causes of increased mucous secretions and figure 141 the causes of airways obstruction.

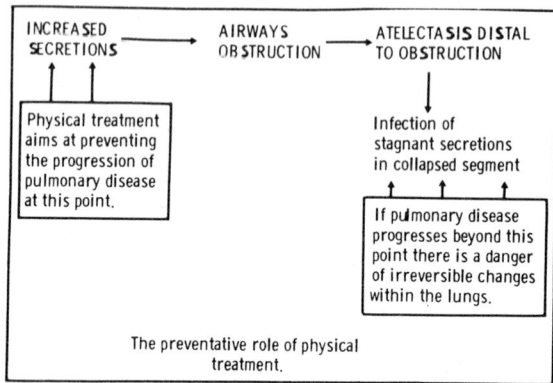

Fig. 139 Preventative role of physical treatment.

There is another aspect of prevention involved in the physical treatment of all children who are at risk of developing disorders of the lower respiratory tract, and who may be seen by the physiotherapist for other reasons. The child who suffers recurrent upper respiratory tract infections may be prevented from developing bronchitis as a recurrent sequela by the use of postural drainage and breathing exercises designed to maintain clear airways. The child with weakness or paralysis of the muscles involved in respiration and the child who is bedridden also needs treatment to prevent the hypostatic pneumonia and segmental collapse which will result if obstruction of the airways by secretions is allowed to occur. The child with severe deformity

404

CAUSES OF INCREASED MUCOUS SECRETIONS

Inflammation of mucosal lining:

        Allergens:-   Asthma
        Infections:-   Pneumonia
                    Bronchitis
                    Bronchiolitis
                    Pertussis

Mechanical irritation:-

                    Foreign body
                    Vomitus

Primary disorder of tracheo-bronchial glands:

        Cystic Fibrosis

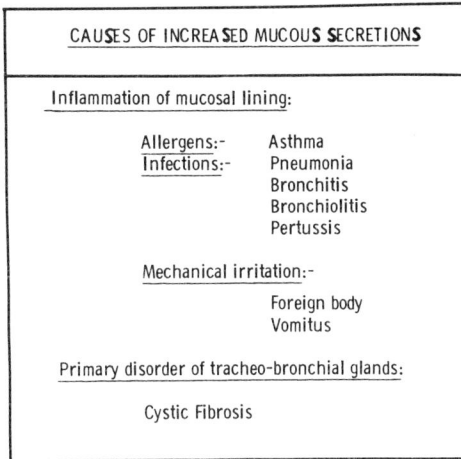

Fig. 140 Causes of increased mucous secretions.

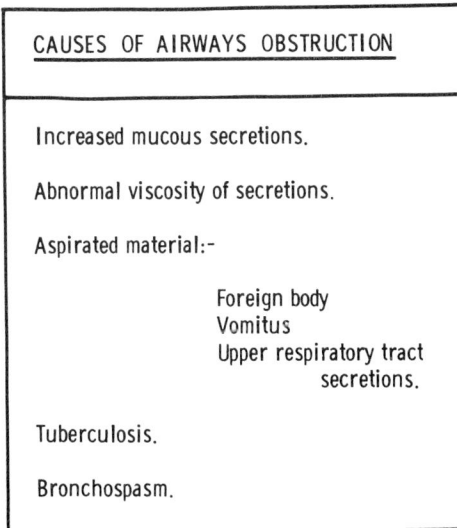

CAUSES OF AIRWAYS OBSTRUCTION

Increased mucous secretions.

Abnormal viscosity of secretions.

Aspirated material:-

                Foreign body
                Vomitus
                Upper respiratory tract
                        secretions.

Tuberculosis.

Bronchospasm.

Fig. 141 Causes of airways obstruction.

involving the thorax, such as occurs in scoliosis and in thoracic myelomeningocele, also requires treatment to maintain the best possible thoracic expansion plus clear airways, and therefore maximum respiratory efficiency.

405

Children who have general surgery usually do not require pre- and post-operative treatment to prevent respiratory complications as do adults in a similar situation. However, the child who undergoes pulmonary or cardiac surgery will require physiotherapy to prevent respiratory complications, and to regain full and effective use of his lungs.

Chapter 1

The Development and Mechanics of Respiration

One of the commonest causes of death in the newborn is respiratory failure. Some understanding of the differences between the fetal, the neonatal and the adult lung is important for the physiotherapist giving treatment to infants and children.

The lungs are not fully developed when the infant makes his first cry. The number of airways and alveoli, and the diameters of the alveoli increase until the child is approximately eight years old, and further increases in terminal air spaces probably occur well into adult life (Kendig 1967). The immature alveoli have not only to increase in size as they mature, but they also have the potential for forming additional alveoli. The physiotherapist must recognize this fact when she treats infants and small children with respiratory disease. The development of the airways and air spaces is dependent to some extent on the demands made upon them, and the presence of disease or the retention of secretions may result in abnormal development. She must also take care that treatment directed at such immature and small airways does not cause damage which will affect the future development and growth of lung tissue.

The embryonic and fetal lung
The embryonic development of the lungs is summarized in figure 142.

The respiratory system arises as a median ventral diverticulum of the foregut called the laryngotracheal groove at about the middle of the fourth week of embryonic life. The lower end of the diverticulum divides into two lung buds. The median stalk of the diverticulum becomes the trachea. The two lung buds will develop into the bronchial tree and respiratory epithelial lining of the lungs. The right lung bud will divide into three branches and the left into two branches. Thus the right lung bud will eventually

PRE AND POST-NATAL DEVELOPMENT OF THE LUNGS	
24 days	Outpouching of gut.
26-28 days	2 primary branches appear - the 2 main bronchi.
8 weeks	Paratracheal mucous glands forming.
10 weeks	Cartilage deposition begins.
12 weeks	Lobes well demarcated. Elastic fibres in walls of main bronchi and trachea. Cartilaginous rings present in lobar and segmental bronchi. Further formation of mucous-secreting glands.
16 weeks	Formation of bronchial divisions nearly completed.
18-20 weeks	Septa now recognisable. Cilia appear on epithelial cells of trachea & main bronchi, and spread towards the periphery.
20 weeks	Cannulisation of airways.
24 weeks	Bronchi now the same as at term. Cartilage formed. Alveolar formation commences.
26-28 weeks	Capillary network proliferates close to the developing airways.

28 weeks	Lung now the most vascular organ in the body. Maintenance of
	  extra-uterine life as depending upon gas exchange is possible
	  at this stage.

28 weeks
to term
	Terminal alveoli appear as outpouchings of bronchioles, and
	  from now to term increase in numbers to form common chambers
	  called alveolar ducts.

BIRTH	Terminal bronchioles are smooth. Terminal air sacs are shallow
	  and wide-mouthed.
	Pulmonary blood flow increases due to mechanical lung expansion.
	Respiratory passages elongate.
	20 million alveoli now present. They become dilated and expand at
	  onset of respiration.

6-8 weeks	Typical sharply curved alveoli can be identified.
Several Months	Terminal air sacs assume cup-like configuration. New alveoli appear proximal to terminal air spaces by transformation of pre-existing bronchioles.
Up to 8 years approximately	Lung growth proceeds with increase in number of bronchiolar divisions, alveoli, alveolar diameters and surface area for gas exchange. Numbers of alveoli and airways increase 10 times from infancy to adulthood. Lung surface area increases 20times. Alveoli number 300 million in adult life.
Up to 40 Years	Further increase in dimensions of terminal air spaces. Bronchiolar and tracheal diameters increase.

Fig. 142 The development of the lungs. (Details from Avery (1968), Langman (1969), and Hamilton, Boyd and Mossman (1972).)

develop three lobes and the left two lobes (Langman 1969).

The size difference between the two lungs is due to the shift of the embryonic heart to the left side of the pleural cavity. The heart's position produces the cardiac notch in the left lung. The relative proportions of larynx and trachea change from the embryonic period to adult life. While the trachea is short and narrow, the larynx is relatively large, and it is not until several months after birth, when the trachea grows at a faster rate than the larynx, that the two structures attain the relative proportions seen in the adult.

The infant's larynx is not a miniature of its adult form. The subglottic cavity below the vocal cords extends backward as well as downward in the neonate. In older children and adults it is almost vertical. An intubation tube must not only be small but also correctly shaped for the airway and introduced correctly. The mucosal lining of the infant's larynx becomes oedematous on minimal irritation and air flow may easily be obstructed.

The lung is a glandular organ with no air spaces in the period before the fetus becomes viable at the twenty-eighth week (Avery 1968). In the fetus the placenta is the organ of gas exchange. On ventilation of the lungs at birth a new vascular bed replaces the vascular bed of the placenta. In the absence of air, the potential airways of the fetus are in contact with a fluid which is partly amniotic, inhaled during in utero respiratory movements, and partly the secretions of submucous glands and goblet cells of the respiratory epithelium. Although respiratory-type movements of the thorax occur in the fetus, this does not occur as a means of gas exchange (Avery 1968). Before birth, the diaphragm is capable of vigorous contraction in a form of hiccup.

The lung at birth

The first breath is a gasp, a contraction of the diaphragm which is probably triggered by tactile and thermal changes (Avery 1968). As the infant takes his first breaths, the alveoli open one after the other in proximal to distal sequence. Good inflation of the lungs occurs with the first loud cry, although for the first 7 to 10 days small areas of lung may remain uninflated. As the infant takes his first breaths air replaces the fluid in the airways. Some of this fluid is extruded from the mouth and nose, but most of it is absorbed into the intestitial tissue of the lung, from whence it is removed by the lymphatic system.

This transition from fluid-filled airways to air-filled airways is potentially hazardous and the principal cause of death in the perinatal period is the respiratory system's failure to function adequately. Success of this transition depends largely on both the presence and the quality of pulmonary surfactant (a mixture of lipo-proteins) which is produced by the alveolar cells. This surfactant lowers the surface tension in the remaining fluid layer which lines the alveoli once air enters the lungs. Before the first breath, the surface tension (Appendix 6) of the partially collapsed alveoli holds the alveolar walls together. Hence a very great effort is needed for the alveoli to inflate.

As air fills the alveoli, surfactant is rapidly released into the alveolar space, forming an interface between the fluid which remains and the newly entered air. It is the presence of surfactant which allows air to remain in the alveoli at all times, and prevents airway collapse.

In neonates whose lungs are deficient in quality or quantity of surfactant more inspiratory effort is needed to produce the appropriate negative pressure within the airways, in other words to retain air at the end of expiration. This extra effort is physically exhausting even for a full-term infant. A premature infant would die without mechanical ventilation to support his breathing.

At birth the alveoli are not present in adult number nor are they fully developed. The airways have a greater relative diameter and the anatomical dead space is correspondingly larger than that of the adult. This is the reason for the preference for administration of oxygen by intubation rather than by tent, taking the gas direct to the respiratory epithelium thus bypassing the dead space of the non-respiratory airways. The respiratory rate of a child also differs from that of an adult (figure 143), gradually approximating to the adult rate during the second decade.

The Mechanics of Ventilation

For air to be inhaled into the lungs and expelled from them, the thorax must increase and decrease in size. This alteration in thoracic volume occurs because of the co-ordinated contraction

NORMAL RESTING RESPIRATORY RATE PER MINUTE		
AGE (YEARS)	BOYS MEAN ± SD	GIRLS MEAN ± SD
0 - 1	31 ± 8	30 ± 6
1 - 2	26 ± 4	27 ± 4
2 - 3	25 ± 4	25 ± 3
3 - 4	24 ± 3	24 ± 3
4 - 5	23 ± 2	22 ± 2
5 - 6	22 ± 2	21 ± 2
6 - 7	21 ± 3	21 ± 3
7 - 8	20 ± 3	20 ± 2
8 - 9	20 ± 2	20 ± 2
9 - 10	19 ± 2	19 ± 2
10 - 11	19 ± 2	19 ± 2
11 - 12	19 ± 3	19 ± 3
12 - 13	19 ± 3	19 ± 2
13 - 14	19 ± 2	18 ± 2
14 - 15	18 ± 2	18 ± 3
15 - 16	17 ± 3	18 ± 3
16 - 17	17 ± 2	17 ± 3
17 - 18	16 ± 3	17 ± 3

Fig. 143 Normal resting respiratory rate from birth to 18 years. SD = One standard deviation of the mean. (From Iliff, A. and Lee, V. A. (1952) Pulse rate, respiratory rate and body temperature of children between 2 months and 18 years of age. *Child Develop.* 23. 237.)

and elongation of the muscles encompassing the thorax. This mechanism is complex and incompletely understood.

The *diaphragm* is not indispensible in adult ventilation, although it usually functions for waking respiration. Adequate ventilation in adults is possible in spite of diaphragmatic paralysis by the use of the accessory muscles of inspiration and the intercostal muscles (Steindler 1955), although activity is very restricted. It is, however, essential during deep anaesthesia when the other muscles of respiration are inactive (Kendig 1967). In the normal person it is the most important of the respiratory muscles, normal resting inspiration being almost entirely due to diaphragmatic contraction. When on inspiration it contracts and

411

descends, the vertical diameter of the thorax is increased. The external intercostal muscles contract to elevate the lower ribs thus further facilitating expansion of the lungs. Their downward pull on the upper thorax is counteracted by the contraction of the scalene muscles. During forced inspiration, such as occurs during effort, the sternomastoid and scaleni muscles contract to elevate the sternum and ribs. On inspiration the descent of the diaphragm tends to pull the lungs downwards and the levator costae and suprahyoid muscles seem to stabilize the trachea and larynx. Resistance to air flow in the upper airway is decreased on deep inspiration by the dilation of the nostrils and by movement of the muscles of the cheek, of the platysma, and of the tongue.

Inspiration requires muscular effort to overcome resistance in the airways and lung elasticity. Normal resting expiration, however, is thought to be a passive process as the muscles of inspiration relax and the lungs recoil. The walls of the thorax relax against the pressure of gravity and the elastic lungs pull inwards on them. The alveoli are prevented from collapsing at the end of expiration by the presence of the fluid, surfactant, which lines their walls. During forced or difficult expiration the abdominal muscles contract strongly, increasing intra-abdominal pressure and thereby aiding elevation of the diaphragm. These muscles are a powerful effector of forced expiration and are strongly used on coughing.

A *cough* results from irritation of the nerve endings in the proximal airways by a foreign body or by accumulated secretions. The diaphragm and intercostals contract and the lungs fill with air. This air is expelled forcefully by relaxation of the diaphragm and contraction of the abdominal muscles, combined with opening of the glottis. The diaphragm and abdominal muscles are therefore essential for an effective cough. The production of mucus is a normal function of the bronchial tree and it is produced by the tracheobronchial glands. It is the action of the cilia in the normal lung which moves this thin layer of mucus upwards to where it can be coughed out. In the infant up to the age of 4 months the mucus appears to be more viscid than in the older child and adult.

The infant's pattern of breathing shows some mechanical differences compared to that of the adult. In the neonate the diaphragm is particularly important for ventilation, especially in the first few days after birth. As the thoracic skeleton contains so much flexible cartilege, contraction of the accessory muscles has little effect. The thorax tends therefore to collapse inwards with each inspiration. Consequently anything that impedes diaphragmatic movement will cause respiratory distress (Roberts and Edwards 1971). In the premature infant this tendency is much greater and may seriously impede ventilation.

SUMMARY

The development of the lungs in the embryonic, fetal and neonatal periods with their continuing development through childhood is briefly described, as are the mechanics of ventilation. It is essential for the physiotherapist to understand the process of development in order to appreciate the importance of physical measures in the prevention and treatment of respiratory disorders in infancy and childhood which are effective in the long term as well as in the short term.

References

Avery, M. E. (1968) *The Lung and its Disorders in the Newborn Infant.* Philadelphia: Saunders.

Kendig, E. L. (1967) *Disorders of the Respiratory Tract in Children.* Philadelphia: Saunders.

Langman, J. (1969) *Medical Embryology.* Baltimore: Williams and Wilkins.

Roberts, K. D. and Edwards, J. M. (1971) *Paediatric Intensive Cure.* Oxford and Edinburgh: Blackwell.

Steindler, A. (1955) *Kinesiology of the Human Body.* Illinois: Thomas.

Further Reading

Bucher, U. and Reid, L. (1961) Development of the intrasegmental bronchial tree. *Thorax*, **16**, 207.

Bucher, U. and Reid, L. (1961) Development of the mucus-secreting elements in human lung. *Thorax*, **16**, 219.

Burns, B. D. (1963) The central control of respiratory movements. *Brit. Med. Bull.* **19**, 7.

Comroe, J. H. (1965) *The Physiology of Respiration*. Chicago: Year Book Medical Publishers.

Comroe, J. H., Forster, R. E., Du Bois, A. B., Briscoe, W. A. and Carlsen, E. (1962) *The Lung. Clinical Physiology and Pulmonary Function Tests*. Chicago: Year Book Medical Publishers.

Cook, C. D., Helliesen, P. J., Kulezycski, L., Banic, H., Friedlander, L., Agathon, S., Harris, G. B. C. and Schwachman, H. (1959) Studies of respiratory physiology in children. *Pediatrics*, **24**, 181.

Crelin, E. S. (1975) *Development of the Lower Respiratory Tract*. New Jersey: Ciba-Geigy.

Davis, J. A. and Dobbing, J. (1974) *Scientific Foundations of Paediatrics*. Philadelphia: Saunders.

de Reuck, A. V. S. and Porter, R. (1967) Ciba Foundation Symposium. *Development of the Lung*. London: Churchill.

Dunnill, M. S. (1962) Postnatal growth of the lung. *Thorax*, **17**, 329.

Emery, J. (1969) Embryogenesis. In *The Anatomy of the Developing Lung*. London: Heinemann.

Hamilton, W. J., Boyd, J. D. and Mossman, H. W. (1972) *Human Embryology*. Cambridge: Heffer.

Herxheimer, H. (1949) Some observations on the co-ordination of diaphragmatic and rib movement. *Thorax*, **4**, 65.

Iliff, A. and Lee, V. A. (1952) Pulse rate, respiratory rate and body temperature between 2 months and 18 years. *Child Develop.* **23**, 237.

Karlberg, P. and Koch, G. (1962) Respiratory studies in newborn infants. III. Development of mechanics of breathing during the first week of life. *Acta Paediat. Suppl.* **135**, 121.

Livingstone, J. L. and Gillespie, M. (1935) The value of breathing exercises in asthma. *Lancet*, **2**, 705.

Mead, J. (1961) Mechanical properties of lungs. *Physiological Review*, **41**, 281.

Polgar, G. and Promadhat, V. (1971) *Pulmonary Function Testing in Children: Techniques and Standards*. Philadelphia, London and Toronto: Saunders.

Shepherd, R. B. (1975) Abnormal growth and development resulting from disease, trauma and deformity. *Aust. J. Physiother.* **21**, 4, 143–150.

Strang, L. B. (1977) Growth and development of the lung. *Ann. Rev. Physiol.*, **39**, 253.

Thacker, E. W. (1971) *Postural Drainage and Respiratory Control*. London: Lloyd-Luke.

Wade, O. L. (1954) Movements of the thoracic cage and diaphragm in respiration. *J. Physiol.* **124**, 193.

Chapter 2

Respiratory Disorders in the Neonatal Period and in Infancy

Respiratory abnormalities are some of the commonest causes of death in the newborn. These abnormalities result from varying causes, infection as in staphylòcoccal and streptococcal pneumonia and bronchiolitis, from congenital abnormalities such as tracheo-oesophageal fistula and congenital heart disease, and from such genetically determined disease as cystic fibrosis. Premature babies may suffer respiratory distress syndrome and other respiratory abnormalities arising from their immature respiratory and circulatory systems.

Generalized atelectasis is seen frequently in premature infants and may be due to a deficiency of the normal alveolar lining layer resulting from the immaturity of lungs which have not progressed to the stage of adequate alveolar formation (Avery 1968). Segmental atelectasis is a more common complication in infants with respiratory infection than in older children (Kendig 1967), because of the relatively undeveloped state of the lungs and the small diameter of the airways. It is difficult for an infant to clear bronchial obstruction because of his hypermobile thorax and undeveloped muscular control. Atelectasis results most commonly from obstruction by mucous secretions in such diseases as bronchiolitis and pneumonia. However, obstruction can also be caused by the inhalation of a foreign body. Young infants have an immature swallowing pattern which allows aspiration of feeds with the possibility of airways obstruction. Atelectasis may result from lack of alveolar patency as seen in infants with respiratory distress syndrome, in which there is no control over surface tension resulting in retraction of the alveolar walls. Obstructive atelectasis is preventable if postural drainage is efficiently and frequently performed on all infants with increased mucous secretions from whatever cause.

It is essential in the treatment of all patients with respiratory disorders for the physiotherapist to consider the brain's need for oxygen, that is the relationship between brain function and respiration. This consideration is particularly important in the treatment of premature and full-term neonates and infants. It appears that acidosis and anoxia may be important factors in the production of lesions of the central nervous system and that there may be some correlation between the severity of these lesions and the length of survival under anoxic and acidotic conditions. The combination of apnoea, cyanosis, hypotension and a sudden drop in haematocrit are recognized as often correlating in pre-term infants with severe intracerebral haemorrhage (Grunnet, Curless, Bray and Jung 1974).

Finer, Boyd and Grace (1978) studied the effects of chest physiotherapy on neonates with various pulmonary disorders, with the specific aim of determining its effect on arterial blood gases. They found that appropriate physiotherapy led to an increase in arterial pO_2 which was sustained.

BRONCHIOLITIS

This is an acute viral infection which affects infants during their first six months of life.

Pathophysiology

Inflammation of the small airways occurs due to the infection, which causes oedema of the bronchial walls, the lumen of which become further obstructed by the excessive secretions from the mucosal lining. If the obstruction is not removed air becomes trapped distally, and atelectasis occurs if this air is completely absorbed. The trapped secretions in the collapsed segment may also become infected. Spasm of the smooth muscles of the bronchiolar walls occurs and is more marked on expiration. Difficulty in expiring air causes hyperventilation of the lungs, and the diaphragm becomes flattened, moving little on inspiration or expiration. If hypoxaemia becomes severe, carbondioxide retention occurs.

Clinical features

The infection begins in the upper respiratory tract. A paroxysmal cough develops. The respiratory rate increases, and because of his distress, the infant uses his accessory muscles of respiration. The chest wall, very mobile in infants, retracts on inspiration because the already flattened diaphragm cannot descend any further and acts paradoxically to retract the lower ribs. Upper thoracic movement is obvious. Crepitations can be heard on auscultation, both on inspiration and expiration, and wheezing is evident on expiration if there is bronchospasm. If carbondioxide retention becomes marked the infant will appear cyanosed. He may become very distressed, with flaring of the nostrils on inspiration, restlessness and opisthotonus. Feeding is usually difficult and insufficient intake of fluid increases the risk, already present, of dehydration.

Treatment

The infant is given oxygen therapy through a plastic head box or a small tent or by endotracheal intubation, and the air is humidified. If there is bronchospasm a bronchodilator is administered before postural drainage is given. Postural drainage with squeezing of the chest wall, vibrations and clapping are done as often as necessary, in order to dislodge obstructive secretions and prevent atelectasis (Chapter 4). The infant may be required to be tube-fed, as respiratory difficulties will increase the likelihood of aspiration of feeds.

PNEUMONIA

This is frequently a fatal condition in the young infant. It may be caused by the aspiration of material such as meconium which may occur just before birth, by the aspiration of regurgitated feeds, or by the inhalation of airborn bacteria or viruses. Regurgitated milk, if aspirated by a newborn baby, particularly if he is premature, may cause severe obstruction of the airways, which may be followed by secondary bacterial pneumonia. Aspiration probably occurs because of the inco-ordination of swallowing mechanisms in the infant, and is therefore particularly likely to occur in premature infants and in infants with brain damage. Aspiration also occurs as a result of the defect in tracheo-oesophageal fistula, and is sometimes the result of the forced feeding of crying infants.

Pathology

Inflammation of the bronchial, bronchiolar and alveolar walls occurs with resultant increase in mucous secretions. Where obstruction is marked atelectasis occurs. Aspiration pneumonia occurs most commonly in the posterior segments of the lungs, particularly of the right upper lobe in infants due to the anatomy of the airways and the habitual horizontal posture. Pneumonia from inhalation of bacteria and viruses is usually diffusely spread throughout the lungs.

Clinical features

The neonate who has aspirated material before birth is slow to establish respiration, will have a low Apgar rating (Appendix 3), and will probably need to be resuscitated. The infant who develops pneumonia later will demonstrate signs of respiratory difficulty, with rapid, shallow, grunting breaths, flaring of the alae nasi and rib recession. He may become cyanosed or have periods of apnoea.

Treatment

This infant must be promptly and vigorously treated. Medical treatment involves the administration of antibiotics, and if necessary oxygen therapy. Physical treatment is directed at clearing the airways by postural drainage and pharyngeal aspiration (see Chapter 4).

TRACHEO-OESOPHAGEAL FISTULA WITH OESOPHAGEAL ATRESIA

The mechanisms of these malformations are still unclear. They are frequently associated with muscular and skeletal anomalies, cardiac lesions and gastro-intestinal abnormalities. The insult to the embryo probably occurs between the second and fourth week after gestation. Oesophageal atresia and tracheo-oesophageal fistula may occur as separate defects but maldevelopment of the trachea and oesophagus in its commonest form results in the oesophagus ending in a blind pouch with a fistula passing between the trachea and the lower oesophagus (figure 144). There are other forms of the defect (Ashcraft and Holder 1976). Mucous secretions and feeds pour into the upper oesophageal pouch, and overflow into the trachea. Gastric contents may also reflux through the distal fistula into the lungs. Crying contributes to this as the closure of the glottis forces air through the tracheo-oesophageal fistula and into the stomach. This allows reflux of the chemical contents of the stomach into the airway, causing a chemical pneumonitis usually located in the right upper lobe.

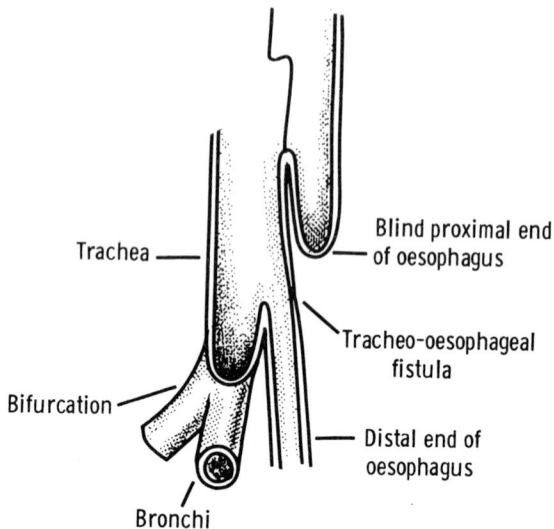

Fig. 144 One type of congenital tracheo-oesophageal fistula with oesophageal atresia.

Treatment

The infant will die in the neonatal period if the condition is not recognized and treated very early after birth. Early treatment is necessary to avoid aspiration and regurgitation pneumonitis. Nurse and therapist must report any neonate who appears to have excessive mucus, who coughs, chokes, regurgitates and becomes cyanotic when being fed. This apparently excessive mucus is regurgitated saliva which cannot be swallowed.

Urgent surgical treatment to divide the fistula and anastomoze the oesophagus is essential. The infant will be referred to the physiotherapist pre and post-operatively to aid drainage of aspirated material and mucous secretions, and to improve aeration of the lungs (Chapter 4).

Pre-operative treatment is essential to improve the infant's chance of surviving surgery and the post-operative period. It includes gastrostomy for gastric decompression and continuous suction of the blind upper pouch. The infant is nursed in semi-Fowler's position.

Following the thoracotomy there is a tendency for right upper lobe collapse. Castilla et al (1971) suggest nursing the infant in prone following surgery to repair oesophageal atresia, and describe a special frame to facilitate nursing care.

IDIOPATHIC RESPIRATORY DISTRESS SYNDROME

This disease is one of the commonest causes of respiratory symptoms and a relatively common cause of death in newborn premature infants. The aetiology is unclear, although there are several theories (Avery 1975). It occurs in premature infants and in infants with diabetic mothers. Its occurrence in premature infants is related to surfactant deficiency. However, other factors, including development of asphyxia in the perinatal period (with resultant damage to the respiratory mucosa), may contribute. At birth these babies have a low Apgar rating (Appendix 3) and require resuscitation. They may demonstrate the flaccidity and frog posture of the premature infant. Respiratory failure may cause death, and cerebral haemorrhage is not uncommon. Not all these infants die. A small percentage, those more mildly affected, and those whose respiratory distress can be controlled, survive.

Pathophysiology

The pathology of this disease is little understood. The appearance of the lungs at autopsy differs according to whether the infant was still or live-born and to the length of time he survived. The lungs usually appear underinflated with areas of atelectasis. Alveoli are often filled with fluid of a high protein content resembling a hyaline membrane. In this case the infant is said to have suffered hyaline membrane disease. There is a decreased amount of surfactant.

The infant shows hypoxaemia and hypercarbia with poor peripheral blood flow (figure 145). The impairment of gas exchange is due to poor perfusion. The deficiency in the surfactant

AETIOLOGY AND CONSEQUENCES OF
RESPIRATORY DISTRESS SYNDROME

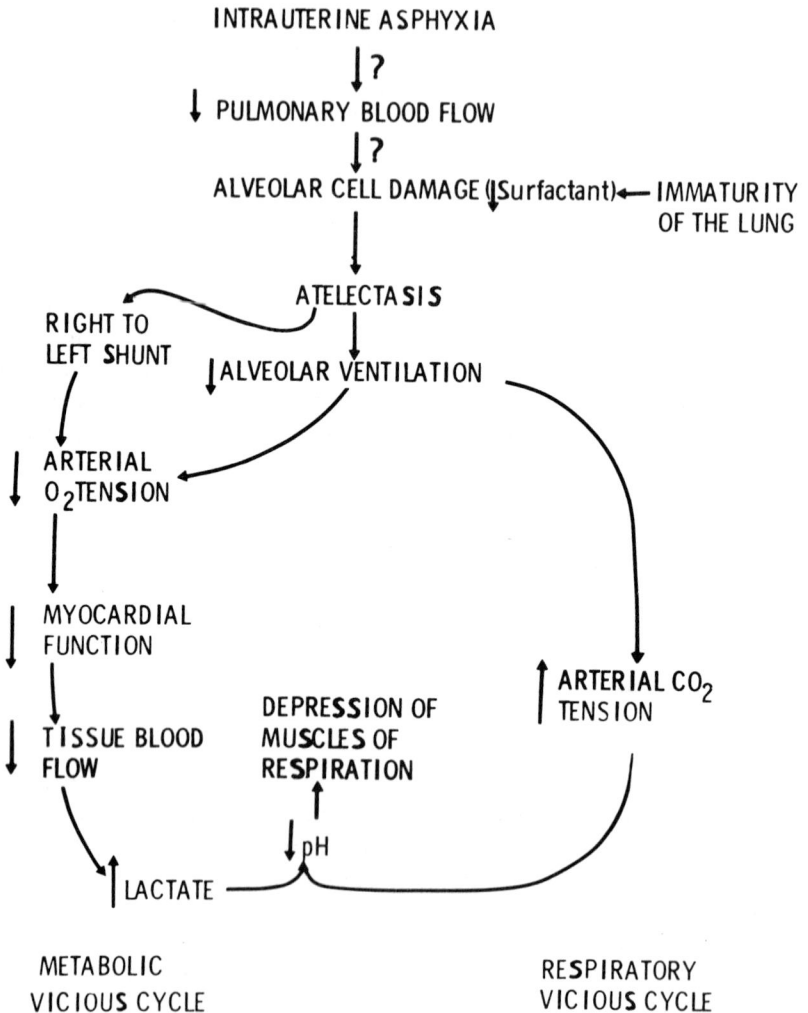

INTRAUTERINE ASPHYXIA

$\downarrow$?

$\downarrow$ PULMONARY BLOOD FLOW

$\downarrow$?

ALVEOLAR CELL DAMAGE ($\downarrow$Surfactant)$\leftarrow$ IMMATURITY
OF THE LUNG

ATELECTASIS

RIGHT TO
LEFT SHUNT

$\downarrow$ ALVEOLAR VENTILATION

$\downarrow$ ARTERIAL
O$_2$TENSION

$\downarrow$ MYOCARDIAL
FUNCTION

$\downarrow$ TISSUE BLOOD
FLOW

DEPRESSION OF
MUSCLES OF
RESPIRATION

$\uparrow$ ARTERIAL CO$_2$
TENSION

$\downarrow$pH

$\uparrow$LACTATE

METABOLIC
VICIOUS CYCLE

RESPIRATORY
VICIOUS CYCLE

Fig. 145 Aetiology and consequences of respiratory distress syndrome.
(From Jones, R. S. and Owen-Thomas, J. B. (1971) *Care of the Critically Ill
Child.* London: Arnold.)

422

allows the alveoli to collapse because of lack of control over the surface tension which it normally provides.

Bronchopulmonary dysplasia has been described (Reilly *et al* 1973) in infants treated for respiratory distress syndrome. It is manifested by bronchospasm, cyanosis, pneumonitis and bronchitis and the infants may have atelectasis, focal air trapping and fibrosis. Philip (1975) comments that immature lungs may develop bronchopulmonary dysplasia when they are exposed to inspired oxygen concentrations over 40% for as little as 3 days via positive pressure ventilation. In other words, it appears that immature lungs react differently from mature lungs in this situation.

Clinical features

Gradually increasing respiratory insufficiency occurs within a few hours of birth. Breathing is difficult and laboured, and the infant demonstrates rapid, shallow, grunting respirations. The intercostal and subcostal spaces are retracted. There are apnoeic periods and central cyanosis, with a tendency to hypothermia. There may be a build-up of secretions.

Treatment

There is considerable controversy about the aetiology and pathology of respiratory distress syndrome, and therefore about the management of these infants.

In general, treatment is directed towards improving ventilation, giving thermal protection, providing for metabolic needs and supporting circulation.

Physiotherapy is designed to clear airways and aerate the atelectactic lungs. The physiotherapeutic management will depend upon the physician's approach to the problem. Treatment is largely supportive, the infant being given oxygen in his incubator. As with all premature infants the body temperature must not be allowed to fall as this will increase his need for oxygen.

The use of respirators for these infants is controversial (Avery 1975). Some surviving infants show the harmful effects of high oxygen and low nitrogen concentrations in inspired air, of endotracheal intubation and positive pressure ventilation (Jones and Owen-Thomas 1971, Philip 1975). The inhalation of a high oxygen concentration by premature infants will lead to retrolental fibroplasia and may cause permanent blindness. Kronskop *et al* (1975) suggest that the early use of continuous positive airways pressure (CPAP) may be protective of the lungs of many infants. They comment that it may prevent the inactivity of surfactant in those infants who weigh 1500 grams or more at birth.

SUMMARY

Some respiratory disorders seen in infants are described. These disorders may be due to the infant's immaturity, or to infection; in rare cases there may be a congenital cause. Early, frequent, and vigorous physical treatment is essential in all cases of respiratory disorder if permanent lung damage or permanent retardation of lung development is to be avoided.

References

Ashcraft, K. W. and Holder, T. M. (1976) Esophageal atresia and tracheoesophageal fistula malformations. *Surg. Clin. North Amer.* **56**, 2, 299.

Avery, M. E. (1975) *The Lung and its Disorders in the Newborn Infant.* 2nd Edit. Philadelphia: Saunders.

Castilla, P., Irving, I. M., Jackson Rees, G. and Rickman, P. P. (1971) Posture in management of esophageal atresia. *J. Ped. Surg.* **6**, 6, 709.

Finer, N. N., Boyd, J. and Grace, M. G. (1978) Chest physiotherapy in neonates: a controlled study. *Physiother. Canada* **30**, 1, 12.

Grunnet, M. L., Curless, R. G., Bray, P. F. and Jung, A. L. (1974) Brain changes in newborns from an intensive care unit. *Develop. Med. Child Neurol.* **16**, 320.

Jones, R. S. and Owen-Thomas, J. B. (1971) *Care of the Critically Ill Child.* London: Edward Arnold.

Kendig, E. L. (1977) *Disorders of the Respiratory Tract in Children.* 2nd Edit. Philadelphia: Saunders.

Kronskop, R. W., Brown, E. G. and Sweet, A. Y. (1975) The early use of C.P.A.P. in the treatment of idiopathic respiratory distress syndrome. *Pediat.* **87**, 2, 263.

Philip, A. G. S. (1975) Oxygen plus pressure plus time: the

etiology of bronchopulmonary dysplasia. *Pediat.* **55**, 44.

Reilly, B. J., Bryan, M. H., Hardie, M. J. and Swyer, P. R. (1973) Pulmonary function studies during the first year of life in infants recovering from the respiratory distress syndrome. *Pediat.* **52**, 169.

Further Reading

Benson, F., Celander, O., Haglund, G., Nilsson, L., Paulsen, L. and Renck, L. (1958) Positive pressure respirator treatment of severe pulmonary insufficiency in the newborn infant. *Acta Anaesth. Scand.* **2**, 37.

Farrell, P. M. and Avery, M. E. (1975) Hyaline membrane disease. *Am. Rev. Resp. Dis.*, **3**, 657.

Field, T. et al (1978) A first-year follow-up of high risk infants. *Child Develop.* **49**, 1, 120–131.

Gregory, G. A. (1971) Respiratory care of newborn infants. *Ped. Clin. N. Amer.*, **19**, 311.

Nelson, W. E., Vaughan, V. C. and McKay, R. J. (1969) *Textbook of Pediatrics.* Philadelphia, London and Toronto: Saunders.

Roberts, K. D. and Edwards, J. M. (1971) *Pediatric Intensive Care.* Oxford: Blackwell.

Silverman, W. A., Sinclair, J. C. and Agate, F. J. (1966) The oxygen cost of minor changes in heat balance of small newborn infants. *Acta Paediat. Scand.* **55**, 294.

Chapter 3

Respiratory Disorders in Childhood

The commonest respiratory disorders of childhood seen by the physiotherapist are asthma, bronchitis, bronchiectasis, asthmatic or allergic bronchitis and cystic fibrosis, and only these will be described at any length. There are, however, other respiratory disorders for which children will be referred to the physiotherapist for treatment. Atclectasis or pneumonia are seen in children who have inhaled a foreign body, following pertussis (whooping cough) and as a complication of other respiratory disorders, such as cystic fibrosis. Atelectasis and pneumonia have been described in Chapter 2.

The infant leads a relatively protected life, hence it is common for respiratory infections to begin when the child first goes to school, and the infections may be recurrent through his early school-going years.

PERTUSSIS (Whooping Cough)

This is a common infectious disease of childhood, and although it usually runs an uncomplicated course, it may be followed by extensive lung collapse or bronchopneumonia. This child will be referred to the physiotherapist for treatment to clear his airways and to assist re-expansion of his lungs.

INHALATION OF A FOREIGN BODY

The embryonic right bronchus is slightly larger than the left and more vertically oriented. These differences become more pronounced as the bronchi mature, and foreign bodies are therefore more likely to enter the right bronchus than the left.

Inhalation of foreign bodies such as peanuts and small toys is common throughout infancy and childhood. If the foreign body is not immediately coughed up it will lodge in the airway causing obstruction. This will be followed by infection in the obstructed segment and eventually by air absorption and collapse of that part of the lung. The foreign body irritates the wall of the airway causing inflammation and mucosal oedema, which further increases the obstruction. Air is trapped distal to the obstruction and the area becomes atelectatic. The accumulated secretions become infected and the child develops the signs of pneumonitis, a fever and cough. The child will be referred for physiotherapy to clear his airways and regain full lung expansion immediately following bronchoscopic removal of the foreign body. Postural drainage given before this may result in obstruction of a vital airway when the foreign body shifts positions, and is therefore contra-indicated.

BRONCHITIS

Clinically bronchitis means many things, and occurs in conjunction with many varied clinical features. It may be more a symptom than a disease entity in itself, occurring, for example, as part of pertussis or cystic fibrosis. The primary problem may exist in the upper respiratory tract with infection spreading from a chronic sinus infection, or from the nose following a common cold. It may also exist in the lower respiratory tract, following on from infection of the trachea, or accompanied by wheezing, or occurring as part of a generalized inflammation of the airways.

It is the acute bronchitis which occurs recurrently in some children, and which may follow on from an upper respiratory tract infection, from measles or another infectious disease, which is described here. It is caused by viral or bacterial infections.

Clinical features

The child develops a cough which may be dry, hacking and painful in the beginning with some fever. Later the cough becomes productive of purulent sputum. Coarse râles or rhonchi (Appendix 6) may be present. If uncontrolled, pneumonia may develop.

Treatment

Antibiotic therapy and postural drainage are the usual means of

427

treatment. Postural drainage need not be specific for certain segments. The child is drained as for the lower lobes (Chapter 4), at an angle of forty five degrees from the horizontal, in prone and side lying, with percussion, vibrations and breathing exercises emphasizing full expiration. His parents are taught how to carry out treatment at home three to four times daily, and it is suggested that this routine be recommenced on any subsequent occasion when the child develops a cough following an upper respiratory tract infection.

This is also an excellent opportunity for teaching nasal hygiene. It is surprising how many older children are incapable of blowing their noses thoroughly, and it is important to spend some time in giving this instruction to any child presenting with a respiratory disorder.

BRONCHIECTASIS

This disease has not been commonly seen in children during the last decade (Kendig 1967, Illingworth 1971). Kendig (1967) suggests that this may be due to the decrease in numbers of children having pertussis and measles and other childhood diseases which were frequently associated with the development of bronchiectasis, plus the effectiveness of antibacterial drugs in preventing and controlling respiratory tract infections.

Bronchiectasis may occur following infectious diseases such as bronchiolitis and pneumonia, as part of Kartagener's syndrome of sinusitis, bronchiectasis and situs inversus, or as part of a genetically determined disease such as cystic fibrosis.

Pathology

As a result of the accumulation of infected secretions and inflammation the bronchial walls dilate causing either cylindrical or saccular dilations (figure 152). The cylindrical form of bronchiectasis is said to be reversible while the saccular form is irreversible. The dilated bronchial walls show, depending on the stage of progression of the disease, loss of elastic tissue and damage to the muscular and cartilaginous walls. This results in loss of the flexibility of the bronchial walls.

Clinical features

The child presents with a chronic cough which is productive of mucus, especially when he first gets up in the morning. In children with severe chronic disease, dyspnoea on minimal exertion, anorexia and haemoptysis may be evident.

Treatment

Medical treatment is aimed at controlling the infection by the use of antibiotics. These children are referred to the physiotherapist for removal of secretions by postural drainage and breathing exercises, and for instruction to the child's mother in the techniques to be used at home (Chapter 4). Medical and physical treatment will be successful in most cases, but if they are not, it may be necessary for surgical removal of the involved section of the lung.

ASTHMA

Children with asthma experience repeated attacks of difficulty with breathing, frequently with considerable respiratory embarrassment. The severity of an attack may range from a mild wheezing to a fatal asphyxia. The aetiology is not clear as it appears there may be many causes even for one patient. Factors such as trauma, change in temperature, stress and fatigue may precipitate an asthma attack. Attacks may come on at night, with little or no warning, or may occur as an obvious result of one of the above factors. There is a large element of fear involved, probably as both cause and effect. During these attacks the child suffers an urgent need for air which varies in degree, and it is not surprising that his appearance is frequently one of extreme anxiety. He demonstrates wheezing on expiration, a tight cough and laboured breathing, and when his cough becomes productive, as it does when the airways resistance is less severe, the sputum is seen to be sticky and tenacious, although it may be coughed up in small plugs. A child whose asthma attack remains unresponsive to treatment after a period of some hours is said to be in status asthmaticus. It should be noted that wheezing does not occur only in asthma, but may be heard in children with obstruction due to an inhaled foreign body, or with bronchiolitis.

Pathology

During an attack there is gradually increasing obstruction of the peripheral airways. Obstruction is rarely complete and it has been suggested (Gandevia 1959) that the term 'airways resistance' is more accurate. This airways resistance is caused by oedema of the inflamed mucous membrane. Spasm of the smooth muscles of the bronchi further decreases the lumen, and increased mucous secretions from the tracheo-bronchial glands cause mucous plugging and further obstruction. The lungs become over-inflated with air which is gasped in by the patient despite the difficulty in expiration. Atelectasis may occur, or complete collapse of a segment, if obstruction of a bronchus or a bronchiole becomes complete.

Physiology

Bronchial and bronchiolar obstruction cause a decrease in the vital capacity and an increase in the residual air. The forced expiratory volume is markedly decreased as demonstrated by the result of pulmonary function tests. In the lungs of children in status asthmaticus so little air is moving in either direction that carbondioxide retention becomes marked. Carbondioxide is the normal stimulus to respiration, acting upon the respiratory centre in the brain stem. When carbondioxide is retained the respiratory centre becomes fatigued and ceases to respond. Respiration is then regulated by oxygen lack, which is detected by the carotid bodies and the aorta. It is this that gives the patient the desperate need for air called air hunger. At this stage, when it is the lack of oxygen only that is driving the patient to breathe, care must be taken in the administration of oxygen, as this may remove the stimulus to breathe. Normally on expiration there is a decrease in the lumen of the airways. In asthma, the increased airways resistance is exaggerated during the expiratory phase due to mucosal oedema, presence of increased secretions and bronchospasm. Air trapping occurs distal to the obstruction. Hence the difficulty the patient experiences in exhaling air.

Allergy

There is said to be an allergic factor present in most cases of asthma in children. It seems that certain substances cause an allergic reaction in the air passages, the allergens having a special affinity for the mucous membranes of the respiratory tract.

430

Allergic children are rarely allergic to only one substance, but are usually found to react to substances as varied as house dust, food and pollen. Some children appear to be prone to allergy from birth, suffering eczema and rhinitis for a few years until they have their first attack of asthma. However, there are some children whose asthma appears to be due to other than allergic reactions, seeming more related to infection, although this also may involve an immunologic reaction.

Clinical features

During an asthma attack the child demonstrates signs and symptoms that result from increased airways resistance causing interference with air exchange. There is a cough which is paroxysmal and nonproductive. Breathing becomes progressively more laboured with shallow inspirations and prolonged wheezing expirations. The child tries to fix his shoulder girdle by bracing his arms and hunching his trunk, thus increasing the effectiveness of his accessory muscles of respiration. The elevation of the thorax results in increased effort, which puts further strain on the respiratory system. He may appear cyanosed. His chest is distended in an antero-posterior direction, and shows little movement. Breathing is mostly abdominal and the ribs, already elevated, flare out on inspiration. If the attack becomes more severe breath sounds are almost inaudible and the cough is suppressed.

At this stage the child is liable to asphyxiate. Signs of right-sided heart failure may be evident. However, the severity of the attack usually decreases and as it does so the cough becomes productive.

Between asthma attacks the child may appear to have normal respiratory function, although he may suffer dyspnoea on minimal exertion. Some children appear in poor health, fail to put on weight, and have poor exercise tolerance. Many are habitual 'upper chest breathers', a method of breathing which both inhibits normal expansion and wastes much energy and have, in addition, poor posture with round shoulders and kyphosis. Some children demonstrate distortions of the chest due to the pressure changes brought about by forced inspiration and expiration. This deformity may be produced early before ossification of cartilaginous junctions occurs.

431

Treatment

The aims of treatment depend on the problems with which each child presents, but the following aims will probably require to be fulfilled with most asthmatic children.

To minimize sensitivity to particular allergens.
To remove as far as possible any predisposing factors.
To decrease bronchial obstruction.
To improve the pattern of breathing, breathing control and exercise tolerance.
To remove excessive secretions from the lungs.
To prevent secondary postural abnormalities and thoracic deformity.

General treatment

A child may undergo hyposensitization to minimize sensitivity to particular allergens, although the effectiveness of this is controversial.

In order to avoid the predisposing causes of his attacks he may have to move to a more agreeable climate, or sleep in a dust-free room. He may be referred for psychotherapy and so may his parents if emotional factors are very evident. In extreme cases he may be sent to a special unit where he can live with other asthmatic children and attend school, away from a home environment which predisposes him to frequent severe attacks. He may, however, only need advice to avoid fatigue and to have sufficient rest.

Corticosteroid therapy will be necessary for some children in order to control frequent attacks, and antibiotics by others in order to counteract infection. Otherwise bronchodilator drugs are prescribed to be taken orally or by spray inhalation when necessary.

Physical treatment

The place of the physiotherapist in the treatment of the asthmatic child is sometimes misunderstood. There have been dogmatic claims made in the past about the effectiveness of certain methods of treatment, although there are probably no completely effective techniques. However, the skilful physiotherapist should be able to work out with each child the way in which she can best help him.

There will be a few children who will not be helped by physical treatment, and these are the children with emotionally-triggered asthma, whose entire environment seems to have built up against them. Most children will derive some benefit from a carefully planned programme of treatment particularly in an improved breathing pattern, improved exercise tolerance, and in the prevention of thoracic and spinal deformity. It is also important to remember two factors. The first is that the lungs of a young child are developing as he grows and secondly, a large number of children with asthma appear to grow out of it by the time they reach adolescence. It is therefore important that the child's breathing pattern and respiratory efficiency are maintained at as normal a level as possible during these essential years of development.

The experienced physiotherapist can also offer considerable psychological support to the child and his family. As Hinshaw and Garland (1965) state: 'Treatment that serves to quiet fear . . . is good treatment.' There is probably considerable value in asthma holiday camps, where a physiotherapist is able to be with the child during his attacks and is able to calm his fears and help him to breathe in a more relaxed manner.

Some of the techniques of treatment which may be of use in overcoming the problems of these children are described below.

To decrease bronchial obstruction and remove excessive secretions from the air passages

Bronchodilator drugs, (for example, salbutamol or isoprenaline) are prescribed by the physician for the relief of bronchospasm. They are administered either from a hand-held apparatus, via a nebuliser attached to an air pump or via IPPB apparatus.

Hand-operated aerosol dispenser. The use of this apparatus must be carefully taught to the child and his mother. This method can only be effective if the child is old enough to co-ordinate an effective inhalation with the operation of the spray mechanism, otherwise the spray will penetrate no further than the mouth. The prophylactic use of sodium cromoglycate (Intal) via a spinhaler enables many children with asthma to lead relatively normal lives. Children over 3 years can inhale effectively, as can some children even younger. A very young child can be taught on an empty spinhaler. The child must be supervised in the use of the spray, as

433

over-use may result in chemical irritation of the airways and other severe complications. There is a limit to the number of times the bronchodilator may be used each twenty-four hours, and this limit must be carefully adhered to.

Nebuliser with mouthpiece. Webber, Shenfield and Paterson (1974) suggest that in the stage of recovery from status asthmaticus, the bronchodilator response is as good using a simple nebuliser as with IPPB. It is also less frightening for young children, and can be used by a young child who cannot yet cope with a spinhaler.

Intermittent positive pressure ventilators. The two machines in common use are the Bennett and the Bird ventilators. The advantage of this method of inhalation is that the aerosol substance penetrates more deeply into the air passages, and it is a suitable method for use with infants and young children. It is also effective for those children who may be too severely dyspnoeic to take a deep enough breath to gain any benefit from the hand-operated spray, such as those who are in status asthmaticus. Use of these ventilators is described in Chapter 4.

Postural drainage. Coughing and postural drainage may aggravate bronchospasm. However, once bronchospasm has been sufficiently relieved, excessive mucous secretions are removed from the lungs by postural drainage. Unless there is a specific area of a lung to be drained, as would occur if there was an area of collapse or infection present, it is usually sufficient to drain the patient in side lying (prone if it is easily tolerated) as for the lower lobes (figure 166). Supine is not usually well-tolerated. There is a tendency for the diaphragm to elevate in supine, due to movement of the abdominal viscera and this increases the patient's breathing difficulties. If the child cannot tolerate the deeply tipped position it may be modified as in figure 146 which is a position of relaxation. Breathing exercises encouraging use of the lower part of the thorax are given, and vibrations on expiration, with encouragement to cough, if they cause no tension or increase in wheezing. Many children find percussion effective in loosening secretions.

Postural drainage techniques are taught to the parents and should be carried out by the child after each asthma attack until the cough is unproductive. There is usually little to be gained from giving postural drainage to a child with unrelieved severe bronchospasm, as the airways obstruction caused by the broncho-spasm will not allow the free passage of secretions and the techniques used may increase the child's respiratory difficulty. However, there are some children who gain relief while lying in a tipped position, and each child must be assessed individually.

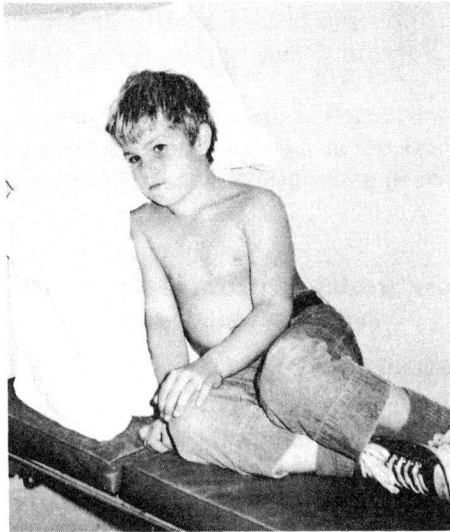

Fig. 146 Position designed to promote relaxation and the elimination of secretions where the patient cannot tolerate the horizontal position.

Some asthmatic children, especially those whose asthma is related to recurrent attacks of bronchitis, require postural drainage as a daily routine at home in order to keep the air passages free from excessive secretions. Others need drain only when necessary following an upper respiratory tract infection, or bronchitis, or an asthma attack. Toddlers may object strongly to the discipline of postural drainage particularly when performed at home. It is better for the therapist to suggest to the parents of a 'chesty' infant that establishing during infancy a routine of daily postural drainage for five minutes will enable the toddler to accept

435

drainage as part of his daily routine of eating, bathing and sleeping.

One two year old patient of the author, who had been on this routine since the age of eight months, would ask his mother for postural drainage whenever he felt he needed it. He seemed to have developed some understanding of the importance of drainage to his subjective well-being. Although he had several attacks of bronchitis and bronchospasm during this period, they cleared up rapidly and he required no further periods of hospitalization.

It is necessary to teach young children how to blow their noses efficiently, one nostril at a time. Allergic rhinitis and sometimes sinusitis, are seen in asthmatic children. Mouth-breathing should be discouraged.

To improve breathing control and exercise tolerance, and to prevent deformity

During an asthma attack

The child is shown what he may do to alleviate his respiratory distress when he has an asthma attack. The success of this depends largely on the physiotherapist's ability to get the idea of self-help across to the child, on the child's age and therefore his ability to understand the situation, and lastly on the ability of his family to control their own anxieties and negative feelings.

The time for him to help himself is when he feels an attack is imminent. Some children are able to lessen the severity of an attack by leaning forwards in a relaxed position with the arms supported on a table, the edge of a bed or railing, and by attempting to breathe quietly with emphasis on depth of inspiration followed by a relaxed expiration (figures 147 and 148). It is not advisable to attempt to alter the rate of breathing as such. The respiratory centre adjusts the rate and depth of breathing to obtain the best ventilation most economically (Gandevia 1959). However, the rate of breathing is also affected by the child's fear, and if this fear can be allayed the respiratory rate may become more efficient. The advantage of suggesting to the child that he can breathe more quietly lies in the allusion to relaxation and in the fact that he is given something positive to think about. If the physiotherapist sees the child when he is in the early stages of an attack, and if she can by her attitude and conversation dispel his fears, she may succeed in convincing him of the usefulness of this approach. If his mother can give him similar support at home, he may be helped considerably. It is probable that this routine has little effect directly upon the respiratory pathophysiology. At least there is no proof that it has. However, if the physiotherapist can

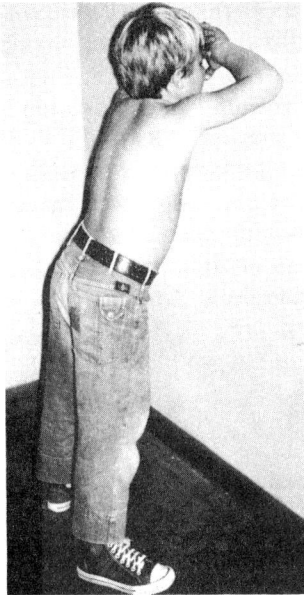

Fig. 147 Position to promote relaxation and control of breathing.

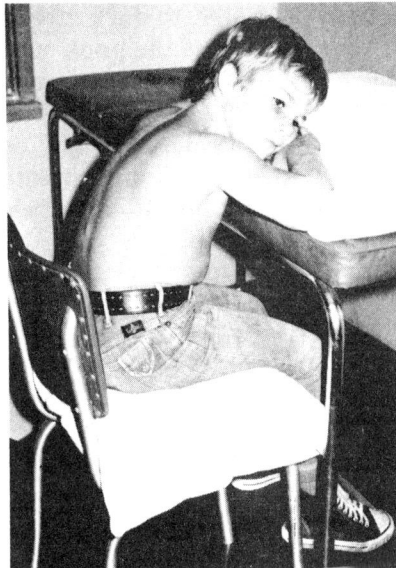

Fig. 148 Position to promote relaxation and control of breathing.

teach the child to relax emotionally, the extra work load which is put on the respiratory system by the tense elevated shoulders and strong contraction of the accessory muscles will be relieved, and this will have an effect on the ventilatory system even if not directly upon the pathophysiology within the lungs themselves. Treatment is an attempt to dispel fear and utilize the individual child's capacity to control to some extent his own body. In the author's opinion, it is always worth while attempting this approach. With some children, circumstances beyond the control of the physiotherapist and the child will render it useless.

Between asthma attacks

It is important that the asthmatic child learns how to avoid dyspnoea on exertion, as this may trigger off an asthma attack. Exercise will induce bronchoconstriction in some children. However, he should not avoid exercise and sport unless it is really necessary. He can be taught to lean against a wall and relax his breathing when he becomes dyspnoeic (figure 149). When possible he should be taught to swim, and encouraged to swim with his face in the water, to duck dive in shallow water to pick up objects from the floor of the pool, and to swim underwater. Swimming has been shown to be preferable to running and bicycling as an exercise, as it results in significantly smaller falls in FEV_1 (Fitch and Morton 1971). Not only does swimming, if properly done, improve co-ordination in breathing, it also improves the child's physical development, and helps prevent secondary deformity, such as kyphosis, rounded shoulders with contracted pectoral muscles, and improves thoracic expansion. Singing lessons accomplish similar aims in some children.

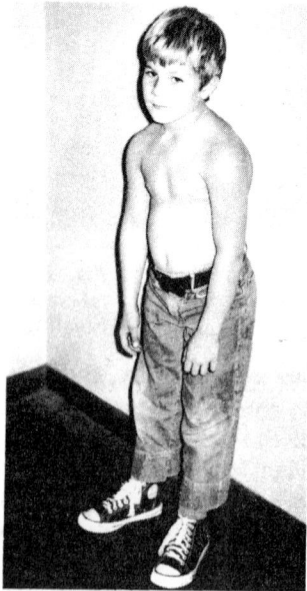

Fig. 149 Position to promote relaxation and control of breathing.

It may be necessary, if swimming is impractical, to give the child one or two exercises to be done at home, which will gain full extension of the thoracic spine, and full length of the pectoral muscles. These exercises must be changed before they become boring. It is most important to remember that the asthmatic child has ahead of him several years of development, and that development cannot proceed normally in the presence of deformity and contracture.

Breathing exercises

The child is taught how to localize his breathing. He is discouraged from expanding only his upper thorax. Each day he should practise for 5 minutes, getting as full and efficient expansion as possible, in a relaxed manner. The aim here is that he should practise the normal pattern of breathing so he understands well enough to attempt it when he feels his respiratory function is threatened. Breathing exercises which emphasize long, forced expiration have no place in the treatment of the asthmatic child. A forced expiratory volume test of a normal person indicates that the amount of air exhaled after the first 2 seconds is negligible. Furthermore, the abnormal breathing of the asthmatic child includes long forced expiration, which is ineffective both because of the normal physiological narrowing of the lumen on expiration, and the pathological narrowing caused by oedema and spasm. Breathing exercises should stress relaxation, an effective deep inspiration concentrating on the diaphragm, which should be followed automatically by a passive relaxed expiration.

Classwork

Once a child and his parents have been taught a home programme and the child is beginning to cope with his problems, he may visit the physiotherapist at monthly intervals and have his treatment with 4 or 5 other children. In this way the physiotherapist is able to see how he is coping with exercise and activities with other children, and can see how effective he is at controlling his breathing in what is a more normal environment than may be present during individual treatment. The children will practise their breathing exercises together, will demonstrate their ability to breathe in a relaxed, normal manner between exercises and games, and there will be time for the physiotherapist to talk to the parents and hear about any difficulties at home. This treatment in a class is not suitable for some children who may need to have more individual contact with the therapist.

For example, if a child comes to the class with bronchoconstriction, he should have individual bronchodilator therapy. Gaskell and Webber (1977) suggest the precautionary measurement of FEV_1 or peak flow rate of each child who attends. The child with low readings would have individual treatment, the administration of a bronchodilator, breathing exercises, with postural drainage if indicated.

The child in status asthmaticus

A child is said to be in status asthmaticus when his asthma is still unrelieved despite usual therapy. Emergency treatment is necessary, and bronchospasm must be relieved as quickly as possible. A child may develop a dangerous degree of carbondioxide retention within a few minutes, and may quickly asphyxiate. He must not be left unattended while so acutely ill.

The administration of a bronchodilator by IPPB or nebuliser with mouthpiece is often very effective. Treatment is given four-hourly during the acute phase. A peak flow chart filled in before and 15 to 30 minutes after treatment gives a picture of the effect of the bronchodilator upon lung function. Postural drainage must be instituted as soon as airway resistance is decreased sufficiently to allow drainage of secretions. The positions used will need to be modified if the child is not able to tolerate a deeply tipped position. Figure 146 shows a possible modification.

CYSTIC FIBROSIS

This is an inherited, generalized disorder affecting the exocrine glands. It is inherited as a Mendelian recessive trait, and is now found to be fairly common in the community (perhaps 1:2,000). The incidence varies within families. For example, in a family of 4 children, 3 may be affected, while in a family of 7 only one may be affected. Some of the children in both families will be carriers, but there is no positive method at the present time for determining which members of the community are carriers. For a child to be born with cystic fibrosis, both parents must be carriers (figure 150).

Pathology

The exocrine glands most frequently and significantly involved are those of the pancreas and of the tracheo-bronchial tree. Glandular secretions are of abnormal viscosity and readily cause obstruction. The salivary glands, nasal sinuses, intestinal and sweat glands are also involved.

The pancreatic defect which is due to obstruction of the ducts, results in failure of the pancreas to secrete the enzymes trypsin, lipase and amylase, which are necessary for the breakdown of fats. Eventually, destruction of the enzyme-producing cells occurs. Interference with fat absorption within the intestine results.

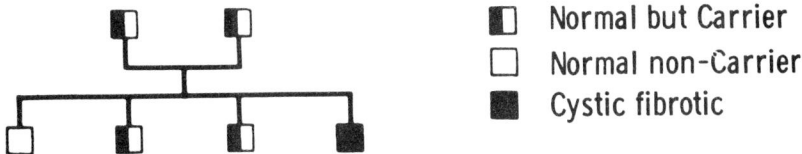

◨ Normal but Carrier
☐ Normal non-Carrier
■ Cystic fibrotic

Fig. 150 Diagram showing the mode of inheritance of cystic fibrosis.

The pulmonary defect is the most serious and difficult to control. Bronchial mucous secretions are normally produced by mucous and serous cells of the submucosal glands, but in the case of cystic fibrosis, in abnormally large quantities. The abnormally thick and sticky mucus causes obstruction of the airways. Pneumonia and recurrent attacks of bronchitis are common and the child may develop a chronic cough. Impacted mucus becomes infected causing further obstruction by producing oedema and stimulating further increase of mucous secretions. Ciliary action is impaired and the normal clearing mechanism in the lungs is ineffective. Obstruction of the smaller airways, if it is complete, will result in atelectasis distal to the obstruction. Bronchospasm may occur with an effect similar to that seen in asthma. If respiratory disease is controlled the pulmonary changes are reversible (figure 139). If disease continues unchecked bronchiectasis may develop due to progressive weakness of the bronchiolar walls. Pockets of mucus in the bronchiectatic sacs are prone to reinfection and lead to further pulmonary damage. The pulmonary lesion may progress to emphysema and eventual right-sided heart failure. The failure to shift mucus will therefore be

441

responsible for severe progressive and irreversible changes within the lungs.

The sweat gland defect results in the excessive secretion of sodium and chloride in the sweat.

Clinical features

The earliest manifestation of the disorder may be meconium ileus in the neonate. Immediately after birth the large intestine is found to be obstructed by thick viscid meconium. In most children the signs of pancreatic insufficiency appear before those of pulmonary insufficiency. The infant passes large quantities of foul-smelling fatty stools, is slow to thrive and gain weight. The pancreatic defect may cause recurrent abdominal pain and constipation.

The respiratory signs vary according to the pathology present at the time. Where there is chronic infection within the lungs the child will fail to thrive, and this failure may be augmented by malabsorption of food within the intestine. If bronchitis or bronchiectasis are present the child will have a cough productive of thick, tenacious and purulent sputum. If infection has caused pneumonia, the cough may be paroxysmal, the breathing rapid and shallow, with the accessory muscles of respiration elevating the thorax on inspiration. If bronchospasm is present, wheezing will be heard. As emphysematous changes develop the thorax may develop a barrel shape. Dyspnoea may be severe. The child is prone to dehydration and heat exhaustion in hot weather because of the sweat gland defect. The disease varies a great deal in severity. Some infants manifest severe symptoms at an early age and the disease proceeds rapidly to death. In others the disease starts in a similar manner, but their condition improves and they manage to live relatively normal lives.

As management of these children improves, more are growing to adolescent and adult life. Their prognosis seems to depend to a large extent on the quality of treatment they receive. If the airways can be kept clear, and if irreversible damage to the lungs can be prevented or kept to a minimum, the prognosis becomes much more optimistic.

Diagnosis

The most reliable test is of the sweat electrolytes. The sweat is

obtained by iontophoresis, and sodium and chloride concentrations are estimated. A sodium content in excess of 60
mEq/1 indicates the presence of cystic fibrosis.

Treatment

There is no cure for this disease. Treatment is symptomatic and
consists of the substitution of animal extract for the absent
pancreatic enzymes, the prevention of irreversible pulmonary
changes, the prevention of heat exhaustion by the addition of
adequate salt to the diet, and the maintenance of good general
health and a sound emotional state both in the child and his
family. The main aim of all treatment is to enable the child to live
as normal a life as possible.

Management of the obstructive pulmonary lesion

Treatment must be adapted to whatever is the stage of pulmonary
involvement, but basically it is directed towards the clearing of
excessive mucous secretions from the airways. This aim should
always be uppermost in the physiotherapist's mind when she
treats these children. Irreversible changes in the lungs must be
prevented if possible, but if they have already occurred, treatment
must aim at maintaining optimum respiratory function. The fact
that irreversible lung changes seem to occur more readily in infants and young children is due to the effect of infection and
retained secretions upon the relatively undeveloped lungs
(Chapter 1).

Methods of clearing secretions

The usual methods of postural drainage alone are not effective in
the treatment of children with cystic fibrosis. The secretions are
thick and tenacious, and therefore difficult to dislodge. They
must be moistened and broken up into smaller particles to
facilitate their removal and the infant who cannot cough effectively must be stimulated to do so.

Inhalation Therapy

The viscosity of the bronchial secretions may be decreased by
several methods.

Mist tent therapy. The child may require to sleep in a tent into which air is passed via a nebuliser, and, if the weather is hot, via a cooling device. An ultrasonic nebuliser is sometimes preferred as it produces extremely fine particles of moisture. The nebuliser contains a liquefying solution, such as propylene glycol in distilled water. For the best effect the mist should be dense enough almost to obscure the child from view. The child is observed carefully on the first few occasions and postural drainage or suction given as the cough becomes productive. Postural drainage must always be given when the child wakes up in the morning. There is a danger of a small child drowning in his secretions if he is not carefully watched in order to determine the effects of this therapy. For this reason, some authorities do not consider this a suitable means of nebulisation therapy for these children.

Intermittent aerosol therapy is considered by many to be preferable to mist tent therapy. It is given via mouthpiece or mask. The mouthpiece is considered to be the more effective but a mask may be necessary for small children and infants. Secretions can be liquidified via a nebulizer attached to a source of compressed air, such as a portable air pump (figure 151). This is also a satisfactory method for use at home. A liquefying agent is used. The child is given this therapy three times a day or as required, and the liquefying of the secretions must be followed by postural drainage. If bronchospasm is present, a bronchodilator is added to the nebulizer. If infection is present, an antibiotic may be given via the nebulizer, but in this case, *after* the postural drainage.

Intermittent positive pressure therapy. Another method of intermittent inhalation is via an intermittent positive pressure ventilator. Its use is controversial and some authorities consider it to be a contraindication in the treatment of most infants and children with cystic fibrosis, due to the possiblity of rupture of the over-distended alveoli in those patients with emphysematous changes. It may be used where there is segmental collapse, in which case the flow rate should be low initially, and only gradually increased. It has been found to increase residual volume after prolonged treatment. For this reason some authors suggest short periods of treatment, with a maximum of 14 days (Matthews *et al* 1964).

Postural drainage

This is an essential method of removing secretions from the lungs and must be accurately and thoroughly done. It should commence as a daily routine *as soon as* the infant is diagnosed as having cystic fibrosis. This is the *only* way of preventing a build-up of

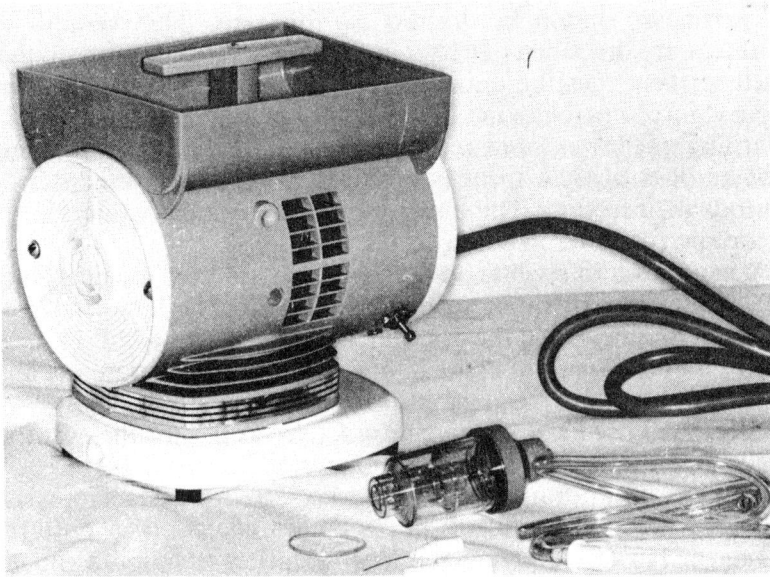

Fig. 151 The Maxi-Myst compressor with nebuliser.
(By permission of Mead Johnson, Crow's Nest, Sydney.)

secretions which will start the patient on the road to gradually deteriorating respiratory function. Tecklin and Holsclaw (1975), in a study on the effects of bronchial drainage on a group of 26 cystic fibrosis patients, found significant increases in peak expiratory flow rate, forced vital capacity, expiratory reserve volume and inspiratory capacity. If the lungs can be kept clear the child will thrive. It is necessary to concentrate on a particular focal area, but all segments may need to be drained at each session. This is time-consuming but essential if the child is to be kept healthy. It is not enough that the physiotherapist herself should be efficient. She must also be able to teach the child's parents the techniques of postural drainage, percussion and breathing and the use of the necessary equipment so they will be efficient at home treatment. It is this aspect of treatment which often becomes the hardest task for the physiotherapist. For the parents to be effective they must understand the child's problems, and some details of respiratory anatomy and physiology should be explained to them. Postural drainage is given twice daily at home with regular visits to the physiotherapist for supervision. Infants in particular should be drained *before* feeds. The methods of drainage are described in Chapter 4. Again it must be stressed that each segment must be drained every day and that the child must have vigorous percussion. The upper lobes may be drained in the morning, the lower lobes and the right middle lobe in the evening. The amount of time spent in drainage must be increased during periods of infection. The upper lobes are the most vulnerable in an infant, the lower in a small child.

When the child reaches adolescence, his need for independence will require the therapist to discuss with him the importance of postural drainage, and the best way this can be organized. He may prefer a good friend to assist him with his daily programme, and he may prefer more frequent visits to the therapist.

Effective nose blowing must be practised as part of the postural drainage routine. Vigorous active exercise is given before and during postural drainage to help loosen secretions. Haemoptysis, provided it is only small, is not a contraindication to postural drainage. However, percussion and vibration techniques should be avoided until the risk of haemoptysis has passed, when it must be vigorously restarted in order to remove old blood which would otherwise cause obstruction.

Breathing exercises

These are given during postural drainage with emphasis on full expansion and expiration, and concentrated in specific areas in order to facilitate drainage of secretions. The child is also given breathing exercises in half lying, sitting or standing after active exercise, with the emphasis on diaphragmatic breathing. Serial chest measurements may be a means of motivating a child who is reluctant to do breathing exercises at home.

General activities

Parents usually need to be given advice about their child's need for exercise and physical activity. Running about and playing active games are useful ways of loosening secretions and stimulating a productive cough. The child who is active will eliminate a certain amount of his secretions himself. Swimming improves breathing control and in the growing child it stimulates skeletal development and co-ordinated muscular action. Infants too small to be active can have their relationship to gravity changed by frequent alteration of bed position.

Methods of treating pancreatic insufficiency and disorder of the digestive tract

The child requires a nutritious diet, with sufficient protein and adequate calories. The physician may refer the parents to a dietician for advice. A substitute for the pancreatic enzymes is taken daily. Good nutrition is also maintained by control of the pulmonary problems. A child with excessive mucous secretions which are allowed to build up will have, understandably, a poor appetite and little interest in food.

Methods of treating the sweat gland defect

The parents must supervise the child's daily salt intake, especially during the hot weather. If insufficient salt is taken with the food, salt tablets should be given.

Psychosocial care

A disease of this nature causes considerable emotional and social problems for parents and child. For the parents there will be anxiety about the genetic nature of the defect, with the risk of subsequent diseased children. There is a large expense involved due to periodic hospital admissions and the cost of equipment for home use. The mother has to bear the burden of the child's home treatment, which is time-consuming and sometimes difficult if the child is rebellious (*see* page 435). The child himself has to endure the visits to the doctor and physiotherapist, the occasional periods of time spent in hospital, interference with school and social life, as well as the terrors and discomforts of respiratory insufficiency. The emotional support for these children and their parents will be similar to that needed whenever a child suffers a chronic disability with a usually fatal outcome.

SUMMARY

Some common respiratory disorders seen in children are described in this Chapter. In the case of cystic fibrosis and asthma, where the physiotherapist may be called upon to take a relatively complex role in the management of the child, details of treatment are given. For specific techniques of physical therapy, the reader is referred to Chapter 4.

References

Fitch, K. D. and Morton, A. R. (1971) Specificity of exercise-induced asthma *Br. Med. J.* **4**, 577.

Gandevia, B. (1959) Pulmonary function and physiotherapy. *Aust. J. Physiother.*, **5**, 87.

Hinshaw, H. C. and Garland, L. H. (1965) *Diseases of the Chest.* Philadelphia: Saunders.

Illingworth, R. S. (1971) *Common Symptoms of Disease in Children.* Oxford and Edinburgh: Blackwell.

Kendig, E. L. (1967) *Disorders of the Respiratory Tract in Children.* Philadelphia: Saunders.

Matthews, L. W., Doershuk, C. F., Wise, M., Eddy, G., Nudelman, H. and Spector, S. (1964) A therapeutic regime for patients with cystic fibrosis. *Pediat.* **65**, 558.

Tecklin, J. S. and Holsclaw, D. S. (1975) Evaluation of bronchial drainage in patients with cystic fibrosis. *Phys. Ther.* **55**, 10, 1081.

Webber, B. A., Shenfield, G. M. and Paterson, J. W. (1974) A comparison of three different techniques for giving nebulised albuterol to asthmatic patients. *Am. Rev. Resp. Dis.* **109**, 293.

Further Reading

Bolton, J. H., Gandevia, B. and Ross, M. (1954) The effects of electrophrenic respiration on asthmatic subjects. *Royal Melbourne Hospital Clinical Research*, **24**, 71.

Bolton, J. H., Gandevia, B. and Ross, M. (1956) The rationale of breathing exercises in asthma, with results of a controlled clinical trial. *Med. J. Aust.* **2**, 675.

Brown, J. (1973) Asthma in childhood. *Med. J. Aust.* **1**, 654.

Campbell, E. J. M. (1958) *Respiratory Muscles and the Mechanics of Breathing.* London: Lloyd-Luke.

Dept. of Child Health (1970) *A Student's Guide to Cystic Fibrosis of the Pancreas.* Sydney: University of Sydney.

Jones, R. S. (1976) *Asthma in Children.* London: Arnold.

Livingstone, J. L. and Gillespie, M. (1935) The value of breathing exercises for asthma. *Lancet*, **2**, 705.

Lorin, M. I., Denning, C. R. (1971) Evaluation of postural drainage by measurement of sputum volume and consistency. *Am. J. Phys. Med.* **50**, 215.

Mascia, A. V. (1974) Rehabilitation of the child with chronic asthma. In *The Child with Disabling Illness,* edited by J. A. Downey and N. L. Low. Philadelphia: Saunders.

Matthews, L. W. and Doershuk, C. F. (1968) *Cystic Fibrosis: Comprehensive therapy. Post-Grad. Med. U.S.A.* **40**, 550.

Matthews, L. and Doershuk, C. (1968) *Cystic Fibrosis: Comprehensive therapy. Post-Grad. Med. U.S.A.* **40**, 550.

Morony, T. (1969) Cystic fibrosis. *Aust. J. Physiother.*, **15**, 4.

Motoyama, E. K., Gibson, L. E. and Zigas, C. J. (1972) Evaluation of mist tent therapy in cystic fibrosis using maximum expiratory flow volume curve. *Pediat.* **50**, 299.

Reid, L. and de Haller, R. (1964) *Lung Changes in Cystic Fibrosis.* London: Chest and Heart Association.

Roberts, K. D. and Edwards, J. M. (1971) *Paediatric Intensive Care.* Oxford: Blackwell.

Ross, M., Gandevia, B. and Bolton, J. H. (1958) The rationale, methods and results of physiotherapy for asthma. *Aust. J. Physiother.*, **4**, 11.

Chapter 4

Specific Techniques of Physical Assessment and Treatment in Infants and Children

METHODS OF ASSESSMENT

Each child is assessed and his history taken by the physiotherapist on the first visit, and he is reassessed during treatment on subsequent visits. Taking a history from the parent enables the physiotherapist to know the answers to such questions as these. Has he a productive cough, and if so are secretions copious, infected or tenacious? Is the cough present constantly, is it worse in the morning or does it recur at intervals? Does he suffer from recurrent respiratory tract infections or rhinitis? Does he develop a cough immediately following an upper respiratory tract infection? Does he have dyspnoea, and if so, when? Is he as active as other children his age? Does he have attacks of wheezing or difficulty with breathing? Do these occur as a result of exertion, emotional strain, or do other factors appear to precipitate these attacks? Do they occur at night or at school? What are the effects of these difficulties on their home life?

The physiotherapist must know what drugs have been prescribed and what advice has already been given to the family by the physician. She will look at the radiographs and the radiologist's reports to see any focal areas of collapse or consolidation, or any other relevant abnormality (figures 152, 153, 154, 155).

The assessment includes an examination of the shape of the child's chest, noting the presence of flared lower ribs, whether the chest is barrel-shaped or asymmetrical, or whether the upper part of the sternum is prominent. She notes his breathing, looking particularly for upper chest breathing, and noting whether the subcostal margins move closer together on inspiration. If the subcostal margins do move closer together this is an indication that the diaphragm is already relatively flattened and on inspiration is moving paradoxically. She notes whether he is a mouth-breather, and if he is, whether he can breathe through his nose when asked. She notes his respiratory rate once she has gained his confidence. She observes whether he is tense or anxious. When he coughs, she notes whether this causes any respiratory embarrassment, whether the cough is paroxysmal, or productive. She needs accurate and if possible first-hand information about the nature and quantity of sputum.

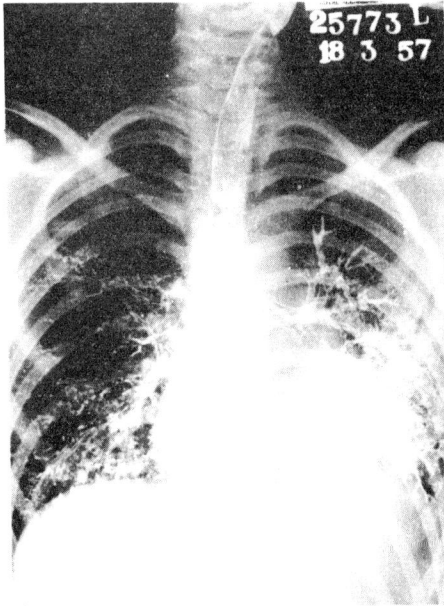

Fig. 152 Radiograph of the lungs of a child with bronchiectasis. Note the crowding of the bronchi in the right lower lobe adjacent to the heart, and the cylindrical dilation of the more distal bronchi, which should normally be narrowing as they reach the pleura. (By permission of the Royal Alexandra Hospital for Children, Sydney.)

451

A hand placed on the chest wall will pick up vibrations due to bronchospasm or accumulated secretions, and will help the physiotherapist to localize areas requiring postural drainage. She will find a stethoscope a useful aid in localizing areas with retained secretions, but she will need a great deal of practice in listening to normal breath sounds before the use of a stethoscope will be of any value (Baskett 1971).

A frightened nervous child may be better assessed on his mother's knee rather than sitting by himself on the treatment bed. It is important that the chest be uncovered eventually for assessment and it is usually less frightening for the child if his mother undresses him.

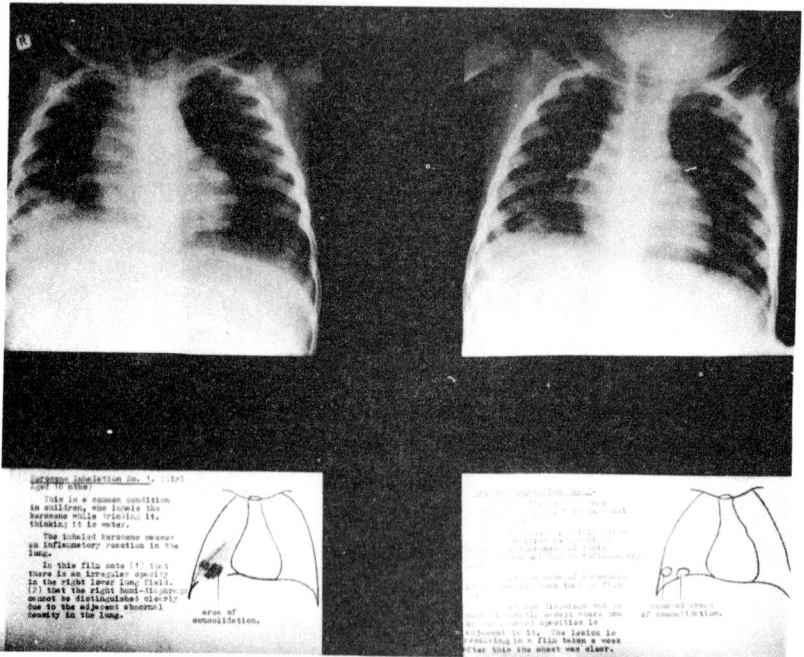

Fig. 153 Radiograph demonstrating the effects of kerosene inhalation in an 18 month old child. (By permission of the Royal Alexandra Hospital for Children, Sydney.)

Measurement of Thoracic Expansion

Measuring thoracic expansion is a method of assessing the range of movement in the thorax. It is important as a means of assessing

452

progress in children with chronic respiratory diseases such as bronchiectasis and cystic fibrosis. It may provide incentive for an older child, but is probably not necessary as a record in a number of children seen by the physiotherapist. In many children, for example those with asthma, it is the way in which they breathe that needs to be assessed and the physiotherapist should record her observations in detail.

These measurements are taken with the patient in the same position each time, half lying, sitting or standing, at the fourth rib

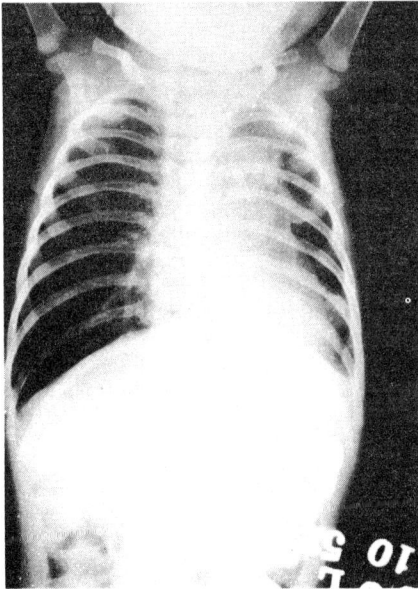

Fig. 154 This radiograph demonstrates collapse of the left lower lobe with emphysema of the remainder of the lungs. Note that the heart and mediastinum have shifted towards the collapse, and the left diaphragm is elevated towards the collapse.
(By permission of the Royal Alexandra Hospital for Children, Sydney.)

453

(at the level of the axillae), at the ninth rib (3 fingers' breadth below the tip of the xiphoid process), and sub-costally. The measurements are taken for a full inspiration and expiration, with the average taken of three attempts.

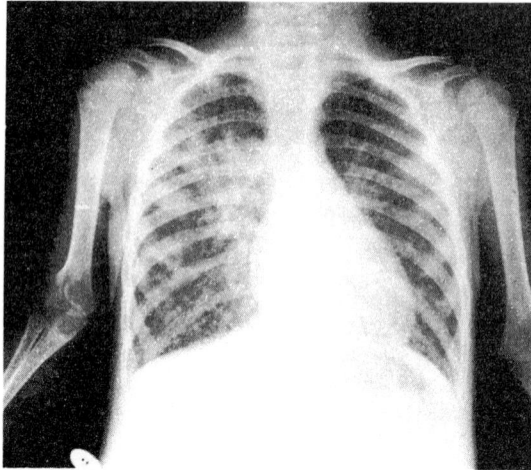

Fig. 155 Radiograph demonstrating bronchopneumonia in the lungs of a child with cystic fibrosis. There are patchy increased densities scattered throughout both lungs.
(By permission of the Royal Alexandra Hospital for Children, Sydney.)

Sputum Collection

The physiotherapist records the amount of sputum at each visit, and the type, whether frothy, tenacious or purulent. The type of cough is also recorded, whether dry and hacking, or paroxysmal, and whether or not it is effective.

If it is necessary to collect a sputum specimen for pathological investigation, the child is asked to cough and spit some sputum into a sterilized glass jar, with his name and the date printed on it. If the child is too young to co-operate, a specimen of sputum can be collected from the back of the throat on the cotton wool tip of a swab stick. A small catheter is inserted to stimulate the cough reflex, the child's cheeks are pressed inwards to prevent him from swallowing and the sputum is removed with a swab stick which is put into a sterilized test tube. Care must be taken not to contaminate the specimen or the collecting device and sterile gloves should be used. A more effective method involves the use of a small plastic container attached to a suction apparatus (figure 156). The container should be labelled with the baby's name, date, time of collection and type of specimen, for example, endotracheal tube or oro-pharyngeal aspirate. It should be sent to the bacteriology department as soon as possible. The sputum can be collected effectively even from an infant in this manner. These are uncomfortable and frightening manoeuvres for an infant or small child, and should be accurately done on the first attempt if possible.

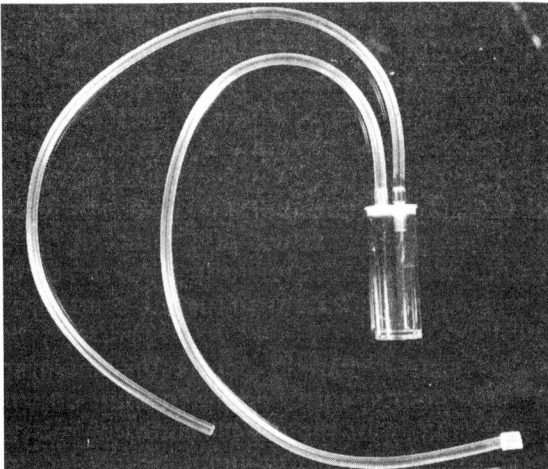

Fig. 156 Mucus extractor.
(By permission of Pharma-Plast (Aust.) Pty. Ltd.)

Assessment of Exercise Tolerance

The child's mother will give an indication of his exercise tolerance if she is asked whether or not he can keep up with other children his age in play activities and in sport. In the case of an asthmatic child a distinction should be made between his exercise tolerance when he is free of bronchospasm as well as when he has bronchospasm. Skipping or jumping on a trampoline is an effective way of assessing exercise tolerance in children with bronchiectasis, cystic fibrosis or asthma. Following two minutes of such activity, the child's respiratory rate, pulse rate, use of accessory muscles of respiration, and any increase in cough or wheeze, are noted. In children who suffer from bronchospasm more specific exercise testing may be necessary as a diagnostic tool. Godfrey (1974) describes the details of this procedure.

Measurement of One Second Forced (or Fast) Expiratory Volume (FEV$_1$)

This test measures the percentage of expiratory vital capacity which can be moved by maximum effort in one second. Children can usually expire more than 90 per cent of the total (Kendig 1968). It is commonly used in children with asthma to estimate the degree of airways resistance, in which case the FEV$_1$ in these children is tested before and after the administration of a bronchodilator. One machine in use is the bellow-type spirometer, the Vitalograph (figure 157), and the use of this machine is described below.

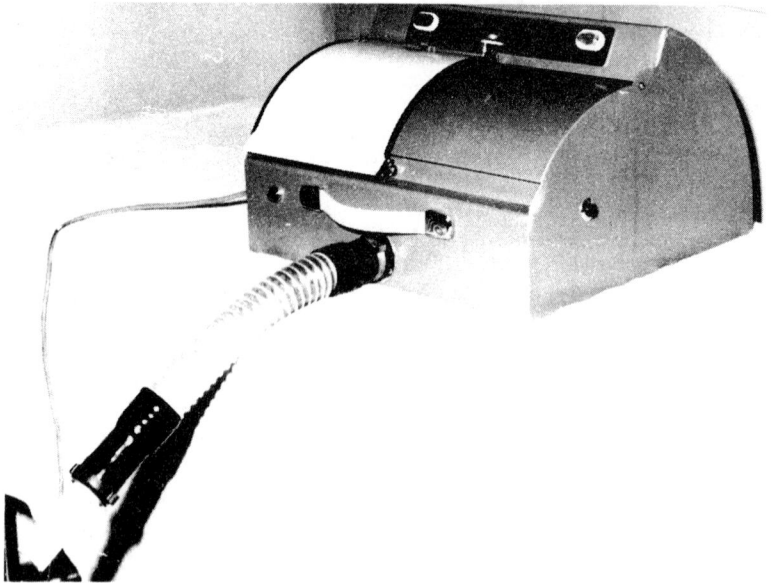

Fig. 157 Vitalograph machine. The starting position of the graph paper is to the right of its present position.
(By permission of Vitalograph Ltd., Buckingham, England.)

456

Method

The child is instructed to take a deep breath, to hold it for a brief period, then to exhale fully through a mouthpiece of disposable cardboard attached to the tubing of the machine. As he exhales, a line is traced on graph paper indicating the volume of air exhaled (figure 158). If the child's FEV_1 is also required after broncho-dilator therapy, the solution is given via a hand-held aerosol spray, and the child is tested again.

The degree of accuracy of this type of test depends upon the child's ability to concentrate and co-operate, and the skill of the therapist in persuading him to perform the test to the best of his ability. It may provide incentive if the child is shown how it is his breath which moves the tracing pen. A small child may try his best if he is told that there is a large balloon inside the machine which he must blow up. Polgar and Promadhat (1971) suggest that the child may be asked to blow out the candles on an imaginary birthday cake, trying to blow out as many of the candles as possible in one breath.

The results of the test are recorded on a card (figure 159). The predicted vital capacity (PVC) for a child his age is taken from a chart and his vital capacity (FVC) is noted from the graph. The percentage of his predicted vital capacity is then calculated $\dfrac{VC}{PVC}$

His FEV_1 is noted from the graph and is measured against his vital capacity $\left(\dfrac{FEV_1}{FVC}\right)$.

In the example given (figures 158 and 159) the child demonstrates a change in his FVC or his FEV_1 following the administration of the bronchodilator.

Measurement of Peak Expiratory Flow Rate (PEFR)

The Wright Peak Flow Meter or Gauge can be used to measure maximum flow over 10 milliseconds at the beginning of expiration. This is a simple portable device which can be used to give information about the reversibility of airways obstruction following administration of a bronchodilator. It does not measure accurately small changes in airways, hence, when this information is required, spirometry is the preferred test. Children as young as 3 years can be taught to use this apparatus.

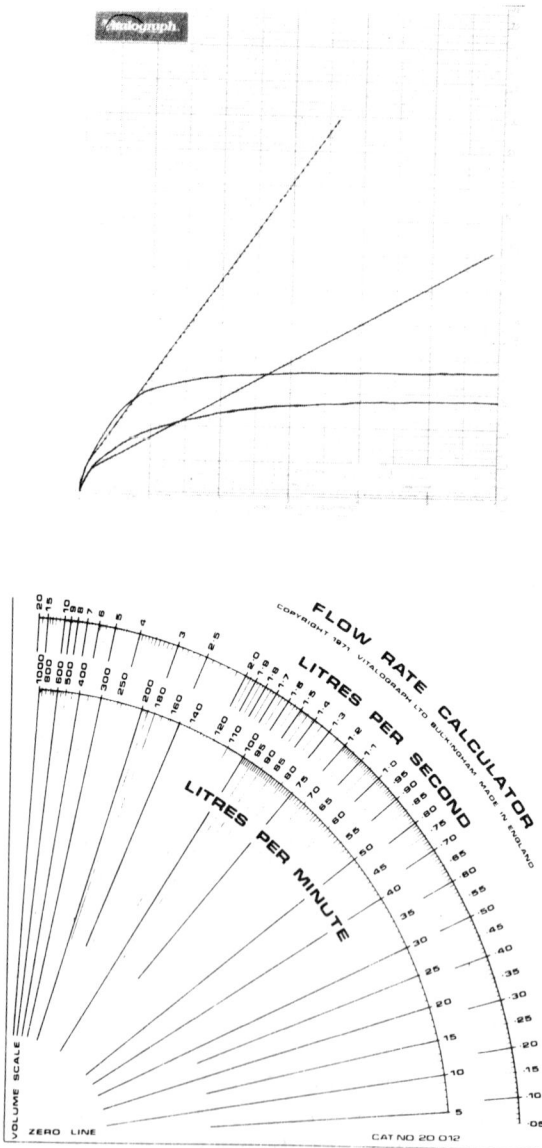

Fig. 158 (a and b) The lower line drawn on the graph paper was made before, the upper line after, the administration of a bronchodilator.
(By permission of Vitalograph Ltd., Buckingham, England.)

H.M.O. _____   NAME

WARD _____ Ht. 130 cm   IDENT. NO.

DATE $7.12.78$ Wt._____   BIRTH DATE $2.7.70$ SEX. M

Provisional diagnosis:

		Pre-Bronchodilator (B.D.)			Post-Bronchodilator (B.D.)	
		Observed A.T.P.S.	Predicted B.T.P.S.	% Predicted	Observed A.T.P.S.	% Predicted
RESULT OF SPIROMETRY	FEV$_1$	950	1750	54 %	1500	86 %
	V C	1400	1875	75 %	1800	96 %
	FEV$_1$: VC ratio	68 %			83 %	
	MMEFR	34	132	26 %	86	65 %
	PEFR	--	-	-	-	-

Explanation of Terms:

V C	= Vital capacity = Litres
FEV$_1$	= Forced expiratory volume in 1 second = Litres per second
MMEFR	= Maximum mid-expiratory flow rate = Litres per second
PEFR	= Peak expiratory flow rate = Litres per minute

Intepretation:

Fig. 159 The result of the ventilatory test as determined from the graph in figure 158.
(By permission of Royal Alexandra Hospital for Children, Sydney.)

POSTURAL DRAINAGE

This is a means of removing excessive secretions from the air passages, and employs the use of gravity to facilitate drainage. Positions are employed which promote the most effective drainage of specific segments of the lungs. These positions are shown in figures 160 to 168. However, although each segment should be drained in the prescribed manner, there are times when the postural drainage position should be adjusted slightly in order to drain the secretions effectively. Thacker (1971) comments that the direction of the airways may be altered by disease.

Drainage may be done on a bed with the necessary elevation gained by lying the child on pillows or by tilting the bed, or over a chair (figure 169). The procedure must be taught to the child's parents as any child attending the physiotherapist for drainage will need to carry out this drainage several times a day at home. It

459

is not a good idea to suggest the child hang over the end of his bed. Drainage positions must be as accurate as possible for the particular segments to be drained, and the child should be comfortable in the position as he will need to co-operate with breathing exercises and coughing. Hanging over the end of the bed is neither accurate nor comfortable. An infant may be drained by tilting his cot or incubator. Alternatively, drainage for an infant may be done preferably on the physiotherapist's lap, or as shown for the older child (figures 160–168). The latter may not be satisfactory as the supporting surface is not firm enough.

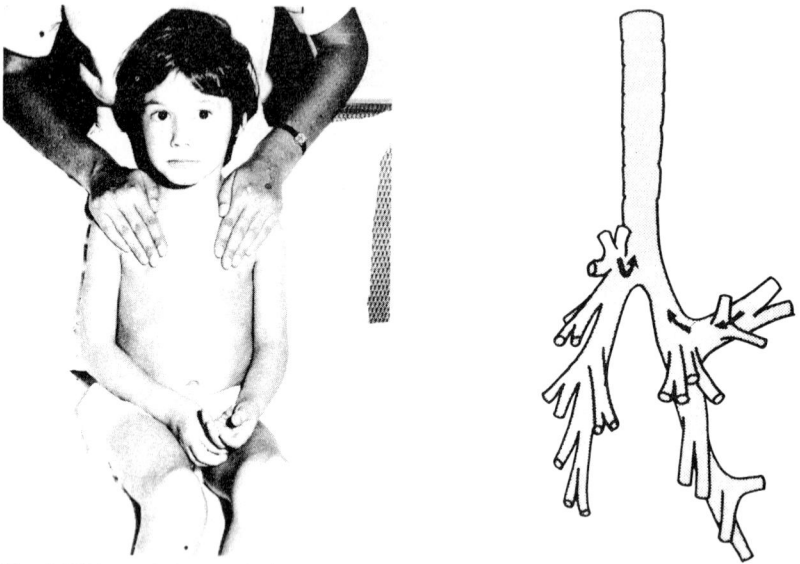

Fig. 160 Upper lobes: apical segments.
Child may lean forwards or backwards to drain the more anterior and posterior areas.

Vigorous activity such as skipping or jumping on a trampoline should precede and interrupt the postural drainage in order to loosen the secretions. This activity may need to be modified or eliminated if the patient's condition contraindicates such exercise.

Each segment in which there is a focus of infection, a collapse or a build-up of secretions must be drained separately until clear. This applies particularly in conditions such as cystic fibrosis, bronchiectasis and pneumonia. Children with bronchitis and asthma, in which there may be no particular focus, can be drained as for the posterior segments of the lower lobes (figure 168). Secretions tend to accumulate towards the bases of the lungs in children who spend their day in an upright position. Infants and bed-ridden children with respiratory disorders tend to accumulate secretions in the upper lobes (particularly the posterior and lateral segments) because of the dependent position of these lobes in the horizontal position, and attention must be paid to clearing these areas. Castilla *et al* (1971) found that a contrast medium instilled

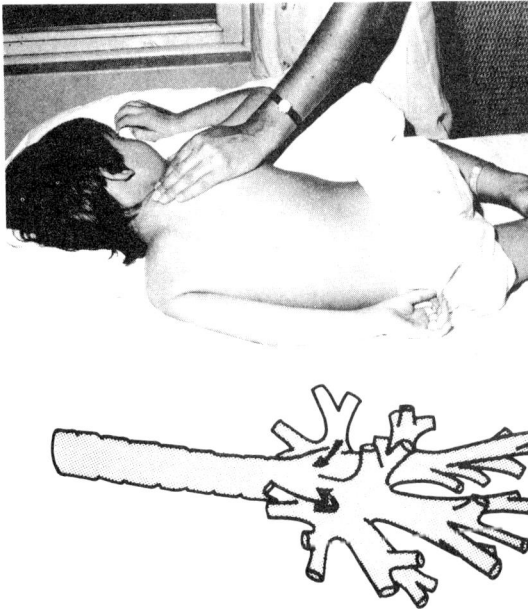

Fig 161 Right upper lobe: posterior segment.
¼ turn from prone. A pillow prevents the child from rolling into prone. To drain the posterior segment of the *left* upper lobe, the child is placed in a similar position but with 2 pillows elevating the head and shoulders on the left side.

into the trachea of an infant lying supine passed first into the right upper lobe. They also found that the angle between the right main bronchus and the right upper lobe bronchus is different in neonates compared to adults. Attention should therefore be paid in particular to the right upper lobe in infants lying supine, and where possible this position should be avoided where the infant is at risk of aspiration.

Children with bronchospasm frequently cannot tolerate a position with head down. The position can be modified as in figure 146. It is of little use to attempt drainage of secretions from the lungs of a patient with unrelieved bronchospasm, as the airways are not patent enough to allow the free passage of mucus. These techniques are used more successfully following the administration by aerosol spray or by intermittent positive pressure respirator, of a bronchodilator.

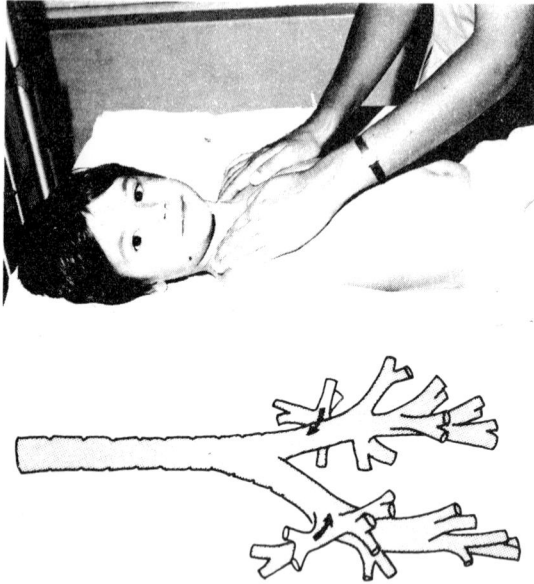

Fig. 162 Upper lobes: anterior segments.
Supine, pillow under knees.

Drainage will not be effective if the child is merely placed in the appropriate position and left alone. He must be percussed and vibrated over his thorax, and be given localized breathing exercises by the physiotherapist or by his mother while he is in the drainage position. It is better for this to be done for a short period of time thoroughly than for him to be left alone for a longer period. He must be reminded to cough while draining, and to blow his nose when necessary.

The physiotherapist will decide with each particular patient the best time of day for drainage to be done, but on waking in the morning and before dinner at night will be the most usual times.

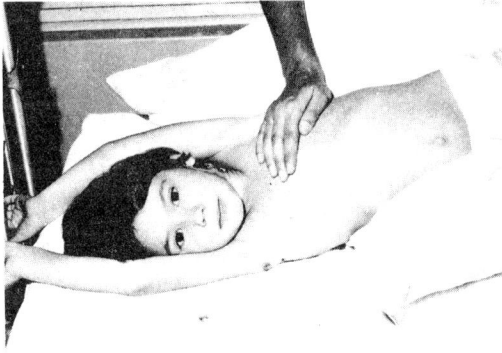

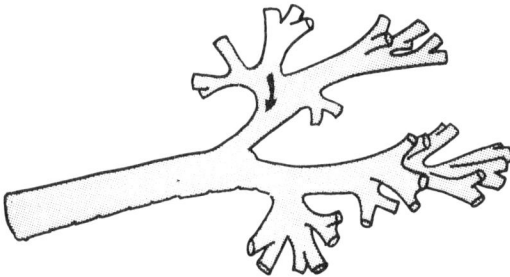

Fig. 163 Left upper lobe: lingular segment.
¼ turn from supine with left side uppermost, 2 pillows under the lower trunk and another pillow to prevent the child from rolling into supine. The thorax should be at an angle of 30° from the horizontal. Alternatively, the bed may be elevated 12″.

This will be decided by the times at which the child is most productive, but the routine of the family should be taken into consideration. The child's chest should be drained until it seems clear.

Percussion and vibration techniques

These techniques, although applied externally to the bony thorax, help loosen secretions within the air passages, and if the child is tilted at the correct angle and coughs effectively the secretions will be removed. *Percussion* is done quickly for maximum vibratory effect on the thorax. *Vibrations* are done, either unilaterally or bilaterally, towards the end of expiration and, according to Thacker (1971), are probably more effective than percussion.

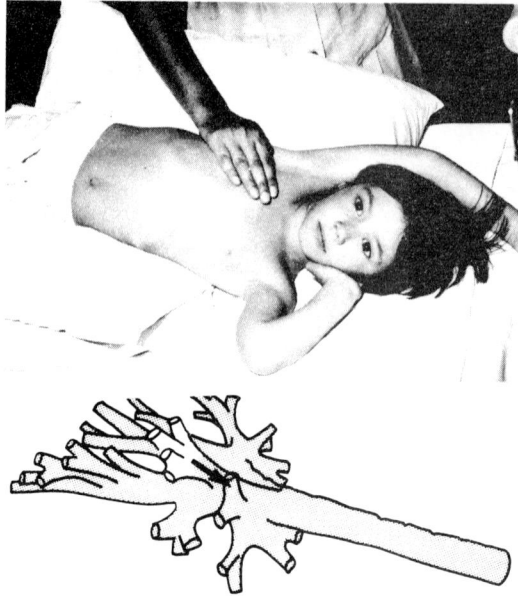

Fig. 164 Middle lobe.
¼ turn from supine with right side uppermost, 2 pillows under the lower trunk and another pillow to prevent the child from rolling into supine. The thorax should be at an angle of 30° from the horizontal. Alternatively, the bed may be elevated 12″.

After each bout of percussion or vibrations the child must be asked to cough. These techniques are interspersed with localized breathing exercises. A small child may have to be taught how to cough. If he places his hand in front of his mouth the sensation of expelled air on his hand may help him to learn the technique. Emphasis must be on a deep inspiration followed by a series of explosive expirations. A child of two to three years can usually be taught to expectorate. Pharyngeal 'tickling' with a small bore catheter will stimulate coughing in infants and young children, as the cough reflex is a protective one. Crying is sometimes an advantage provided it is not prolonged, as it ensures the infant takes deep breaths. In the author's opinion the therapist should work hard at treating the infant and young child without provoking crying, and she should discuss her strategy with the parents.

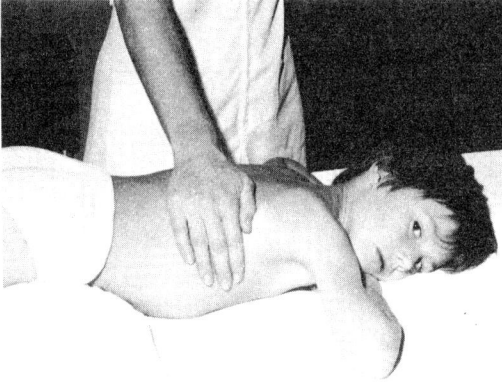

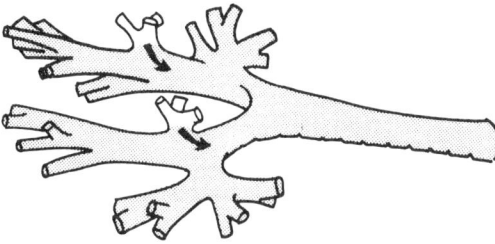

Fig. 165 Lower lobes: apical segments.
Prone, pillow under the abdomen.

Talking to the infant with her face close enough for him to see her, reassuring him that he is alright, combined with percussion which starts off very gently, will enable the infant to accept more vigorous percussion. It is not fair to send the parents home with an upset infant who they know will continue to be upset. Parents should also be shown ways of comforting the infant and helping him to comfort himself, by talking to him, putting a hand on his chest, holding his hands gently to help him quieten himself.

Rib springing may also provoke a cough from an infant (see below). Care should be taken by the physiotherapist to avoid being directly in front of the child when he coughs, as this may result in inhalation of infected material by the physiotherapist herself.

465

Percussion and vibrations are also given to small infants but with care not to use too much force or pressure. In the treatment of a small premature baby one finger on top of another will give sufficient vibration. However, treatment must still be vigorously done. It is extremely important to remove secretions quickly from

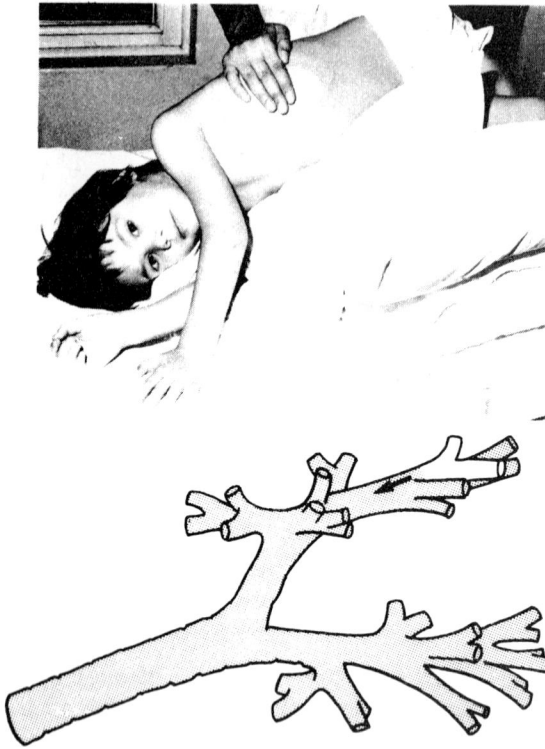

Fig. 166 Left lower lobe: lateral segment.
Side lying, thorax at an angle of 45° from the horizontal. Alternatively the bed may be elevated 18–20″.

an infant's lungs, as obstruction of the tiny airways occurs rapidly with subsequent deterioration in the infant's condition. The physiotherapist must take care not to be ineffectual in these treatments. Vibrations and percussion are contraindicated in infants and children with tuberculosis or a tendency to haemorrhage.

Breathing exercises and coughing

Breathing exercises may be done bilaterally or unilaterally, and are localized to a particular area or concentrated on diaphragmatic movement. A child with excessive secretions in the right lower lobe is encouraged by the pressure of the physiotherapist's hands to localize his breathing to the lower part

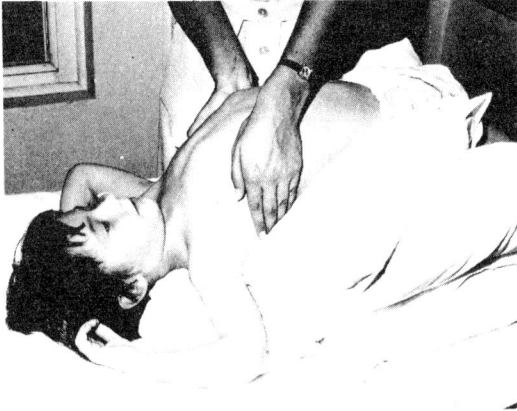

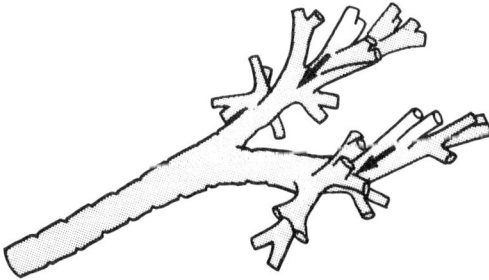

Fig. 167 Lower lobes: anterior segments.
Supine, thorax at an angle of 45° from the horizontal. This child should have another pillow to support the pelvis and take the strain from the abdominal muscles. Alternatively the bed may be elevated 18–20″.

of the right side of his thorax. He does as full as expiration as possible without effort, as this will facilitate further drainage. A few breaths are followed by a cough and by a short rest. A deeper inspiration may be encouraged in an infant or unconscious child

467

by manual pressure on the thorax called rib springing. In the infant whose ribs have not yet developed the normal bucket-handle action, rib springing must be done more horizontally.

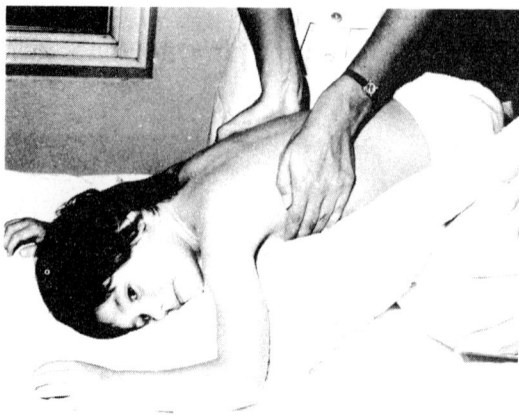

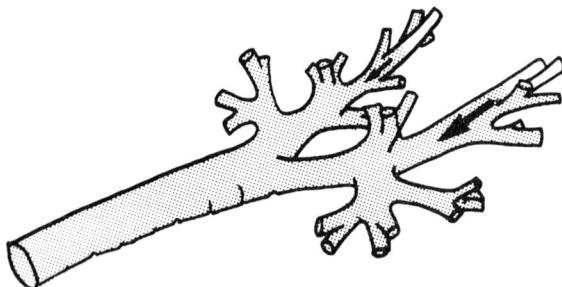

Fig. 168 Lower lobes: posterior segments.
Prone, thorax at an angle of 45° from the horizontal. This child should have an extra pillow under his pelvis. Alternatively the bed may be elevated 18–20″.

Clearing the upper respiratory tract

If the child is to breathe in through his nose, his nose must be clear. When necessary he must be taught to blow his nose correctly one nostril at a time. Most children need to be reminded of this.

Teaching parents

It is not sufficient for the physiotherapist to demonstrate the above techniques to the child's parents. At the first visit, they are shown the methods required and the mechanism of drainage and the reasons for the techniques are explained. The parent practises the techniques in front of the physiotherapist. Most parents feel clumsy on attempting vibrations, percussion and breathing exercises for the first time, and the physiotherapist must be encouraging. Percussion can be practised on a pillow if necessary.

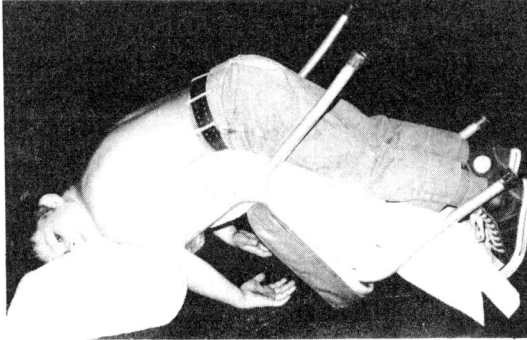

Fig. 169 Alternative method of draining the posterior segments of the lower lobes which may be more conveniently used at home.

At each subsequent visit the parent does some of the treatment with the physiotherapist, who can then judge how successful her teaching has been. A printed sheet with pictures of the various drainage positions, and some details of the other techniques should be available for parents.

In summary, postural drainage involves tilting of the thorax to facilitate drainage from a particular segment of a lung, plus breathing exercises, effective coughing, percussion and vibration techniques to loosen the secretions. *It must be noted that merely tilting the thorax does not imply drainage will take place.*

BREATHING EXERCISES

Breathing exercises may be given with any one of several objectives. They may be given in order to maintain or restore more normal breathing, to aid in the expulsion of excessive secretions from the lower airway, and to maintain or regain thoracic mobility. They are usually done voluntarily by the patient with the physiotherapist or the child's mother guiding the thoracic movement, or in the case of the infant or unconscious child techniques are used which facilitate better expansion. For whatever reason breathing exercises are being given, the method is similar, involving expansion of the lungs in as normal a pattern as possible.

Traditionally the physiotherapist has guided rib movement in order to expand particular areas of the thorax either unilaterally or bilaterally by upper costal, lateral basal or posterior basal as well as diaphragmatic breathing. Whether the effect on the lungs, that is the actual expansion of the lungs, alters with pressure on different parts of the thorax has not been proved. However, where maintenance of mobility of the thorax itself is required breathing exercises to the above areas will certainly have a mobilizing effect. If an attempt is being made to restore more normal breathing in, for example, a child who has excessive movement of the upper thorax, or who pulls his abdomen in on inspiration, emphasis must be on relaxation, a quiet inspiration with shoulders relaxed, followed by a relaxation of the respiratory muscles which will result in expiration.

When breathing exercises are being used as an adjunct to drainage of secretions, emphasis is on as full an expiration as possible, as this has an expulsive effect on the mucus to be removed. Breathing exercises may need to be avoided or modified in the presence of certain conditions. Where there is a lung abscess postural drainage may be performed but breathing exercises should be avoided. A child with emphysema can be given breathing exercises by blowing bubbles, the expiration against some resistance maintaining airways patency more effectively in emphysematous lungs than the normal relaxed breathing exercises.

If the patient is an infant or young child, or is unconscious and unable to co-operate, voluntary breathing exercises cannot be given. However, movement of air through the lungs can be encouraged by firm manual pressure on the chest during the expiratory phase. In the case of a small infant, it is necessary to give stability to the thorax with one hand in order to give pressure over a particular area of the lung. This is also done in the appropriate postural drainage position if it is also required to aid expulsion of excess mucus from the airways.

Breathing exercises will be done as part of home treatment where appropriate, the child's mother being taught the necessary techniques. Some authorities advocate the use of a belt to enable an older child to do his breathing exercises unaided.

INTENSIVE CARE

Infants and children will be placed in an intensive care unit if they are unconscious, or in respiratory distress, if in the case of neonates they are of low birth weight, and following thoracic or cranial surgery. Intensive care implies a situation in which special and continuous care is given the child by physician, nurse and therapist. Temperature, pulse and respiratory rate are recorded more frequently than usual and technical tests to determine the oxygen and carbondioxide concentrations of the blood will be carried out as often as necessary.

The seriously ill infant or child is nursed in the horizontal position if he is comatose or receiving positive pressure ventilation. If there is respiratory failure and the child is breathing without mechanical assistance, or if he has a tracheo-oesophageal fistula or gastro-oesophageal reflux, he is nursed with his head and shoulders elevated. If he is nursed horizontally, he is turned from side to side approximately every two hours (Jones & Owen-Thomas 1971). The infant may be nursed in an incubator or a tent. Both the infant and child may be tracheostomized and ventilated via a positive pressure ventilator or ventilated by endotracheal intubation. However, he may not need such continuous respiratory assistance, requiring instead frequent visits from the physiotherapist to drain excess secretions from his lungs and to improve aeration by breathing exercises and in some cases by the administration of bronchodilator or mucolytic substances via an aerosol apparatus. The therapist must remember that there is an urgent need for her treatment to be effective, and it will not be effective if she does not appreciate the need for treatment to be vigorous and frequent.

An important factor to be remembered during treatment of infants with respiratory distress is the effect of cooling on oxygen consumption, which is said to be lowest when the abdominal skin temperature is 36 degrees C (Silverman, Sinclair and Agate 1966). The therapist must therefore take care not to allow the infant's skin to cool off during treatment. This applies particularly to the treatment of an infant in an incubator.

There is considerable stress for children undergoing cardiothoracic surgery and for those who are admitted into an intensive care unit. The problems of the child in hospital are discussed briefly in Section I, Chapter 1.

It is the author's opinion that infants and children requiring intensive care should be treated only by physiotherapists with experience in this field, and that until they become proficient they should only work under the guidance of someone who has experience.

CARE OF THE INFANT OR CHILD FOLLOWING CARDIAC SURGERY

Infants and children undergo cardiac surgery for such congenital defects as Fallot's Tetralogy, transposition of the great arteries, persistent patent ductus arteriosus, coarctation of the aorta or septal defects.

Pre-operatively the physiotherapist may need to institute treatment to clear the airways, as many infants and children requiring cardiac surgery have excessive secretions. Also important are the explanations and demonstrations to the child and his parents which will prepare them for the immediate post-operative period. The therapist must build up a good relationship with the child and parents at this stage.

Modified postural drainage, gentle percussion and vibrations and stimulation to cough are given when necessary. By clearing his chest in this way the therapist is aiming to decrease the risk of post-operative complications (Thoren 1954), thereby decreasing the time the child will need to be hospitalized.

Even at 16 to 18 months many children can be taught deep breathing by blowing balloons, paper toys and pinwheels. This will prepare the child for the breathing exercises he will do post-operatively.

Rockwell and Campbell (1976) stress the importance of pre-operative family education in anticipating and avoiding the detrimental effects of hospitalization and surgery on children who are unprepared. They describe a pre-operative visit to the intensive care unit, and aids such as tape recordings, glove puppets and colouring books.

472

Post-operatively the child when he goes to the intensive care unit may be intubated using IPPV or continuous positive airways pressure (CPAP).

On CPAP the infant breathes spontaneously against positive pressure. This appears to assist the airways to remain patent, and to increase the functional residual capacity or FRC (Gregory *et al* 1975). When moving the child, care must be taken to ensure the tubing remains in a dependent position behind the child's head. Otherwise condensation from the humidified air could drain into the respiratory tract.

An infant after hypothermia will be kept warm by an overhead radiant heat warmer. Pericardial drains carry blood to underwater seal drainage bottles. Frequent checks of blood gases and electrolytes are made to assess progress.

Should physiotherapy be necessary to clear his chest, the child is turned into side lying and given gentle percussion or vibrations. In infants, even a small amount of mucus can block off a large amount of lung.

Effective and regular suction may be necessary, and the physiotherapist must be very alert to changes in the infant's condition.

Removal of secretions may be difficult and *manual hyperinflation* or 'bag squeezing' may be necessary. The tracheostomy or endotracheal tube is disconnected from the ventilator, one operator, who must be highly skilled in the technique, squeezes the bag slowly, then releases it quickly. The bag should be squeezed during inspiration or the air will inflate the stomach. The other operator compresses the chest with her hands just before the bag is released. The combination of high expiratory flow rate and chest compression assists movement of secretions towards the main airways where they can be coughed up.

The chest should be 'splinted' when the child coughs. Coughing may need to be stimulated by the therapist, by either a soft tube down through the nose and into the larynx or by gentle lateral pressure on the trachea (which is soft and pliant in infants and young children) to bring the walls into apposition.

Following extubation, physiotherapy may be given several times a day for a couple of days, with the aim of clearing the airway. Not all children require this treatment but the therapist should check the child's condition regularly as changes may occur rapidly.

Children who are not intubated are also turned into side lying and the chest is cleared as above.

Where there are no complications, children are usually allowed out of bed on the second or third day, and go home on the seventh to tenth day, with instructions to continue deep breathing exercises and active play. Some children need stimulation to move, others do not, and run around freely as soon as they are allowed up.

EMERGENCY CARE

Changes in the infant or child's condition may be sudden and the physiotherapist must be observant of the patient's respiratory rate and colour at all times during treatment. Deterioration may be rapid in the small child and collapse quickly occurs. Should a cardio-respiratory arrest occur, and this will be evidenced by the absence of pulse and respiration, the physiotherapist must remain calm, lying the child flat, and calling medical or nursing help by whatever means are used in the unit. There are certain procedures which the experienced physiotherapist will use, including suction of the airway if blockage by secretions appears the cause of respiratory arrest, and administering oxygen and commencing external cardiac massage if there is cardiac arrest, but it is not within the scope of this book to describe these procedures in detail.

CARE OF THE INFANT IN AN INCUBATOR

Infants are nursed in incubators (figure 170) if they are premature, or if they are neonates of low birth weight or with any acute respiratory illness. The advantages of an incubator are the maintenance of even temperature, the ease with which the infant can be observed, and by which an oxygen–air mix can be circulated. Humidity is provided and may be added to by the nebulisation of water. The disadvantages are the ease with which the incubator becomes contaminated, both by the infant himself and by the arms and sleeves of staff handling him through the portholes. An added problem with infants in incubators is their isolation from the outside world and the unrelenting nature of the bright environment to which they are exposed for 24 hours a day.

The physiotherapist must avoid undue handling of the infant, and take care not to contaminate the incubator when she puts her hands and arms through the portholes. Opening the incubator causes a loss of heat and oxygen and allows pathogenic organisms to enter. The infant is nursed uncovered so his respiratory rate and depth and his colour can be easily observed. Chilling must be avoided as it may lead to sclerema, and as described above, a lowering of the temperature will cause an increase in the need for oxygen. Similarly, over-heating will also lead to an increase in oxygen consumption. The amount of oxygen is carefully monitored by the physician, particularly in low birth weight premature babies, who may develop retrolental fibrodysplasia and blindness as a result of an excessive oxygen intake.

Postural drainage is given by elevating the mattress within the incubator. Percussion is given by the fingers rather than with the whole hand if the infant is very small. Gentle over-pressure is given on expiration to aid the elimination of secretions.

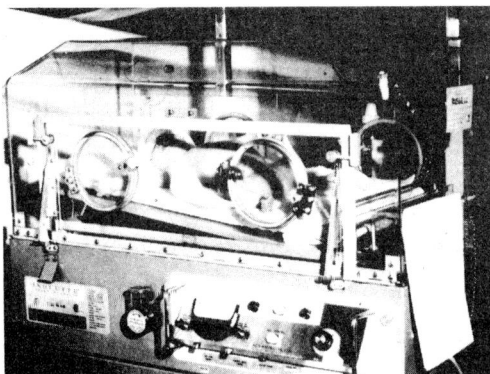

Fig. 170 Baby nursed in incubator. Note the portholes through which the baby may be handled.
(By permission of R. Samios.)

VENTILATION THERAPY

Artificial ventilation may be given by an intermittent positive pressure or an intermittent negative pressure apparatus. In the case of positive pressure ventilation, it may be given via a mouthpiece, a face mask, a tracheostomy tube or an oral or nasal

475

endotracheal tube. Positive pressure ventilation may be used to administer drug therapy direct to the airways or to administer humidified air/oxygen to a respiratory distressed child although the value of this type of ventilation in infants and young children is controversial and considered by some to be positively harmful. It is generally considered to be contraindicated in the treatment of children with cystic fibrosis, except in selected cases, due to the possibility of rupture of over-distended alveoli. However, this form of ventilation is commonly used to maintain ventilatory function in a child with paralysis of the respiratory muscles, following poliomyelitis, polyneuritis or curare paralysis in the treatment of tetanus, or a flail chest due to multiple rib fractures. Alternatively, the child with paralysis of the respiratory muscles may be ventilated by intermittent negative pressure in a tank respirator or by a cuirass-type ventilator.

It is beyond the scope of this book to describe in detail the management of an infant or small child requiring this type of therapy. Only the major points will be mentioned. Pressures produced in the thorax by artificial ventilation are different from those of normal respiration. Roberts and Edwards (1971) and Jones and Owen-Thomas (1971) describe the types of ventilators commonly in use, the mechanics of artificial ventilation, and the methods of endotracheal intubation and tracheostomy which may be required.

Some Specific Points in management

Application by face mask or mouthpiece

If a face mask is used it must be a good fit (there are several sizes available) and must be held firmly over the child's mouth and nose in order to prevent leakage of air around the sides of the mask (figures 171 and 172). If a mouthpiece is used, the child must be old enough to understand the need for firm lip closure again to prevent the leakage of air (figure 173). Humidification of air, normally performed by the upper respiratory tract, is provided by the fluid in the nebuliser, which will be either sterile water or a mucolytic or bronchodilator substance prescribed by the physician. The child may sit in a chair, or lie in a position which will facilitate postural drainage. The airways of small children are narrow, and where there is bronchospasm they are narrower still, so a low flow rate is used and pressure over 15 cms of water pressure is usually not prescribed. The upper limits of pressure which are safe to use in all circumstances are not known. The child, who preferably has already been taught breathing exercises, may be given these exercises while using the ventilator, but if he is inexperienced, he must be encouraged to take deep breaths with the machine.

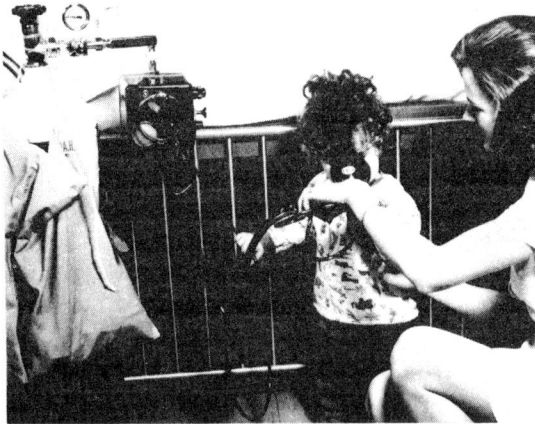

Fig. 171 Child being shown the use of the intermittent positive pressure respirator. (By permission of R. Samios.)

The tracheostomized or intubated child

Endotracheal intubation involves the insertion of a tube into the trachea via the nose or mouth (figure 174). It is usually inserted via the nose in infants and children to avoid the tubing being bitten. Tracheostomy, which involves the passage of a tube directly into the trachea, is the preferred method of providing an artificial airway if this airway will be required for any length of time, for example, longer than one week. It is performed under general anaesthesia, a tube is inserted into the trachea and held in place by tapes around the neck. The advantages of artificial ventilation by these means include the enabling of any upper airways obstruction to be bypassed, the reduction of anatomical dead space thereby reducing the amount of respiratory effort necessary, an increase in alveolar ventilation, the facilitation of aspiration of secretions and the passage of bronchodilators, oxygen and moisture. The dangers include lack of natural humidification, inability to cough effectively, inability to speak which is particularly frightening for a child, increased risk of infection, and asphyxia if the tube becomes blocked. Following tracheostomy inco-ordination of the larynx may occur (Roberts and Edwards 1971).

Importance of artificial humidification. This is required whenever the nose is continually bypassed during artificial

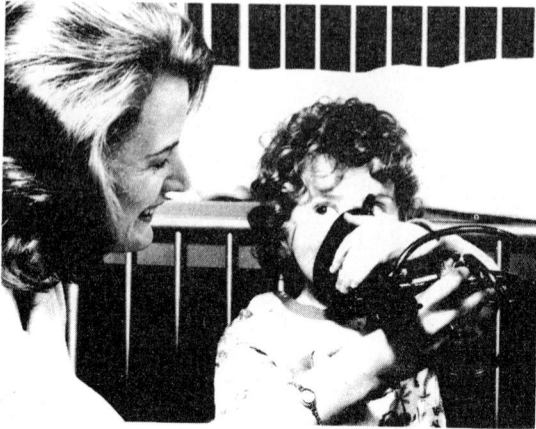

Fig. 172 Child is encouraged to hold the mask firmly over his mouth and nose. (By permission of R. Samios.)

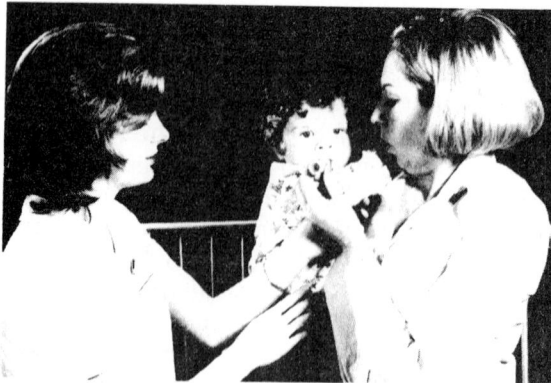

Fig. 173 The child's mother encourages him to hold the mouthpiece firmly between his lips.
(By permission of R. Samios.)

ventilation, whether by an endotracheal tube or a tracheostomy. The nose normally heats air to approximately 35 degrees centigrade, and adds water vapour to it. If a humidifier is not added to the circuit of the ventilator, bronchial secretions become thick and inspissated, the cilia of the cells of the bronchial mucosa cease working and sputum retention occurs (Roberts and Edwards 1971). The efficiency of the humidifier must be checked by the physiotherapist on each visit, to ensure that it is filled with water and that the temperature is correct.

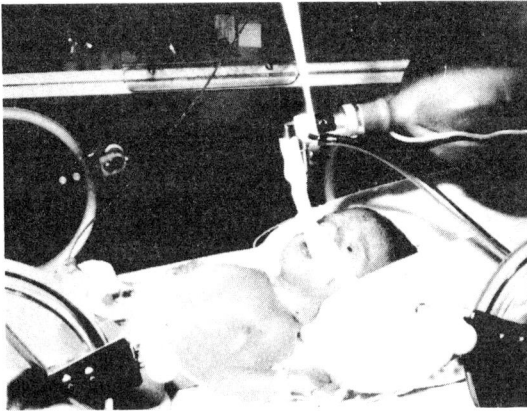

Fig. 174 Nasal endotracheal intubation of an infant in an incubator following cardiac surgery.
(By permission of R. Samios.)

Postural Drainage. It is most important that secretions are not allowed to accumulate in the lower airways, and postural drainage is given to children on ventilators either to drain specific segments of the lungs or by elevating the foot of the bed in order to get a more overall drainage. Following cardiac or cranial surgery, drainage may have to be given in the child's nursing position as elevation of the foot of the bed may be contraindicated. Consideration should be given to the child's position throughout the day. Secretions will accumulate in the posterior segments if the child is nursed in supine, and in the lateral segments if he is side lying. Side lying with two hourly turning is a position frequently adopted for nursing, and postural drainage may be given if necessary two hourly to whichever side the child is turned.

479

Vibrations and percussion are given, with pressure on expiration, and secretions are removed by aspiration as described below.

Throughout treatment the condition of a child on a ventilator is checked by observing his colour, respiration rate and depth, and pulse rate. If his condition is being monitored, the physiotherapist must be experienced enough to interpret the signs shown by the monitors. When the child is removed from artificial ventilation, and he will be slowly weaned from this, the main aim of the physiotherapist must be to restore normal respiratory function.

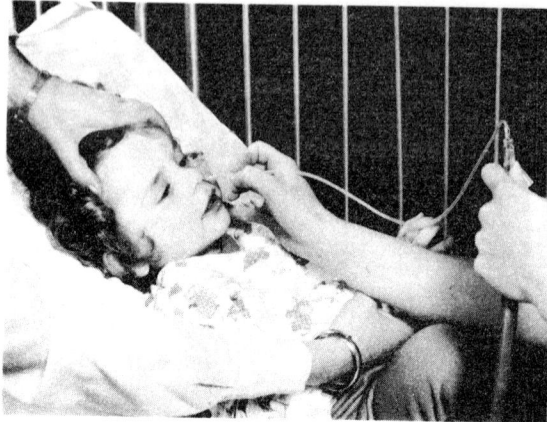

Fig. 175 Nasopharyngeal aspiration. The child is restrained at his head and hands.
(By permission of R. Samios.)

Techniques of aspiration or suction. In order to remove accumulated secretions from the airway, which will be necessary if only because of the child's depressed cough reflex, a rubber catheter is inserted into the airway and suction employed. This must be done at all times quickly and gently. The catheter must be the correct size for the child's airway, that is, not so large that it causes trauma to its walls. Nasal suction should only be done when necessary and not as a routine, as this procedure easily causes trauma to the nose and is most unpleasant. The nasal passage is horizontal and runs parallel to the roof of the mouth, and this is the direction in which the catheter should be passed (figure 175). It must be emphasized that suction as a general rule is not bronchial. Bronchial suction may need to be performed on some children where blockage is suspected, but will only be done as requested by the physician and then only by specially trained staff. Whether the catheter is passed via the naso-pharynx or via the tracheostomy, it must not pass down the airway too far, such as to the carina, as damage to the mucosal lining and infection of the lower air passages, especially if the technique is not strictly aseptic, will readily ensue. In most cases it is sufficient for the catheter to be passed only as far as the pharynx, as this will be sufficient to stimulate a cough reflex. There must be one other person present to restrain the child as aspiration is a frightening procedure.

While the catheter is being introduced the suction is occluded by the therapist, then released while the catheter is slowly withdrawn. The routine is repeated until the therapist, by listening to the sound of the air passing through the trachea and pharynx, can be certain that no further secretions are accumulating. This procedure must be strictly aseptic. The physiotherapist must be gowned and in some cases masked, and should be sure that the catheter does not touch any object outside the airway as it will then be no longer sterile.

CARE OF THE UNCONSCIOUS CHILD

A child may be unconscious for a significant period of time as a result of head injury, following neurosurgery, encephalitis or meningitis. He may have been rendered paralysed by tubocurarine (curare) as part of the management of his tetanus. He requires special care from the physiotherapist in order to prevent contractures which may occur due to posture, the effects of gravity, and the effects of spasticity. Mobility must be maintained in order to avoid the effects of a relative stagnation of the circulatory system on the nutrition of bones, muscles and viscera. Respiratory efficiency must also be maintained, and he may need to be artificially ventilated by endotracheal intubation or tracheostomy.

Following neurosurgery, it is important to prevent the buildup of carbondioxide in the body as this has a harmful effect on brain function, causing dilation of cerebral vessels and an increase in cerebral oedema. There will then follow an increase in intracranial pressure, which will jeopardize the child's chances of recovery from the brain injury.

General physical techniques will include passive movements of trunk and limbs, with emphasis on gaining full range, and as much trunk movement, particularly rotation, as possible; positioning and frequent turning in order to avoid pressure areas on spine, sacrum, pelvis, elbows, heels and malleoli, to prevent pooling of secretions, and in the case of the spastic child, to avoid positions which stimulate abnormal tonic reflex activity. The risk of pressure areas may be further minimized if the child sleeps on a ripple mattress or a sheet of sheepskin. Care must be taken in picking up and handling the hypotonic infant and child in order to avoid causing damage to soft tissues. It must be remembered that these patients may be unable to move in response to painful stimuli.

Specific techniques, such as postural drainage, assisted breathing exercises and pharyngeal aspiration of mucous secretions will be needed on a preventive basis in all these children, but may at times need to be done intensively should respiratory infection or distress supervene.

PARTICULAR PROBLEMS IN MANAGING THE CHILD WITH TETANUS

There are special problems when a child has tetanus. His voluntary muscular system will be paralysed by the administration of tubocurarine in order to prevent spasm. This will necessitate that he be tracheostomized and ventilated by positive pressure apparatus dispensing an oxygen-air mix. His main problems at this stage are likely to arise from his diminished or absent cough reflex, and the possibility of aspiration of vomitus or saliva. He will therefore require endotracheal suction at times, and this must be done with great care and only as necessary, as even this small stimulus may cause an increase in blood pressure and pulse rate, and cardiac irregularities.

SUMMARY

This Chapter describes the physical methods used by the physiotherapist in the treatment of respiratory disorders in infants and children. Basically these involve techniques for draining excess secretions and for aerating the lungs. Some techniques, such as the aspiration of secretions from the trachea of small infants, and the care of infants and children in intensive care units, require considerable skill and experience, and should not be attempted by the inexperienced physiotherapist unless under supervision.

In the case of the child with chronic respiratory illness, it is essential that parents be taught techniques for draining and aerating the lungs and clearing the upper respiratory tract, so treatment commenced and supervised by the physiotherapist continues regularly at home. The teaching of parents is sometimes difficult and time-consuming, but without their well-trained help no regime of treatment will be successful.

References

Baskett, P. J. F. (1971) The clinical assessment of the respiratory system by the physiotherapist, including reference to the use of the stethoscope. *Physiotherapy*, **57**, 7.

Castilla, P., Irving, I. M., Jackson Rees, G. and Rickham, P. P. (1971) Posture in management of esophageal atresia. *J. Ped. Surg.* **6**, 6, 709.

Godfrey, S. (1974) *Exercise Testing in Children.* New York and London: W. B. Saunders.

Gregory, G. A., Edmunds, L. H., Kitterman, J. A., Phibbs, R. H. and Tooley, W. H. (1975) Continuous positive airways pressure and pulmonary and circulatory function after cardiac surgery in infants less than three months of age. *Anaesthesiol.* **43**, 426.

Jones, R. S. and Owen-Thomas, J. B. (1971) *Care of the Critically Ill Child.* London: Arnold.

Kendig. E. L. (1967) *Disorders of the Respiratory Tract in Children.* Philadelphia and London: Saunders.

Polgar, G. and Promadhat, V. (1971) *Pulmonary Function Testing in Children: Techniques and Standards.* Philadelphia: Saunders.

Roberts, K. D. and Edwards, J. M. (1971) *Paediatric Intensive Care.* Oxford: Blackwell.

Rockwell, G. M. and Campbell, S. K. (1976) Physical therapy program for the paediatric cardiac surgical patient. *Phys. Ther.* **56**, 6, 670.

Silverman, W. A., Sinclair, J. C. and Agate, F. J. (1966) The oxygen cost of minor changes in heat balance of small newborn infants. *Acta Paediat. Scand.* **55**, 294.

Thacker, E. W. (1971) *Postural Drainage and Respiratory Control.* London: Lloyd-Luke.

Thoren, L. (1954) Post-operative pulmonary complications: Observations on their prevention by means of physical therapy. *Acta Chir. Scand.* **107**, 193.

Further Reading

Coran, A. G. (1973) Resuscitation following cardiopulmonary arrest. In *Surgical Pediatrics*, edited by S. L. Gans. New York: Grune and Stratton.

Gaskell, D. (1970) The Bird Mark 7 ventilator. *Physiotherapy*, **56**, 8.

Gaskell, D. (1971) *Postural Drainage at Home.* London: Brompton Hospital.

Gaskell D. and Webber, B. A. (1977) *The Brompton Hospital Guide to Chest Physiotherapy.* London: Blackwell.

Jackson, B. (1964) Problems in management of IPPR in the newborn. *Med. J. Aust.* **6**, 183.

Lough, M. D., Doershuk, C. F. and Stern, R. C. (1974) *Pediatric Respiratory Therapy.* Chicago: Year Book Publishers.

Mushin, W. W., Rendell Baker, L., Thompson, P. W. and Mapleson, W. W. (1969) *Automatic Ventilation of the Lungs.* Oxford and Edinburgh: Blackwell.

Wade, O. L. (1954) Movements of the thoracic cage and diaphragm. *J. Physiol.* **124**, 193.

Appendix I

Tests for Normal Postural Reflex Activity and Automatic Reactions to being moved

Except where reference is made to a specific author, the references for the following tests are Gesell and Amatruda (1947), André-Thomas, Chesni and Dargassies (1960), Peiper (1963) and Illingworth (1970). Appendix 7 illustrates the times at which these reflexes and reactions can be elicited in normal babies.

AMPHIBIAN REACTION

This is tested with the infant in prone. The examiner rotates the pelvis away from the table a short distance. This is followed by flexion and abduction of the leg on the same side. This reaction can be elicited from birth. It will be absent in hypotonic babies, and in those very hypertonic babies who have increased extensor tone in the legs, in which case the leg will remain extended instead of flexing and abducting. The response may be delayed in the moderately hypertonic baby, the leg extending at first, but flexing after a few moments. Care must be taken not to confuse a passive movement into flexion with the normal active response.

AUTOMATIC STANDING AND WALKING

The examiner holds the baby with his feet on the table. The baby responds by straightening his legs and standing, although he needs support as he has not yet developed balance reactions (figure 9). If his body is inclined forward he will take a few steps, lifting his legs high and putting his feet down firmly. He may get one leg caught behind the other, and this should not be confused with the scissoring associated with hypertonus, when the legs are internally rotated and the feet plantarflexed (figure 176). These reflexes are seen in newborn babies, and can be elicited, although with

485

diminishing response, until four to six weeks of age. They will be absent in hypotonic and severely mentally retarded babies.

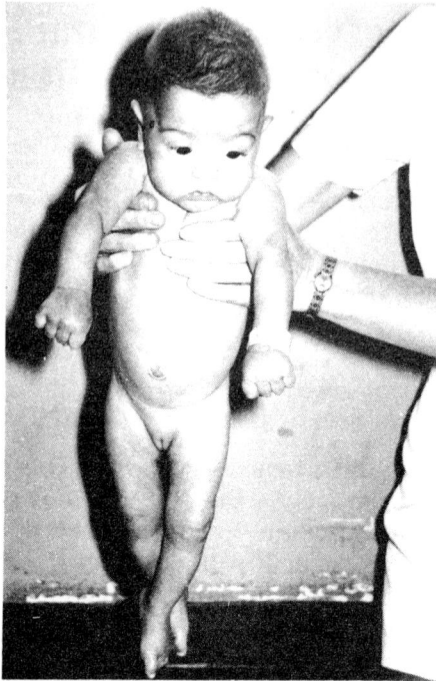

Fig. 176 Spastic quadriplegia. Note the extended, adducted legs and the plantarflexed feet.

CROSSED EXTENSOR RESPONSE

This is tested with the baby in supine. The examiner holds one leg extended and firmly strokes the sole of the foot from heel towards the toes. The infant responds by flexing the contralateral leg into abduction, then by adducting and extending the leg as though to push the stimulus away. This response is present from birth until four to six weeks of age. Absence or persistence of this reflex may indicate a pathological state. It will be absent or delayed in a hypertonic baby with extension spasticity in his legs. It will also be absent in a hypertonic baby who may have insufficient tone to react. It may persist beyond its normal span in brain-damaged babies causing problems in standing and walking as the baby develops.

GALANT REFLEX

The baby is tested in prone or ventral suspension. The examiner runs a finger parallel to the spine from the last rib to the iliac

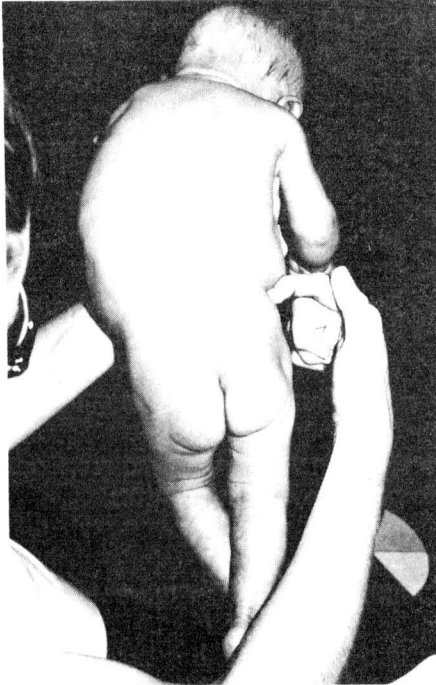

Fig. 177 Galant reflex (trunk incurvation reflex) is positive on the right side.

crest. The baby responds by side flexing towards the stimulus (figure 177). This reflex is present at birth and can be elicited for six to eight weeks. It may be absent in some very hypotonic babies, and may persist in hypertonic and particularly athetoid babies, either symmetrically or asymmetrically. Its persistence makes sitting balance difficult or impossible to maintain, and the baby cannot develop symmetrical movement as any lateral stimulus forces him into this asymmetrical posture.

MORO REFLEX

The examiner holds the baby with his head and trunk supported. He withdraws support from the head, letting it drop back into his hand. This sudden loss of head control backward startles the baby and he responds by extending his arms in a wide embracing movement, hands open and fingers abducted. His legs may also extend, although this response varies. The movement is usually accompanied by a wail from the baby. The reflex is present at birth. After the first few weeks the arms extend and abduct less widely, and the reflex can usually no longer be elicited after two to three months (Mitchell 1960). This reflex will be absent or diminished in hypotonic and in severely mentally retarded babies. It will be asymmetrical in a baby with hemiplegia or obstetrical paralysis. If it persists, as it may do in a brain-damaged baby, it makes the development of milestones such as balance in sitting impossible. In the hypertonic baby the reaction may be decreased due to limitation of extension by the flexor spasticity in the arms.

PROTECTIVE SIDE TURNING OF THE HEAD

This is tested in prone. The examiner holds the baby's head gently face downward on the table, then releases it. The baby responds by turning his head to one side to protect himself from smothering. This reaction is present from birth. It may be absent in hypotonic babies and in the severely mentally retarded. It may also be absent in very hypertonic babies where a positive tonic labyrinthine reflex causes an increase in flexor spasticity.

RIGHTING REACTIONS

These are responsible for the baby's ability to maintain his head and body in relation to space, and to maintain the relationship of various parts of his body to each other (Bobath and Bobath 1955).

Neck Righting Reflex

This is tested in supine. It is a proprioceptive reflex elicited by stretching of the neck muscles. The examiner holds the baby's head and rotates it to one side. The trunk follows the head, rolling in one piece with no rotation within the trunk. This reflex is present at birth and is most evident at three months, after which it becomes less reliable, until it can no longer be elicited at five months. It may be absent in hypotonic babies. In hypertonic babies the response will be abnormal. The trunk may follow the head but the shoulder girdle will remain retracted and the baby will not bring the arm forward.

Labyrinthine Righting Reflex

This reflex is tested by observing the position of the baby's head in relation to his body when he is held in supine and prone and when he is tilted laterally in the vertical position. A normal newborn baby demonstrates a head lag when he is pulled to sitting, although he makes some attempt to hold his head, and does not allow it to fall back limply into extension as does a brain-damaged or mentally retarded baby (figure 6). By four months he holds his head in line with his body when he is pulled to sitting (figure 7). By five to six months he will lift his head in supine in anticipation of being pulled to sitting (figure 8). A newborn baby held in ventral suspension will allow his head to fall into some flexion (figure 178), but not into the completely flexed position of the brain-

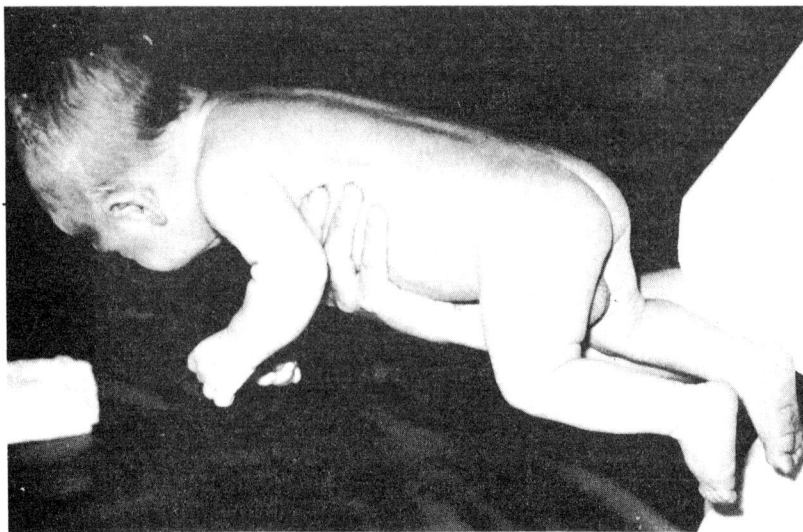

Fig. 178 Aged 6 weeks in ventral suspension. Note the head held in line with the body, which is normal finding at this age. Compare with baby in figure 32.

damaged or mentally retarded baby (figure 32). By eight weeks he will hold his head in line with his body. By four months he will lift his head at an angle of 90 degrees from the floor when he is lying in prone (figure 10).

Body Righting Reflex

This reflex follows on from and modifies the neck righting reflex. For the development of skilled movement it is necessary that the total body movement which is seen at the stage of the neck righting reflex is altered by the development of rotation within the body axis. When the body righting reflex appears, between five and seven months, the baby is able to rotate his trunk. The reflex may not develop in a mentally retarded baby or in the presence of brain damage where the baby retains the primitive neck righting reflex, or where trunk spasticity is marked.

PLACING REACTIONS

The examiner holds the baby so the dorsum of the foot or anterior aspect of the leg touches the edge of the table. The baby responds by flexing his leg and placing the foot flat on the table. A similar reaction can be found in the hands, the hand being placed on the table in response to a touch on its dorsal aspect. These reactions can be elicited from birth (Zapella 1963). They may however be absent in hypotonic babies, and in babies with extensor hypertonus of the legs, whose legs extend, adduct, and plantarflex. Similarly, the baby with flexor spasticity in the arms will be unable to lift his arm and extend the wrist and fingers. These responses will be asymmetrical in a spastic hemiplegic baby, and this test is useful in detecting hemiplegia in a baby who shows few other signs of abnormality.

LANDAU REACTION

This is tested with the baby held in ventral suspension. The normal baby from four to five months responds to ventral suspension by extending head, trunk and, by six or eight months, the legs. The examiner flexes the baby's head which is followed by flexion of the trunk and legs. When the head is released, the limbs, head and trunk usually return to their extended positions. This reaction may be absent in hypotonic and severely mentally retarded babies who maintain a flexed position when held in ventral suspension. It will be absent in hypertonic babies who have not developed sufficient extension tone. It may appear to be present in a hypertonic baby but as a manifestation of his abnormal increase in extensor tone. However, this baby's legs will be adducted, internally rotated and plantarflexed. There is no alteration in position when the head is flexed forward, extension being maintained elsewhere.

PARACHUTE REACTION

The baby is held at the trunk and lowered head first towards the ground. He responds by extending his arms and putting out his hands towards the floor as though to save himself. It can be elicited in this way after six months, but is more evident at nine months, and continues throughout life. The reaction will be absent in hypotonic, brain-damaged or mentally retarded babies. The hypertonic baby's response to falling forward may be an increase in the abnormal pattern of retraction and flexion in the arms which will inhibit the protective response. The spastic hemiplegic baby will respond asymmetrically.

This reaction is also tested in sitting, when the baby is pushed gently forward, sideways and backward. He catches his balance in response to this push by putting out one or both hands toward the floor. A normal baby demonstrates this reaction forward at six months, sideways at eight months and backward at twelve months.

EQUILIBRIUM REACTIONS

These reactions are automatic responses to loss of balance. They may be tested in prone, supine, sitting and standing. In *prone* and *supine* the tests are performed on a balance board or on a table which is tilted slowly to one side. The child will react by flexing his trunk and head sideways away from the pull of gravity, abducting the arm and leg on the side to which he has flexed. The full response in supine involves an element of rotation which occurs as side flexion becomes extreme.

491

In *sitting* and *standing* the child is tilted slowly to one side, then forward and backward, and as he loses balance he will protect himself by movements of his trunk and limbs (figures 179 and 180). These reactions develop first in prone and supine at six months, in sitting at nine months and in standing at approximately fourteen months. Equilibrium reactions will not develop effectively in the presence of such primitive reflexes as the Moro reflex, or where there is marked hypertonus or hypotonus. They will be slow to develop in mentally retarded children.

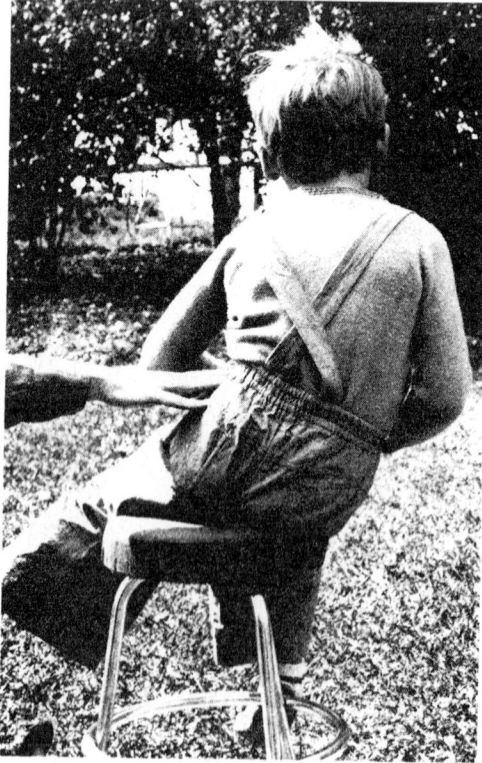

Fig. 179 Normal equilibrium reactions in sitting. Note the lateral movement of the head and trunk.

TONIC NECK REFLEXES

Asymmetrical Tonic Neck Reflex

This is tested in supine. It is a response elicited by stretch applied to the neck muscles. The baby's head is turned to one side. The examiner both watches and feels the response in the limbs. The arm and leg on the face side are seen to extend while those on the occiput side flex (figure 181). There may not be an actual movement, but only an increase in tone felt by slight resistence to flexion of the limbs on the face side and to extension on the occiput side. Normal babies in their first two to three months are often seen to lie in this 'fencing' position for short periods, but it is a fleeting, not a persistent response, and cannot be regarded as a

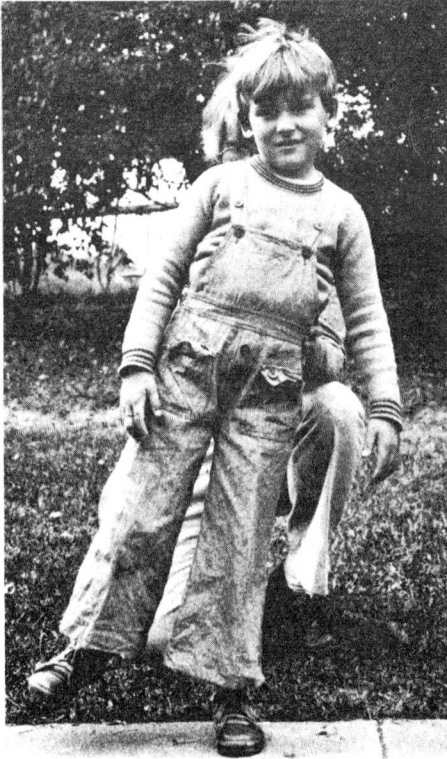

Fig. 180 Normal equilibrium reactions in standing. Note the lateral movement of the head and trunk.

493

reflex. If the posture is persistent, or if it is a stereotyped response to rotation of the head, it is abnormal. It may dominate the baby's motor function to such an extent that the hand cannot be taken to the mouth. It may be seen in either spastic or athetoid babies. In cases of severe athetosis it also affects the trunk causing it to flex to the occiput side (Bobath and Bobath 1955).

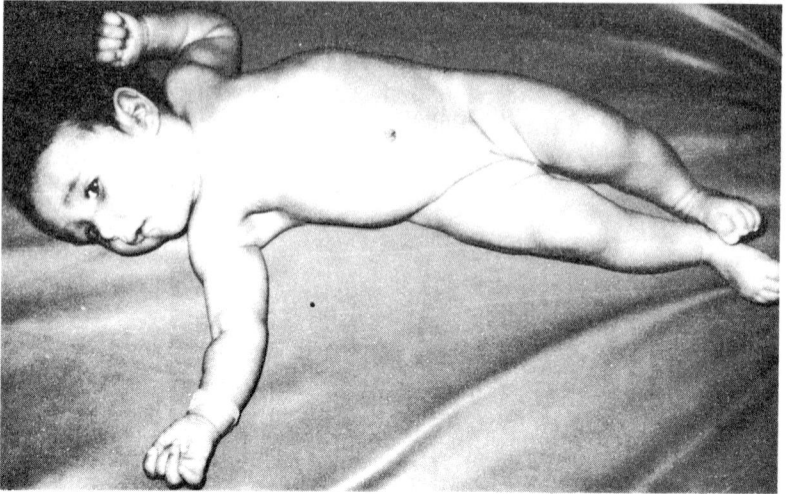

Fig. 181 Asymmetrical tonic neck reflex to the right.

Symmetrical Tonic Neck Reflex

This may be tested in four point kneeling. It is elicited by stretch applied to the neck muscles. When the examiner extends the baby's head the arms will extend while the legs flex. If he then flexes the head, the arms will collapse into flexion and the legs will extend. The influence of this reflex is seen in the normal baby when he pushes up on his hands to kneeling. However, if it occurs in the stereotyped manner described above it is abnormal and will prevent the baby from developing milestones such as crawling. He will be at the mercy of his head movement, unable to move effectively because the position of his head decides the position of his limbs. This reflex may be seen in spastic and athetoid babies (Bobath and Bobath 1955).

References

André-Thomas, Chesni Y. and Dargassies, S. S.-A. (1960) *The Neurological Examination of the Infant.* London: Heinemann.

Bobath, K. and Bobath, B. (1955) Tonic reflexes and righting reflexes in the diagnosis and assessment of Cerebral Palsy. *Cerebral Palsy Bulletin*, **16**, 5.

Gesell, A. and Amatruda, C. S. (1947) *Developmental Diagnosis.* New York: Hoeber.

Illingworth, R. S. (1970) *The Development of the Infant and Young Child.* London: Livingstone.

Mitchell, R. G. (1960) The Moro reflex. *Cerebral Palsy Bulletin*, **2**, 135.

Peiper, A. (1963) *Cerebral Function in Infancy and Childhood.* London: Pitman.

Zapella, M. (1963) *Placing reactions in the newborn.* Develop. Med. and Child Neurol. **5**, 497.

Appendix 2

Name	Date
Date of Birth	Place of Birth
Address	Medical Officer
Prenatal & Birth History	
Drug Therapy & Time Elapsed Since Last Dose	Time Elapsed Since Last Feed
Supine: Observation of Posture & Movement	
Basic Tone & Reaction to Stimulation	
Neck Righting Reflex	Body Righting Reflex
ATNR	Ankle Clonus
Head Control when pulled to sitting	
Equilibrium Reactions	
Prone: Observation of Posture & Movement	
Basic Tone & Reaction to Stimulation	
Protective Side Turning of Head	Head Control
Amphibian Reaction	Galant Reflex
Equilibrium Reactions	
Ventral Suspension: Observation of Posture & Movement	Parachute Reaction Downwards
Landau Reaction	

(a) Infant Assessment Chart

<u>Sitting</u>: Observation of Posture & Movement	
<u>Parachute Reaction</u>: Forward Sideways Backwards	Equilibrium Reactions
<u>Standing</u>: Automatic Standing	Automatic Walking
Held in Standing	
<u>Manipulation</u>: Tonic Reaction of Finger Flexors	Approach to Object
Hands to Mouth	Hands to Midline
Type of Grasp	Type of Release
Transfer Hand to Hand	Hand Regard
<u>Oral Function</u>: Rooting Reflex	Bite Reflex
Gag Reflex	Sucking Reflex
Tone in Oral Region	Tongue Movement
Vocalisation	Feeding
<u>Other Reactions</u>: Placing Reactions of Feet	Placing Reactions of Hands
Moro Reflex	
Emotional Response to Examiner	Visual Response to Bright Light
<u>Parents' Comments</u> Feeding	Dressing
Bathing	Sleeping
<u>Main Problems</u>:	

Name	Date
Date of Birth	Place of Birth
Address	Medical Officer
Prenatal & Birth History	
Basic Tone & Reaction to Stimulation	
Hearing	Vision
Emotional & Mental State	
Contracture & Deformity	Drug Therapy & Time Elapsed Since Last Dose
Social Background	
Reflex Activities Neck Righting Reaction	Amphibian Reaction
Landau Reflex	Moro Reflex
Parachute Reactions	Placing Reactions
Tonic Reflexes	
Equilibrium Reactions	
Supine: Observation of Posture & Movement	
Rolling	
Pulled to Sitting: Head Control	
Sitting Up	Crook lying Bridging

(b) Child Assessment Chart

Prone: Observation of Posture & Movement	
Head Control	
Forearm Support	Extended Arm Support
Reaching Out	Effect on Bending Knee
Progression Along Floor	
To Prone Kneeling	To Sitting
Sitting: Long Sitting	Sitting on Stool
Side Sitting	Pivoting
Sitting to Standing	
Prone Kneeling: Observation of Posture & Movement	
Crawling	Reaching Out
To Sitting on Stool	To Standing Up
To Upright Kneeling	
Upright Kneeling: Observation of Posture & Movement	
Walking on Knees	To Half Kneeling
Half Kneeling: Observation of Posture & Movement	To Standing
Standing: Observation of Posture & Movement	
Weight Transference: Stride, walk & step standing	

DYSLEXIA

The inability to recognize conventional graphic symbols. The patient demonstrates various disturbances in reading and writing.

LATERALITY

The ability to use one side better than the other. The term is usually used to indicate foot or hand preference.

Suggested Reading

Abercrombie, M. L. J. (1964) *Perceptual and Visuomotor Disorders in Cerebral Palsy.* London: Heinemann.

Cratty, B. J. (1967) *Developmental Sequences of Perceptual Motor Tasks.* New York: Educational Activities Incorporated.

Critchley, M. (1966) *The Parietal Lobes.* New York: Hafner.

Kephart, N. C. and Roach, E. G. (1966) *The Purdue Perceptual Motor Survey.* Columbus, Ohio: Merrill.

Touwen, B. C. L. (1972) *Laterality and dominance.* Develop. Med. Child Neurol. **14**, 747.

Appendix 5

The following relaxation and facilitation techniques are described by Knott and Voss (1968). They are useful in the treatment of children with musculo-skeletal or peripheral neurological disorders, whose problems of movement result from muscle weakness or contracture. They are described here in isolation, but are frequently used in combination, techniques of relaxation followed by techniques of facilitation, according to the patient's needs. They are not intended to be learnt by the student in a purely theoretical manner, but are included in this Appendix in order that the student may use these descriptions in conjunction with practical instruction.

RELAXATION TECHNIQUES

Contract-Relax

The part is moved passively to the point in its range where limitation of movement occurs. The patient then contracts *isotonically* the muscles which are causing the limitation against maximal manual resistance from the therapist. The patient is then asked to relax, and when the therapist feels relaxation occur, she takes the part once more to the point in its range when limitation occurs. This is performed several times, and it is hoped that increase in range of movement will occur due to relaxation and therefore lengthening of the muscles antagonistic to the movement required.

Hold-Relax

The part is moved passively to the point in its range where limitation of movement occurs. The patient then contracts *isometrically* the muscles which are causing the limitation against maximal manual resistance from the therapist. The patient is then

Rhythmic Stabilization

The patient holds isometrically with the agonists and antagonists against maximal resistance, and co-contraction is gradually built up between the two (Knott and Voss 1968). The therapist must be careful to change the direction of resistance slowly, allowing the patient to maintain the co-contraction.

The above techniques are applicable where it is necessary to increase the ability of particular muscle groups to contract, and where increased strength of a movement is required. Rhythmic stabilization is also effective as a means of building up co-contraction in a part, and therefore stability.

Reference

Knott, M. and Voss, D. E. (1968) *Proprioceptive Neuromuscular Facilitation*. London: Ballière, Tindall and Cassell.

asked to relax, and when the therapist feels relaxation occur, the patient takes the part actively in the opposite direction. It is important with this technique that the therapist increase resistance gradually while the patient holds the part isometrically, and that the therapist's resistance at no time breaks the patient's hold.

The above techniques may be used instead of passive stretching, where limitation of range of movement is due to contracted soft tissues. Following acute injuries, where movement may be painful, care must be taken that isotonic contraction is within the painfree range, and that isometric contraction is done carefully with resistance applied gradually in order to make sure no movement occurs. The student should note that 'maximal' resistance does not imply that the therapist should use excessive resistance, but that she should grade her resistance in order to allow the patient to contract with *his* maximum effort, which may not be very great in the presence of muscle weakness.

FACILITATION AND STRENGTHENING TECHNIQUES

Repeated Contractions

The patient is asked to contract the agonistic muscle isotonically against maximal manual resistance given by the therapist. The response of the agonist is facilitated by repeated stimulation of the stretch receptors, the patient attempts to contract the muscle immediately following and in response to a short sharp stretch applied to the muscle. If the patient can respond sufficiently he is asked to hold isometrically in various parts of the range of movement.

Slow Reversal-Hold

The patient contracts isotonically in the pattern antagonistic to the pattern required, then reverses and contracts isotonically in the agonistic pattern. Both movements are given resistance throughout the range with care that the therapist changes her resistance slowly and avoids jerkiness. During the movement in the agonistic pattern the therapist may ask the patient to hold in parts of the range against maximal resistance, and repeated contraction may also be given in order to encourage a stronger, more controlled movement.

Standing on One Leg	
Hopping	Jumping
Gait	
Function: Dressing	Washing
Toileting	
Sensation: Stereognosis	Position & Movement Sense
Two Point Discrimination	
Hand Function: Tonic Reaction of Finger Flexors	Approach to Object
Use of Hands in Midline	
Type of Grasp	Type of Release
Manipulation of Large Objects	of Small Objects
Transfer Hand to Hand	Hold Object Thro' Range of Movement
Oral Function: Sucking Reflex	Bite Reflex
Gag Reflex	Swallowing
Tone in Oral Region	Tongue Movement
Feeding	
Vocalisation-Speech	
MAIN PROBLEMS:	

Prone: Observation of Posture & Movement	
Head Control	
Forearm Support	Extended Arm Support
Reaching Out	Effect on Bending Knee
Progression Along Floor	
To Prone Kneeling	To Sitting
Sitting: Long Sitting	Sitting on Stool
Side Sitting	Pivoting
Sitting to Standing	
Prone Kneeling: Observation of Posture & Movement	
Crawling	Reaching Out
To Sitting on Stool	To Standing Up
To Upright Kneeling	
Upright Kneeling: Observation of Posture & Movement	
Walking on Knees	To Half Kneeling
Half Kneeling: Observation of Posture & Movement	To Standing
Standing: Observation of Posture & Movement	
Weight Transference: Stride, walk & step standing	

Appendix 4

AGNOSIA

The inability to recognize the relevance of sensory stimuli. *Visual agnosia* denotes the inability to recognize objects seen. *Auditory agnosia* denotes the inability to appreciate the significance of sounds. *Tactile agnosia* (astereognosis) denotes the inability to identify objects felt.

APHASIA (DYSPHASIA)

Expressive or motor aphasia is an inability to express thoughts in words. The patient understands spoken words, but although he knows what he wants to say he cannot find the appropriate words. *Receptive or sensory aphasia* is an inability to appreciate the significance of words, whether spoken or written, as symbols. The patient does not comprehend the words although he hears them.

APRAXIA

The inability to do a willed voluntary movement despite the fact that the motor and sensory pathways concerned in the control of the movement are intact. For example, the child may be unable to put out his hand on request, although he will put it out for a biscuit.

DYSARTHRIA

A disorder of articulation due to inco-ordination of the muscles of speech. There is a lack of control over lips and tongue. The patient has a good understanding of speech, as well as the ability to use words correctly.

Appendix 3

	EVALUATION OF THE NEW BORN INFANT ONE MINUTE AFTER BIRTH (APGAR)				
SCORE	HEART RATE	RESPIRATORY EFFORT	REFLEX RESPONSE	MUSCLE TONE	COLOUR
2	Over 100	Good strong cry	Cough, cry or sneeze	Well flexed	Pink all over
1	Under 100	Irregular weak cry	Grimace	Some flexion of extremities	Extremities blue, body pink
0	Absent	Absent	Absent	Flaccid	Blue or pale

Apgar Chart

APGAR TEST

This is a method of evaluating the condition of a newborn infant in the first few months of life suggested by Apgar. It summarizes the vital clinical findings in the immediate post-natal period. The method of scoring at one minute is shown above. The score is also recorded at five minutes, which gives an assessment of the infant's rate of recovery. An infant in optimal birth condition will score the maximum of ten. A score of three or less indicates a markedly asphyxiated infant. Many of the signs are decreased or absent in the presence of asphyxia. Its predictive value is unproven.

DYSLEXIA

The inability to recognize conventional graphic symbols. The patient demonstrates various disturbances in reading and writing.

LATERALITY

The ability to use one side better than the other. The term is usually used to indicate foot or hand preference.

Suggested Reading

Abercrombie, M. L. J. (1964) *Perceptual and Visuomotor Disorders in Cerebral Palsy.* London: Heinemann.

Cratty, B. J. (1967) *Developmental Sequences of Perceptual Motor Tasks.* New York: Educational Activities Incorporated.

Critchley, M. (1966) *The Parietal Lobes.* New York: Hafner.

Kephart, N. C. and Roach, E. G. (1966) *The Purdue Perceptual Motor Survey.* Columbus, Ohio: Merrill.

Touwen, B. C. L. (1972) *Laterality and dominance.* Develop. Med. Child Neurol. **14**, 747.

Appendix 5

The following relaxation and facilitation techniques are described by Knott and Voss (1968). They are useful in the treatment of children with musculo-skeletal or peripheral neurological disorders, whose problems of movement result from muscle weakness or contracture. They are described here in isolation, but are frequently used in combination, techniques of relaxation followed by techniques of facilitation, according to the patient's needs. They are not intended to be learnt by the student in a purely theoretical manner, but are included in this Appendix in order that the student may use these descriptions in conjunction with practical instruction.

RELAXATION TECHNIQUES

Contract-Relax

The part is moved passively to the point in its range where limitation of movement occurs. The patient then contracts *isotonically* the muscles which are causing the limitation against maximal manual resistance from the therapist. The patient is then asked to relax, and when the therapist feels relaxation occur, she takes the part once more to the point in its range when limitation occurs. This is performed several times, and it is hoped that increase in range of movement will occur due to relaxation and therefore lengthening of the muscles antagonistic to the movement required.

Hold-Relax

The part is moved passively to the point in its range where limitation of movement occurs. The patient then contracts *isometrically* the muscles which are causing the limitation against maximal manual resistance from the therapist. The patient is then

asked to relax, and when the therapist feels relaxation occur, the patient takes the part actively in the opposite direction. It is important with this technique that the therapist increase resistance gradually while the patient holds the part isometrically, and that the therapist's resistance at no time breaks the patient's hold.

The above techniques may be used instead of passive stretching, where limitation of range of movement is due to contracted soft tissues. Following acute injuries, where movement may be painful, care must be taken that isotonic contraction is within the painfree range, and that isometric contraction is done carefully with resistance applied gradually in order to make sure no movement occurs. The student should note that 'maximal' resistance does not imply that the therapist should use excessive resistance, but that she should grade her resistance in order to allow the patient to contract with *his* maximum effort, which may not be very great in the presence of muscle weakness.

FACILITATION AND STRENGTHENING TECHNIQUES

Repeated Contractions

The patient is asked to contract the agonistic muscle isotonically against maximal manual resistance given by the therapist. The response of the agonist is facilitated by repeated stimulation of the stretch receptors, the patient attempts to contract the muscle immediately following and in response to a short sharp stretch applied to the muscle. If the patient can respond sufficiently he is asked to hold isometrically in various parts of the range of movement.

Slow Reversal-Hold

The patient contracts isotonically in the pattern antagonistic to the pattern required, then reverses and contracts isotonically in the agonistic pattern. Both movements are given resistance throughout the range with care that the therapist changes her resistance slowly and avoids jerkiness. During the movement in the agonistic pattern the therapist may ask the patient to hold in parts of the range against maximal resistance, and repeated contraction may also be given in order to encourage a stronger, more controlled movement.

Rhythmic Stabilization

The patient holds isometrically with the agonists and antagonists against maximal resistance, and co-contraction is gradually built up between the two (Knott and Voss 1968). The therapist must be careful to change the direction of resistance slowly, allowing the patient to maintain the co-contraction.

The above techniques are applicable where it is necessary to increase the ability of particular muscle groups to contract, and where increased strength of a movement is required. Rhythmic stabilization is also effective as a means of building up co-contraction in a part, and therefore stability.

Reference

Knott, M. and Voss, D. E. (1968) *Proprioceptive Neuromuscular Facilitation*. London: Ballière, Tindall and Cassell.

Appendix 6

The amount of resistance that the flow of air meets in the airways depends on the size and the number of these airways. Airways resistance is therefore greater in infants than in children, and greater in children than in adults, as the airways increase both in size and number between infancy and adult life. The term 'increased airway resistance' is used by some authors to describe the interference with airflow which occurs in bronchospasm or emphysema, this term being thought more accurate than the word 'obstruction' used by some authorities.

APNOEA

This word denotes a temporary cessation of respiration. It commonly occurs as temporary apnoeic spells in premature infants who take a sequence of breaths followed by a period of apnoea. Its significance is not understood although it is possibly due to immaturity. It is unusual after 36 weeks gestational age. Prolonged apnoeic attacks (of more than twenty seconds duration) occur if aspiration and obstruction of the larynx or trachea has occurred, in the presence of hyaline membrane disease, pneumonia and any condition in which the infant or child suffers respiratory distress. These attacks may be very serious and may lead to death. Avery (1968) suggests a tactile stimulus such as turning the infant or slapping his feet will often result in more regular respiration.

CROUP

This term is used to describe upper airways infections by viruses or Haemophilus influenzae, which cause acute laryngo-tracheobronchitis or epiglottitis. The child demonstrates inspiratory stridor, a non-productive cough and is febrile and ill. He is nursed in a humid atmosphere in a special tent, and may need to be intubated if his condition does not improve or if it deteriorates.

DYSPNOEA

Difficult or laboured respiratory effort in infancy is found in aspiration syndromes, emphysema, atelectasis, tracheo-oesophageal fistula, congenital heart disease and other conditions. In premature babies the commonest cause of dyspnoea is hyaline membrane disease. Dyspnoea on exertion occurs in older children with asthma, emphysema, pneumothorax, massive atelectasis, congenital heart disease or in the presence of severe thoracic deformity such as kyphosis or scoliosis. Extreme dyspnoea is accompanied by flaring of the alae nasi, and use of the accessory muscles of respiration. It is caused by increased stimulation of the respiratory centre by abnormal oxygen, carbondioxide or pH factors in the blood.

RALES

Sounds produced by air bubbling through fluid in the airways. They are otherwise called crepitations. When the fluid is in the alveoli they are described as fine, and when secretions are in the trachea or major bronchi they are termed coarse.

RHONCHI

Harsh breath sounds heard on either inspiration or expiration, and produced by obstruction of the airways. This may be due to bronchospasm, blockage of a foreign body or by accumulated secretions, or oedema of the mucous membrane.

RESPIRATORY ACIDOSIS AND ALKALOSIS

A condition in which the arterial pH is below the normal range is called respiratory acidosis. Where the arterial pH is greater than normal the condition is called respiratory alkalosis. These disturbances are due to alveolar hypoventilation or hyperventilation, which will lead to an accumulation or a washing out of carbondioxide.

RESPIRATORY FAILURE

This may be seen following several causes (figure 182) and is said to be present if the patient's $PaCO_2$ is above the normal limit, or if he is hypoxic, that is with a decreased PaO_2. However, the criteria for respiratory failure vary according to the child's disease and his age. There is an increase in respiratory rate and effort in order to maintain alveolar ventilation and blood gas tensions despite increasing obstruction.

CAUSES OF RESPIRATORY FAILURE

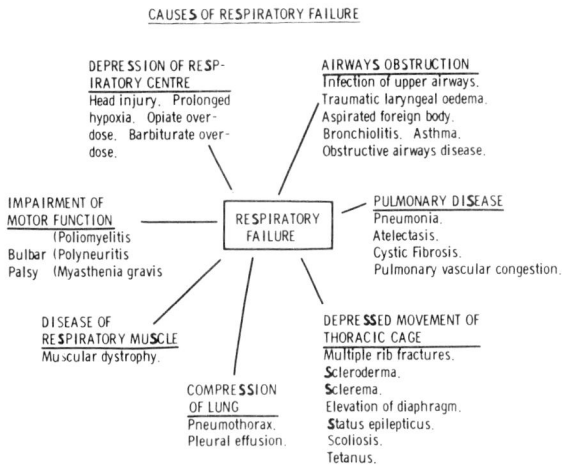

DEPRESSION OF RESP-
IRATORY CENTRE
Head injury. Prolonged
hypoxia. Opiate over-
dose. Barbiturate over-
dose.

AIRWAYS OBSTRUCTION
Infection of upper airways.
Traumatic laryngeal oedema.
Aspirated foreign body.
Bronchiolitis. Asthma.
Obstructive airways disease.

IMPAIRMENT OF
MOTOR FUNCTION
(Poliomyelitis
Bulbar (Polyneuritis
Palsy (Myasthenia gravis

RESPIRATORY
FAILURE

PULMONARY DISEASE
Pneumonia.
Atelectasis.
Cystic Fibrosis.
Pulmonary vascular congestion.

DISEASE OF
RESPIRATORY MUSCLE
Muscular dystrophy.

COMPRESSION
OF LUNG
Pneumothorax.
Pleural effusion.

DEPRESSED MOVEMENT OF
THORACIC CAGE
Multiple rib fractures.
Scleroderma.
Sclerema.
Elevation of diaphragm.
Status epilepticus.
Scoliosis.
Tetanus.

Fig. 182 Causes of respiratory failure in infants and children.

STRIDOR

Stridor is usually inspiratory and indicates laryngeal or pharyngeal obstruction. Persistant stridor will occur in the presence of a congenital abnormality of the larynx.

SURFACE TENSION

Liquids have a property called surface tension. The surface of a liquid tends to contract to the smallest possible area, which is illustrated by the tendency of liquid to form drops when placed on a solid surface. A bubble of fluid behaves similarly except that the interior of a bubble is air which can be compressed. The surface tension of a bubble tends to collapse it while compression of the air within the bubble creates pressure to resist collapse. Hence a state of equilibrium is reached, with the pressure of air within the bubble equalling the pressure created by surface tension. Within a bubble the pressure created by surface tension is inversely proportional to the radius of the bubble.

The law of physics is expressed by the La Place equation, $P = 2T/r$, where P is the pressure within the bubble, T is the surface tension and r is the radius of the bubble.

Alveoli with a fluid layer covering their surface are virtually tiny bubbles except they are not intact as they open into alveolar ducts. This makes it difficult for intra-alveolar air pressure to resist collapse. Pulmonary surfactant lowers the surface tension in the fluid layer.

WHEEZING

Wheezing is due to narrowing of the airway and is heard usually on expiration. High-pitched rhonchi are heard on auscultation. Wheezing nearly always signifies bronchospasm. It occurs in asthma, asthmatic or allergic bronchitis, following inhalation of a foreign body, and in bronchiolitis.

Appendix 7

DEVELOPMENTAL REACTIONS

	1	2	3	4	5	6	7	8	9	10	11	1 Year	2 Years
PRIMITIVE REACTIONS													
Moro	+	+	+	+/-									
Galant	+	+											
Primary Standing	+	+											
Automatic Walking	+	+											
Tonic reaction of finger flexors	+	+	+/-										
Tonic reaction of toe flexors	+	+	+	+	+	+	+	+					
Placing reaction of hands				+	+	+							
Placing reaction of feet	+	+	+	+									
Neck righting	+	+	+	+	+/-	+/-	+/-	+/-	+/-				
Rooting	+	+	+/-	+/-									
Sucking	+	+	+	+/-									
RIGHTING REACTIONS													
Body righting on body						+	+	+	+	+	+	+/-	+/-
								Optical righting					
Labyrinthine righting	+/-	+	+	+	+	+	+	+	+	+	+	+	+
Landau					+/-	+	+	+	+	+	+	+	+/-
Parachute - forwards						+	+	+	+	+	+	+	+
sideways									+	+	+	+	+
backwards										+	+	+	+
EQUILIBRIUM REACTIONS													
In supine							+	+	+	+	+	+	+
In prone						+	+	+	+	+	+	+	+
In sitting								+	+	+	+	+	+
In four foot kneeling					.				+	+	+	+	+
In standing												+/-	+/-

RESPECT THE CHILD
BE NOT TOO MUCH HIS PARENT
TRESPASS NOT ON HIS SOLITUDE

—*Emerson*

Index

Acceptance, 289–91
Achilles tendon, 210, 213, 314–15
Adduction tenotomy, 253
Aerosol therapy, 433, 444, 462
Agnosia, 63, 149, 502
Airways resistance, 507
Allergic reaction, 430–1
Allergic rhinitis, 436
Amelia, 288, 291, 298–304
Amphibian reaction, 485
Anterior horn cells, 19, 51, 63, 64
Anti-burnscar elastic pressure
    supports, 393
Antigravity posture, 133
Anxiety, 5, 40, 290
Apgar chart, 501
Apgar rating, 421
Apgar test, 501
Aphasia, 502
Apnoea, 507
Apparatus, checking, 283
Apraxia, 63, 502
Arm strengthening, 278
Arnold-Chiari malformation, 258
Arthrogryposis multiplex
    congenita, 251–4
  aetiology, 251
  management, 251
  physical treatment, 252–3
  surgical treatment, 253
Asphyxia, 501
Aspiration, 480, 482
Assessment, 450–7

brachial plexus lesions, 201–3
cerebral palsy. *See* Cerebral
    palsy
developmental disorders, 161
general procedure, 450–2
limb deficiencies, 298
mental retardation, 164
minimal brain dysfunction,
    153–4
muscular dystrophy, 324–5
muscular torticollis, 340–1
poliomyelitis, 188–90
spina bifida, 283–4
talipes calcaneo-valgus, 234
talipes equinovarus, 215
tone, 89, 107, 202
Assessment chart
  child, 498
  infant, 496
Associated movement, 60, 74
Associated reactions, 59, 60, 75,
    111, 123
Astereognosis, 111
Asthma, 404, 429–40, 461
  allergy, 430
  clinical features, 431
  general treatment, 432
  inhalation therapy, 433–4
  pathology, 430
  physical treatment, 432
  physiology, 430
  treatment, 432
  treatment to decrease bronchial

Asthma—*cont.*
    obstruction and remove
    excessive secretions from the
    air passages, 433-6
    treatment to improve breathing
    control and exercise
    tolerance, and to prevent
    deformity, 436-40
Asymmetrical tonic neck posture,
    34
Asymmetrical tonic neck reflex,
    57, 75, 91, 493
Ataxia, 62, 70, 79, 112, 123, 125,
    149
Atelectasis, 403, 416, 418, 423,
    441
Athetoid, 126
Athetosis, 61, 70, 76-8, 112, 117,
    149, 164
    choreo, 78
    dystonic, 77
    with spasticity, 77
Auditory agnosia, 502
Auditory imperception, 149
Aversion responses, 175

'Bag squeezing', 473
Balance, 155, 163, 165, 170,
    175-6, 276
Balance control, 25
Balance development, 133
Balance problems, 291
Balance stimulation, 303-4
Balance tests, 154
Barlow's sign, 239
Basal ganglia, 17, 20, 51, 61
Bathing, 97
Behavioural management, 156
Behavioural problems, 154, 155,
    393-9
Biofeedback, 130, 156
Bite reflex, 94, 128
Bladder behaviour, 266-8
Blindness, 132

Body alignment, 118
Body image, 110
Body righting reflex, 490
Bow legs (genu varum), 309, 311,
    312-13
Bowel training, 268
Brachial plexus lesion, 51, 200-5
    assessment, 201-3
    description, 200
    prognosis, 201
    treatment, 203-4
Brain, 14
    pathophysiology, 56-63
Brain growth spurt, 52
Brain stem, 16, 18, 71
Brazelton Neonatal Behavioural
    Assessment Scale, 132
Breathing, 77
Breathing control, 129, 436
Breathing exercises, 326, 362,
    404, 429, 434, 439, 446, 462,
    464, 467, 469-71, 482
Bronchial tree, 403, 407
Bronchiectasis, 404, 428-9, 453,
    460
Bronchiolitis, 416-18
Bronchitis, 404, 427-8, 435, 441,
    460
Bronchoconstriction, 438, 440
Bronchodilator, 457, 458, 462,
    471
Bronchodilator drugs, 433
Bronchodilator therapy, 440
Bronchopneumonia, 454
Bronchopulmonary dysplasia,
    423
Bronchospasm, 433-5, 456, 462
Burn physiology, 385
Burn size estimation, 385
Burns, 384-400
    active movement, 389
    cigarette, 384
    contracture, 392
    electrical, 384

emotional and behavioural complications, 393
first degree, 385
flame, 384
fluid loss, 385–6
hand, 391
hypertrophic scarring, 391
immediately post-burn period, 387
limb elevation, 388
physical treatment, 388
post-burn period, 387–99
respiratory complications, 386
second degree, 385
skin grafting, 389–91
splinting, 392
superficial, 385
third degree, 385
wound depth, 385
wound healing, 391

Calcaneus, 211
Calipers, 282
Cap and jacket splinting, 348–51
Capsulotomy, 253
Cardiac failure, 319
Cardiac surgery, after-care, 472–4
Cardio-pulmonary arrest, 386
Cardio-respiratory arrest, 474
Cardiothoracic surgery, 472
Cauda equina, 63
Central nervous system, 3
    development, 52–6
    malformations, 161
Cerebellum, 16, 17, 51, 53, 61–2
Cerebral contusion, 142
Cerebral cortex, 16, 17, 51, 53
Cerebral palsy, 51, 66–141
    aetiology, 70
    assessment of infant, 80–98
    assessment of mildly handicapped children, 111–12
    assessment of premature babies, 97–8
    assessment of tone, 89–91
    assessment of young child, 98–112
    assessment procedure, 83–4, 98
    assessment record, 82
    characteristics of types, 70–2
    definition, 67
    development and treatment, 120
    hand function test, 91
    management, 80
    neurodevelopmental treatment, 112–14
    observation of posture, movement and reflex activity, 84, 100
    oral function tests, 93
    parent's comments, 95
    physical management, 112–35
    surgery, 129–30
    tone assessment, 107
    treatment, 114–19
    treatment criteria, 69
    treatment objectives, 69
    treatment systems and techniques, 68–70
    variety of problems, 67
Cerebrospinal fluid in myelomeningocele, 258
Chailey Chariot, 265, 266, 278, 300
Chewing, 128
Child abuse, 5–6
Choreo-athetosis, 78
Chromosomal abnormalities, 160
Chronic alveolar hypoventilation, 326
Clonus, 154
Clumsy child, 71, 112, 149
Co-contraction, 72–3, 76
Cognitive development, 178
Cold application, 374
Communication, 40
Concussion, 142

Conductive education, 130
Congenital hemivertebra, 340
Congenital vertical talus, 316–18
Continuous positive airways
  pressure (CPAP), 424, 473
Contract-relax, 504
Contraction
  isometric, 504
  isotonic, 504
  repeated, 505
Contractures, 74, 293–4, 320,
  327–31, 392
Cortical responses, 284
Corticosteroid therapy, 432
Cough, 412, 464, 465, 467, 472,
  473
Counselling, 290
Cranial asymmetry, 338
Crash helmets, 282
Crawling, 101, 278
Creatine-phosphokinase (CPK),
  322
Crossed extensor response, 486
Croup, 507
Crutches, 282
Crying, 40
Cryoprecipitate, 379
Curvature of the spine, 355
Cystic fibrosis, 416, 440–8, 453,
  454, 460
  clearing secretions, 443
  clinical features, 442
  diagnosis, 442
  general activities, 447–8
  inhalation therapy, 443–4
  inheritance of, 440
  management of obstructive
    pulmonary lesion, 443
  pathology, 441
  psychosocial care, 447
  treatment, 443

Deformity following paralysis,
  195

Deformity prevention, 203
Denis Browne hip splint, 243, 249
Denis Browne night splints, 229
Denis Browne splints, 225–8, 272,
  360
Depression, 335
Deprivation, 4–5
Dermatomyositis, 369–70
Desensitization, 128, 175
Development, 3–6, 292–3
  and treatment, 120
Development stimulation, 165
Developmental delay, 131
Developmental disorders,
  assessment, 161
Developmental reactions, 20, 511
Diaphragm, 409, 411
Digestive tract disorder, 447
Diplegia, 71, 72, 74, 102, 104,
  106, 107, 115, 125
Discipline, 8
Dominance tests, 154
Down's syndrome, 51, 78, 164,
  166, 172, 178
Dressing and undressing, 96, 299
Drug therapy, 156
Duchenne type dystrophy. See
  Muscular dystrophy
Dysarthria, 502
Dysgraphia, 149
Dyslexia, 149, 503
Dysmelia, 288
Dysphasia, 502
Dyspnoea, 508
Dystonic attacks, 79

Electromyographic studies, 44,
  322
Emergency care, 474
Emotional problems, 334, 393–9
Emotional response, 5
Emphysema, 404
Encephalitis, 51, 52, 182
Encephalomyelitis, 182

Endocrine disorders, 160
Endotracheal intubation, 423, 477
Environment effects, 3
Equilibrium reactions, 491
Erb-Duchenne-Klumpke type
   paralysis, 200
Erb's palsy, 200–5
Escherichia coli, 182
Exercise tolerance, 455
Eye control, 177

Facial asymmetry, 338
Facilitation, 115, 117, 118, 125,
   505–6
Fear, 10, 290
Feedback, 14–15, 61
Feeding, 36, 95, 161, 166–7, 300
Fine-motor control, 151
Flaccidity, 70, 78–9, 126
Flat foot (pes planovalgus), 309,
   311, 314–16
   painful, 316
   peroneal spasm causing, 316
'Flower pot' apparatus, 304
Foam wedge, 277
Forced (or fast) expiratory
   volume (FEV), 456–7
Foreign body inhalation, 426
Four-foot kneeling, 103
   to upright kneeling, 103
Fractures, 310
Frejka pillow, 242
Functional residual capacity
   (FRC), 473

Gag reflex, 94, 128
Gait, 105
Galant reflex, 487
Gastro-oesophageal reflux, 471
Gastrostomy, 421
Genetic disorders, 160
Genetic factors, 51
Genu valgum (knock knees), 309
   311–12

Genu varum (bow legs), 309, 311,
   312–13
Gleno-humeral joint, 61
Grasp, 33
Grasp development, 34, 38
Grasp reflex, 33, 91
Group activity, 155
Group therapy, 178, 439–40
Guillain-Barré's syndrome, 51,
   183, 196
Gymnastics, 8

Haemarthrosis, 379
Haemophilia, 379–80
Haemophilus influenza, 182
Halo-pelvic tractions, 361
Hamstrings, 329, 331
Hand function, 376
Hand function test, 91, 108
Head control, 21–2, 76, 163, 167,
   261, 276–8, 344
Head injuries, 142–6
   early features, 142
   immediate effects, 142
   incidence, 142
   treatment, 143–4
Head lag, 22
Head righting, 150, 353
Head rolling, 168, 342
Head turning, 488
Heart disease, 416
Heat aplication, 373
Heated wax, 374
Hemiplegia, 71
Hemivertebra, 340
Hip dislocation, 237–50, 269, 272
   aetiology, 237–8
   bilateral, 239
   description, 237
   diagnosis, 238–42
   management, 242–9
   physical treatment, 249
   radiograph, 238

Hip dislocation—*cont.*
  treatment, 242
  unilateral, 239
Hip instability tests, 239–42
History-taking, 84, 99
Hold. relax, 331, 504
Home treatment, 5, 6, 113
Hospitalization, 7
Humidification, 478
Hyaline membrane disease, 421
Hydrocéphalus, 258–9, 276
  surgical control, 261
Hydrotherapy, 376
Hyperactivity, 150–1, 156
Hypercarbia, 421
Hyperkinesis, 127
Hypertonus, 56, 60, 72, 76, 94, 485
Hypertrophic scarring, 391
Hypothermia, 473
Hypotonus, 76, 94, 117, 126, 161, 168, 251, 315, 482
Hypoxaemia, 421

Ileal loop diversion, 267
Ileocutaneous ureterostomy, 267
Iliopsoas transplant, 253, 272
Ilio-tibial tract, 331
Incubator, 474–5
Infections, 182–99
Inflammatory disorders, 366–83
  home treatment, 378
  stimulation of mobility,
    strength and function, 374–7
  treatment of, 370–2
Inhalation of foreign body, 426
Inhibition, 114, 118, 128
Inspiration, 412
Institutions, 4–5
Intensive care, 471
Intermittent positive pressure
    therapy, 434, 444, 462, 473
Intracranial haemorrhage, 142
Iridocyclitis, 368

Jobst anti-burnscar support, 393
Joint position sense, 109
Joint range tests, 202
Joints, inflammatory disorders, 366–83

Key points, 115, 117
Kinaesthetic system, 150
Klippel Feil Syndrome, 340
Klumpke's paralysis, 200
Knock knees (genu valgum), 309, 311–12

Labyrinthine righting reflex, 489
Landau reaction, 490
La Place equation, 510
Laryngotracheal groove, 407
Larynx, 409
Lateral movement, 176
Laterality, 503
Lead poisoning, 51
Learning difficulties, 154
Leggings, 172
Limb deficiencies, 288–306
  acceptance, 289–91
  assessment, 298
  deformities associated with, 293–4, 302
  development, 291
  exploration ability, 296
  loss of surface area, 294
  management, 296–8
  mobility, 298–302
  muscle strength and endurance, 302
  physical therapy, 298–304
  prehension, 296
  problems involved, 289–95
  prosthesis, 294–5, 297, 302
Locomotion, 277
Locomotion development, 24–32
Lung abscess, 470
Lung development, 407–10
Lung function, 40

Manipulation development, 34–9
Manipulative activities, 377
Manual hyperinflation, 473
Maxi-Myst compressor, 445
Mechanical aids, 334
Medial plaster splints, 223–5
Meningitis, 51, 52, 182, 261
Meningocele, 256
Meningococcus, 182
Mental backwardness, 321
Mental deficiency, 51
Mental retardation, 160–81, 264
  aetiology, 160–1
  assessment, 164
  effect on motor development
    and movement, 161–4
  incidence, 161
  management, 164–8
  treatment, 165
  use of term, 160
Mental subnormality, 262
Metabolic disorders, 160
Microcephaly, 51
Milwaukee brace, 194, 359
Minimal brain dysfunction, 71,
  147–59
  aetiology, 147–8
  assessment, 153–4
  description of, 148–52
  diagnosis, 148
  management, 154–6
Mist tent therapy, 444
Mobilization, 234, 252, 380
Monoplegia, 71
Moro response, 33, 74, 488
Motor assessment, 164
Motor behaviour, 81, 149
Motor control, 14
Motor development, 112, 117,
  122, 161–4, 202, 284, 291–3,
  322
Motor performance, 178
Motor problems, 151
Motor skills, 155

acquisition, 119
development, 41
Movement, 13–47, 161–4
  abnormal associated, 74
  abnormal patterns, 58
  assessment, 283
  automatic nature of, 15
  neurophysiology, 13–20
  normal, 13–20, 42, 70
Movement control, 13, 14
Movement development, 8,
  20–42, 170, 176
Movement disorder, 275
Movement patterns, 17
Movement stimulation, 8, 277
Movement tests, 202
Muscle biopsy, 322
Muscle chart, 188, 269, 283, 325
Muscle fibres, 16, 19, 64
Muscle imbalance, 74
Muscle length, 189
Muscle spindles, 63
Muscle tone, 15, 16–20
Muscle weakness, 193, 251, 319,
  320, 327
Muscular activity, 44
Muscular dystrophy, 161, 319–37
  assessment, 324–5
  child requirements, 335
  clinical features, 322
  contracture, 327–31
  deformity, 327–31
  description, 319–21
  diagnosis, 322
  management, 324
  parental involvement, 333–5
  pathology, 322
  prevention of immobility and
    inactivity, 332
  preventive treatment, 326
  splinting, 332–3
  supportive treatment, 333
  surgery, 332–3
Muscular torticollis, 338–54

Muscular torticollis—*cont.*
  active correction, 344–6
  aetiology, 338
  assessment, 340–1
  differential diagnosis, 339–40
  home treatment, 346–7
  parental involvement, 346–7
  pathology, 339
  prognosis, 340
  surgical treatment, 352–3
  treatment methods, 340, 342
  treatment rationale, 341–2
  use of term, 338
Myelination, 53
Myelomeningocele, 256–7, 276, 283
  cerebrospinal fluid in, 258
  clinical features, 259–60
  lumbosacral, 259
  pathology, 257–9
  problems involved and their management, 260
  skin in, 258
  spinal cord in, 257–8
  surgical repair, 261
  treatment objectives, 284
  vertebrae in, 258

Nasopharyngeal suction, 388, 390
Nebulization therapy, 434, 444
Neck righting reflex, 488
Nerve cell recovery, 189
Neurodevelopmental treatment, 112–14
Neurological signs, 154
Neurological syndromes, 182
Neurones, 19, 62
Neurosis, 5

Obesity, 334
Obstetrical paralysis of the upper limb, 200
Occupational therapist, 113
Oesophageal atresia, 419–21

Oral function 40
Oral function tests, 93, 108, 154
Oro-facial dysfunction, 127–9
Osteoporosis, 368
Over-protection, 289
Overflow, 60
Oxygen consumption, 471
Oxygen therapy, 423–4

Pain relief, 372–5
Pancreatic defect, 441
Pancreatic insufficiency, 447
Parachute reaction, 34, 35, 87, 491
Paralysis, 4, 194–5, 275, 278, 279
Paralytic scoliosis, 193
Paraplegia, 72
Parapodium, 279, 280
Parental advice, 155
Parental involvement, 95, 113, 121–2, 131, 135, 165–6, 193, 262, 269, 285, 289, 290, 329, 333–5, 346–7, 378, 468
Patience, 9
Pavlek harness, 245
Peak expiratory flow rate (PEFR), 457
Perception, 110
Perceptual defects, 71
Perceptual stimulation, 176–8
Percussion, 463–6, 472, 475, 480
Percutaneous faradic stimulation, 283
Peripheral neuropathy, 196–7
Peripheral system, 64
Peroneal spasm, 316
Perseverant actions, 133, 162
Perthes' disease, 309, 311
Pertussis, 426
Pes planovalgus (flat floot), 309, 311, 314–16
Pharyngeal 'tickling', 464
Phocomelia, 288–90, 295, 299, 301, 303, 304

Physiotherapist, approach to child, 7
Pin-prick test, 284
Placing reactions, 490
Plagiocephaly, 338, 340
Plasma administration, 379
Plaster cast removal, 10
Plaster hip spica, 245-8
Plaster splints, 273
Play, 97, 162
Pneumococcus, 182
Pneumonia, 403, 404, 416, 418-19, 441, 460
Poliomyelitis, 51, 52, 183, 315
  assessment, 188-90
  clinical features, 184-5
  management, 185-96
  paralysis, 194-5
  paralytic stage, 184-7
  pathology, 184
  physical treatment, 190-3
  preparalytic stage, 184, 185
  recovery stage, 185, 187-8
  vaccination, 183
Poor posture, 309
Posterior plaster splint, 229
Post-rotary nystagmus, 150
Postural development, 377
Postural drainage, 388, 404, 429, 434-6, 443, 445-6, 459-69, 470, 472, 475, 479, 482
Postural reactions, 70
Posture control, 16-20
Prehension, 134
Prehension development, 32-9
Prematurity, 42
  assessment, 97-8
Primitive reactions, 74, 75
Prone position, 167-70
Prone scooter, 265, 300
Proprioception, 274
Proprioceptive system, 150
Prosthesis, 294-5, 297, 302
Pseudohypertrophy, 320

Psoas muscle, 73, 253
Pulmonary disorders, 417, 441
Quadriplegia, 71, 72, 74, 114, 486
Questionnaires, 122
Radio-ulnar joints, 73
Rales, 508
Recreation, 334
Reflex activity tests, 485-95
Reflex inhibiting patterns, 114
Reflexes, 18, 19, 33, 85-8, 93, 94
Rejection, 6, 289, 290
Relaxation, 435, 436, 437, 470, 504
Respiration, 175, 407-15
Respiratory acidosis, 508
Respiratory alkalosis, 508
Respiratory complications, 386, 406
Respiratory disorders, 403-6, 453
  in childhood, 426-49
  in neonatal period and infancy, 416-25
Respiratory distress, 421-4, 471
Respiratory failure, 326, 407, 509
Respiratory function, 362, 377
Respiratory function tests, 325
Respiratory infection, 319
Respiratory movement, 283
Respiratory problems, 127, 185
Respiratory system, 3
Respiratory tract, 403, 404
Respiratory tract clearance, 468
Rest, 373, 380
Retardation, 4
Retrolental fibroplasia, 424
Rheumatoid arthritis, 366-9, 375
Rhonchi, 508
Rhythmic stabilization, 506
Rib springing, 465, 468
Righting reactions, 488
Rigidity, 56, 70
Risser jacket, 361

Risser turnbuckle jacket, 361
Rolling over, 100, 277
Rooting reflex, 93
Rossfeld prone board, 330
Rotation, 123

Scalds, 384
Scar hypertrophy, 392
Scleroderma, 370
Scoliosis, 333, 355–65
  aetiology, 357
  congenital, 357
  description, 355–6
  general mobility and strength,
    363
  idiopathic, 357
  paralytic, 357
  physical treatment, 362–3
  pre- and post-operative
    treatment, 363
  respiratory function, 362
  splinting, 359–62
  structural, 355
  surgery, 362
  treatment, 357–63
  use of term, 355
Sensation tests, 154
Sensori-motor defect, 71
Sensori-motor development, 21,
  164
Sensori-motor disorders, 52
Sensori-motor integration, 178
Sensori-motor reactions, 53
Sensori-motor system, 15
Sensory discrimination, 152
Sensory feedback, 130, 295
Sensory integrative dysfunction,
  152
Sensory integrative functions, 153
Sensory loss, 273–5, 284
Sensory perception, 110
Sensory problems, 151
Sensory stimulation, 176–8
Sensory system, 14

Sensory testing, 108, 284
Separation effects, 4
Serum enzymes, 322
Shame, 290
Shasbah trolley, 265
Shrewsbury splint, 279, 281, 282
Sinusitis, 436
Sitting, 102, 175, 292, 492
  to standing, 43
Sitting up
  from prone, 101
  from supine, 101
Skin in myelomeningocele, 258
Skin grafting, 389–91
Sleeping, 96–7
Slow reversal-hold, 505
Social development, 178
Social responses, 161
Social skills, 155
Soft tissue, inflammatory
  disorders, 366–83
Spasms, 60, 77, 117, 124, 126,
  374, 375, 380
Spastic hemiplegia, 58
Spasticity, 56, 58, 60, 61, 69, 70,
  72–6, 122, 149, 164, 258
  moderate, 75–6
  patterns of, 73
  severe, 72–5
  with athetosis, 77
Speech, 77, 162
Speech defects, 149
Speech development, 40
Speech mechanisms, 129
Speech therapist, 113
Spina bifida, 255–87
  assessment, 283–4
  child in, 263–6
  classification, 255–7
  deformity, 268–73
  grading of paralysis, 275
  parents in, 262
  primary developmental defect,
    255

sensory loss, 273-5
social and psychological
factors, 262
See also Myelomeningocele
Spina bifida cystica, 51, 256-7,
271
See also Myelomeningocele
Spina bifida occulta, 255
Spinal cord, 18-20, 51, 53, 63,
257-8
Spinal muscular atrophy, 319
Spine curvature, 333
Splinting, 129, 193-6, 203-4,
219-29, 234-6, 242-8, 252,
272-4, 278, 279, 281, 282,
312, 332-3, 348-51, 359-62,
376, 378, 388, 392
Sputum collection, 454
Stability, 126
Standing, 25, 28, 134, 171, 172,
277, 279-81, 300, 485, 492
from sitting, 105
from upright kneeling, 104
Status asthmaticus, 434, 440
Stereognosis, 109
Stereotyped actions, 162
Stereotypic behaviour, 133
Sternomastoid muscle, 342-4
Sternomastoid tumour, 338-42,
346, 352
Still's disease, 366-9
Strapping, 219-23, 272
Stretching technique, 342-4,
346-7, 505-6
Stridor, 509
Stroke, 52
Subarachnoid haemorrhage, 142
Subdural haematoma, 142
Suckling reflex, 93, 96
Suction technique, 480
Supine position, 168
Surface tension, 509-10
Swallowing, 128, 129
Sweat gland defect, 442, 447

Swimming, 175, 282, 311, 332,
362, 363, 376
Symmetrical tonic neck reflex,
494
Synergies, 73
Synkinetic movement, 60

Tactile agnosia, 502
Tactile sensitivity, 134
Talipes calcaneo-valgus, 233-6,
272, 273
active correction, 236
aetiology, 233
assessment, 234
management, 233
physical treatment, 234-6
prognosis, 233
Talipes equinovarus, 209-32, 269,
272
active correction, 230
aetiological factors, 209
arthrogrypotic type, 212
assessment, 215
conservative treatment, 215
deformity, 210-14
incidence, 209
management, 214
mobilization, 216
mobilization precautions, 218
mobilization technique, 216-18
pathological anatomy, 210-13
physical treatment, 215-31
plantarflexion degree, 210, 211
postural, 209, 212
prognosis, 214
surgical management, 231
types, 209
Talus, 211
Tapping, 125
Taylor's brace, 194
Tay-Sachs disease, 78
Tenotomy, 352
Tension, 40
Tetanus, 481, 482

Thalidomide syndrome, 288–90
Thomas' posterior spinal support, 193
Thoracic expansion measurement, 452–4
Thoracotomy, 421
Tolerance, 9
Tone
abnormal, 70
assessment, 89, 107, 202
increase in, 60
testing, 94
Tongue, 128
Tongue movement, 40
Tongue vibration, 167
Tonic labyrinthine reflexes, 18, 72, 101
Tonic neck reflexes, 18, 57, 72, 493–4
Touch testing, 109
Tracheo-oesophageal fistula, 416, 419–21, 471
Tracheostomy, 477
Traction, 253
Traction bands, 361
Transverse myelitis, 197
Trauma, 51, 63
Trendelenburg sign, 242
Trunk control, 292
Trunk extension, 277
Tubocurarine, 481, 482
Tumours, 52
Two-point discrimination, 109, 111

Unconscious child, care of, 481–2
Upright kneeling, 103

Ventilation mechanics, 410, 471
Ventilation therapy, 471, 475–81
application by face mask or mouthpiece, 476
management, 476
tracheostomized or intubated child, 477–81
Vertebrae in myelomeningocele, 258
Vestibular dysfunction, 149–50
Vestibulo-spinal tract, 18
Vibration, 128, 130–1, 388, 463–6, 472, 480
Visual agnosia, 502
Visual perceptual function, 154
Vitalograph, 456
Vitamin deficiency, 51
Vocalization, 41, 77, 95
Volkmann's ischaemia, 51
Von Rosen splint, 243

Walking, 25, 28, 43, 105, 277, 278, 280–2, 303, 485 See also Locomotion
Wallerian degeneration, 184
Warm packs, 373
Weight bearing, 170
Weight traction, 242
Weight transfer, 168
Werdnigg-Hoffman's disease, 78, 315
Wheel-chair, 281, 333
Wheezing, 510
Whooping cough, 426
Wright peak flow meter or gauge, 457